The Nurse in Popular Media

T0197883

The Nurse in Popular Media

Critical Essays

Edited by
MARCUS K. HARMES,
BARBARA HARMES *and*
MEREDITH A. HARMES

McFarland & Company, Inc., Publishers
Jefferson, North Carolina

ISBN (print) 978-1-4766-8418-5
ISBN (ebook) 978-1-4766-4546-9

LIBRARY OF CONGRESS AND BRITISH LIBRARY
CATALOGUING DATA ARE AVAILABLE

On the cover: *Carry on Doctor*, 1967, shown:
Barbara Windsor (Rank Film Distributors of America/Photofest)

Printed in the United States of America

McFarland & Company, Inc., Publishers
Box 611, Jefferson, North Carolina 28640
www.mcfarlandpub.com

Table of Contents

Introduction

Barbara Harmes,
Meredith A. Harmes *and*
Marcus K. Harmes

"Beneath the bosom of every woman beats the heart of a nurse" said the British comedian Benny Hill, an observation made in a comedy sketch on how to meet women. As the sketch continues, nurses do indeed appear, young, glamorous, in a cap and uniform but with skirts cut daringly short, and they promptly proceed to ignore their "patient," Benny Hill, who is feigning a fainting fit to get attention and sympathy. Several points lurk within the comedy, including (as may be expected of Benny Hill) an association of the nursing profession with amorousness and sexual availability, the association of nursing with women, and the immediate resort to stereotypes that make nurses highly visible and recognizable in popular awareness but often in ways detached from reality (McAllister and Brien, 2020). As Linda Hallam notes, "nurses have been constructed as whores and prostitutes since Victorian times," or at least as sex objects (Hallam, 2000: 77). Many of the essays in this collection note the resort to stereotypes in the construction of nurses and nursing activity, stereotypes that often draw on the traditional uniform of the nurse, whereby the cap, the starch and the collars evoke a sense of "cleanliness is next to godliness," but where this purity interacts with possibilities of danger, transgression or dirt (136; Pittard, 2013: 168). As suggested by Barbara Melosh (1987: 57), the angel, the handmaiden, the all-American girl and the "castrating bitch" are all possibilities in the way media presents nurses, but Melosh also notes the importance of where and how nurses have represented themselves, as authors and content creators, crafting their own more consistent impressions.

Perhaps one of the earliest instances of nursing and media coming together is the Edison phonographic recording of Florence Nightingale's voice, made at her house in London in 1890. The cylinder preserves her quavering voice commenting "When I am no longer even a memory, just a name, I hope my voice may perpetuate the great work of my life. God bless my dear old comrades of Balaclava and bring them safe to shore." Although that is the only recording of her voice and there are no moving images of her, Nightingale was already readily identifiable. Nightingale herself realized that how she appeared, what people thought she looked like, and how people wished to portray her were all contested spaces. She noted the disparity between what she had really been like in the filthiness of Scutari compared with the popular impression of her in the wards, and she said "Good public! It knew nothing of what I was really doing in the Crimea" (in McDonald, 2006: 232). It is striking that even the most singly iconic representation of nursing, Nightingale as the Lady with the Lamp, is of unknown provenance. In addition, the image itself, regardless of its source, is at odds with the actuality of Nightingale the administrator and statistician; one contemporary noted the existence of the "plaster saint" version of Nightingale compared with the "resolute and masterful" person she actually was (Bostridge, 2015). Nightingale's image has continued to resonate and she appears in various guises throughout this collection, from nursing saint to futurist. Arguably, every primly uniformed nurse in cap and cape was a physical and visual embodiment of Nightingale and her hope that nursing would be a suitable career for respectable women. Nightingale featured on the British ten pound note as the Lady with the Lamp. But even this image was unstable, and by the end of the 20th century Nightingale was even competing with the hitherto overlooked Mother Mary Seacole, who literally took a place on a pedestal that more logically belonged to Nightingale, when Seacole was honored with a statue at St Thomas's Hospital in London.

Nonetheless, Nightingale as a name, an identity and a stock image endures. At the time of writing, the COVID-19 pandemic has given a new and tragic impetus to nurses in media. The coordinated clap for the National Health Service (NHS), and above all the reams of footage of nurses and other care givers struggling to deliver medical care in overstretched hospitals are on every television screen, as are the names and the mortality statistics for nurses who have died from contracting coronavirus while performing their work. Nightingale herself has in various ways returned to the wards. The British government's emergency hospitals carry her name. Writing in the *Nursing Times*, Jo Stephenson drew out meaningful parallels to Nightingale not only in nursing practice (such as Nightingale's insistence on hand hygiene, the need for nurses to have appropriate equipment and for patients to have constant monitoring) but also in popular consciousness, as she could adroitly use the media. In turn, the higher profile of nursing leadership during the COVID pandemic is reminiscent of her impact on governments, her high profile and her ability to use her influence.

The intersection between nurses and popular media is longstanding. Florence Nightingale died in 1910, and British Pathé's coverage of the 1920 centenary service of her birth is a very early instance of nurses appearing on film. Jumpy footage shows a cavalcade of nurses, all women, pouring out of Westminster Abbey in caps, capes, sensible boots, and with scarcely a man to be seen. Nightingale was the subject of a silent film biography by 1915 and thereafter film, television, theatre and live performance and other media have showcased the nurse and the nursing profession. The familiarity of the nurse is inherently visual; the iconography of nurse in cap, cape and uniform remains current in pop culture realms from the stripper to the memories of the matron of the *Carry On* films, even though that iconography, especially the cap, has disappeared from real world nursing.

A parade of nurses, good, bad or otherwise, has appeared on both cinema and television screens. Ratched and Wilkes torment and maim, the Matron presiding over the hospitals of the *Carry On* films vainly tries to keep order in a comedic shambles.

The interactions between the actual and the fictional, the capacity of the nurses of popular culture to mirror, distort, or inspire the nurses of the real world warrants further attention. Does seeing a nurse on screen inspire people to enter the profession? To what extent is gender disparity in the profession attributable to mediated distillations? If nurses are the caring profession, why are there so many nurses in horror films? If Florence Nightingale was a secular saint, why is the profession's iconography appropriated by the stripper and the porn actress?

Collectively, the essays address these points and more. They interact with media of different types, including film and television, as well as archives preserving audience reactions, the press, museum collections of nursing outfits, tools and the documentary traces of their education and corporate lives, as well as ephemera such as picture postcards and portrait photographs. Notably but unsurprisingly, the essays are almost all about women. They include women as saviors, victims, survivors, as the embodiment of the perfect nurse or as the grotesque perversion of an ideal. Actual nurses, from Florence Nightingale to Judy Hill, the nurse at the center of 1972 air crash and cannibalism incident in Canada, are examined alongside fictional nurses from the Anglican sisters of Nonnatus House in *Call the Midwife*, the nurses interned in *Tenko* and the Matron of the *Carry On* films.

In Section One: Contested Heroines, Richard Bates' essay on Florence Nightingale in film and television opens this collection. While the stock nature and the wide dissemination of the Lady with the Lamp imagery was noted previously, Bates notes that surprisingly, Nightingale has rarely been the subject of feature films, and has been played by well-known actresses who nonetheless would not consider those performances the highlights of their careers. Examining the few films about her, Bates locates differences in tone and emphasis even in this small number, finding that they embody conflicting impulses to condemn or celebrate Nightingale, in ways reminiscent of broader cultural discourse about her. While Nightingale remains chiefly famous for her work in the Crimean War, Mark Aldridge considers a fictionalized account of nurses based on the realities of internment in World War II. His study of the BBC's *Tenko*, a female-led ensemble drama set in a Japanese prisoner of war camp, focuses on the characters of two young women nurses and an older female doctor to explore the shifting power dynamics as they carry out their professional responsibilities out of the hospital and in the prison camp.

Shifting from fiction to nonfiction, the actual nurse Judy Hill, who died in an air crash in Canada in 1972 and was cannibalized by a crash survivor, is the subject of Travis Hay's essay, which uses the specific incident of the air crash as a focal point for a wider ranging analysis of how cultural archetypes of the Arctic nurse intersect with the actualities of post-colonial disparities in health care in Canada. The next essays consider fictional nurses in different conditions of strain and challenge. *The Doctors and the Nurses* (1962–1965), later called *The Nurses* (1965–1967) is discussed in Caitlin Fendley's essay with a specific focus on viewer feedback to a controversial episode in which a nurse became a patient in her own hospital seeking sterilization. The episode's focus on the nurse as patient and the study of viewer reactions to her treatment opens a window into the debates taking place in the United States on voluntary female sterilization, and examining this character illuminates the later acceptance and popularity of this procedure in the 1970s. *M*A*S*H*, a film and television series set during the Korean War but resonating with the Vietnam War, is the subject of detailed scrutiny in Susan Hopkins' study of the character Major "Hot Lips" Houlihan, the head of nursing. Interpreting the writing and performance of this character as a nurse seeking to impose high standards but constantly under duress from sexist and misogynistic antagonists, Hopkins places the treatment of this nurse and nursing in a troubling trajectory, from the 1970s to contemporary revenge porn.

Section Two: Seeking the Ideal, contains essays where the images and paraphernalia of nursing have been judged and curated and been the subject of competitions, often in pursuit of the ideals of a type of nurse. While many essays discuss film and television, media has wider meanings, including the collections that can be built from the uniforms, tools, and educational and corporate lives of nurses that are left to posterity. Jeannine Uribe writes of the Museum of Nursing History, Inc., located in the St. Benilde Tower at La Salle University in Philadelphia, Pennsylvania, and its varied collections of timeworn objects. From these, Uribe accounts for the demographic changes that drive processes of donation and acquisition and the meaning that can be taken and organized via curation from media such as textbooks and yearbooks.

Another type of ephemera, the postcard, is the focus of Julia Hallam's essay, which examines examples from the turn of the nineteenth and twentieth centuries from the Zwerdling Collection in the U.S. National Library of Medicine. The cards capture in time representative examples of the "ideal" of nurse, meaning a white woman, but also preserve the various enduring stereotypes of the battle-ax and the saucy nurse that have recurred in representations of nurses in the mass media. Interpreting similar stereotypes, the essay by Marcus K. Harmes, Barbara Harmes and Meredith A. Harmes moves forward in time from Hallam's to postwar British popular culture. There, the cheekiness of Victorian postcards re-emerged in the bawdy comedy of the *Carry On* films. However this humor based on stereotyped nurses sits alongside more serious iterations of nursing such as *Emergency Ward 10*, and this essay sets the presentation of nursing education, training and practice in popular media against the reforms taking place in actuality, seeking the points of intersection, as different agencies have sought to improve training and raise standards. In this section on ideals and their recurring stereotypes, Sarah Chaney's essay examines the interwar competition to find the typical British nurse, one which was centered on the media of the photograph as nurses everywhere sent in images of themselves prim and starched in their uniforms. She considers these images and the types of nurse and nursing they foregrounded against a wider range of archival sources to explore what they represented of class-based expectations and efforts to make nursing a middle class occupation. Another type of ideal is examined by Morag Martin's essay on the popular *Call the Midwife*. Martin studies the nostalgia inherent in the Docklands and 1950s settings and the portrayal of the Anglican sisters as a utopian community. However Martin considers the tensions within this world as the sisters interact with both the new National Health Service and their superiors in the Church of England. Finally, the unusual (in English-language literature) perspective of Estonian nursing is considered in the essay by Merle Talvik, Taimi Tulva, Ülle Ernits and Kristi Puusepp. Florence Nightingale is re-examined this time from the perspective of her cultural and practical impact on Estonian nursing and the development of the archetype of a "Queen of Nursing."

Moving from the idealized to the horrific in Section Three: When Nurses Go Wrong, Victoria N. Meyers' essay opens the section with a wide-ranging analysis of nurses in films of the 1960s and 1970s. She locates in these films and their nurses signs of a widespread cultural pessimism and rejection of authority that are related to changes within nursing and changes in attitudes to nursing. Marcus K. Harmes, Meredith A. Harmes and Barbara Harmes explore the appearances of nurses in horror films, considering the high levels of agency granted to nurses and the peculiar liberation of the nurse from a subordinate role to a dynamic and powerful position through the enactment of horror. Ronja Tripp-Bodola considers similar films and fictional nurses including Nurse Ratched in a theoretically rich analysis of nurses as sites of abject monstrosity and the qualities in nursing that modulate into this horrific type. Tatiana Prorokova-Konrad studies *Nurse 3D* in her essay, looking at this horror film using an interpretation based on many of the similar stereotypes explored in other essays, including the angel of mercy, the caring mother and the sex object. Thinking especially of the last of these and its use in *Nurse 3D*, she argues that sexually objectifying nurses is of course a form of oppression, but especially so for bisexuality and lesbianism, as the objectification is, at its core, something created and consumed by heterosexual men.

References

Bostridge, M. (2015) *Florence Nightingale: The Woman and Her Legend*. Penguin.

Hallam, J. (2000) *Nursing the Image: Media, Culture, and Professional Identity*. Psychology Press.

McAllister, M., and Brien, D.L. (2020) *Paradoxes in Nurses' Identity, Culture and Image: The Shadow Side of Nursing*. Routledge.

McDonald, L. (2006) *Florence Nightingale on Society and Politics, Philosophy, Science, Education and Literature: Collected Works of Florence Nightingale, Volume 5*. Wilfrid Laurier University Press.

Melosh, B. (1987) Nursing Illusions: Nurses in Popular Literature. In: Buhle, P. (ed.) *Popular Culture in America*. University of Minnesota Press, pp. 57–72.

Pittard, C. (2013) *Purity and Contamination in Late Victorian Detective Fiction*. Ashgate.

Contested Heroines

Florence on Film

Representations of Nightingale
in Cinema and on Television

RICHARD BATES

Introduction

Given Florence Nightingale's ongoing reputation as a pioneering heroine of nursing, public health care, and statistics, it is perhaps surprising that she has not turned up on our screens more often. Hollywood made its sole Nightingale biopic in 1936; the last cinematic portrayal of her anywhere was released in 1951. For seventy years, the only feature-length representations of Nightingale on screen have been in a handful of British and American made-for-TV movies; she has otherwise been limited to children's television and walk-on roles in programs about other famous figures. This is a relatively meager haul in the context of Nightingale's cultural status, especially in the United Kingdom. Nightingale regularly appears on lists of the greatest ever Britons, sometimes at the top (Fox-Leonard, 2015). She continues to feature in the British school curriculum and in nursing education courses around the world. In 2020 her name was quickly mobilized during the Covid-19 pandemic in England, with the creation of seven emergency "Nightingale hospitals." Yet Nightingale's total of three cinematic biopics and a handful of television portrayals contrasts with the far more numerous representations of comparable historical figures such as Winston Churchill, Queen Victoria, or Queen Elizabeth I. No female director has ever taken on Nightingale as a central subject; none of the actresses who have played her would consider the role an especially significant one in their career.

This relative absence of screen depictions seems even more unusual given the plethora of representations of Nightingale that have appeared in other media. From the 1850s onwards, Nightingale has generated an avalanche of cultural production, from paintings, engravings, newspaper profiles, *cartes de visite*, and books, to commemorative crockery, figurines, ornaments, and trinkets (Crawford, Greenwood, Bates and Memel, 2020: 143–178; 229–238). The first years of her fame produced a great deal of poetry, including Henry Wadsworth Longfellow's famous *Santa Filomena*, which cemented Nightingale's image as the "lady with the lamp" (Longfellow, 1857). There were children's books, popular songs, music hall performances, and marionette theatre productions recreating Nightingale's role in the Crimean War. In the twentieth century there were a number of stage and radio plays (see Kalisch, 1983: 185–187, 274–278), while a Florence Nightingale Museum opened at St Thomas' Hospital, London, in 1989. Since Nightingale's death in 1910, influential biographies have appeared at regular intervals (Cook, 1913; Strachey, 1918; O'Malley, 1931; Woodham-Smith, 1950; Smith, 1982; Small, 1998; Gill, 2004; Bostridge, 2009), and Lynn McDonald has overseen the publication of a monumental sixteen-volume *Collected Works* (McDonald, 2001–2012).

This essay will briefly discuss each of the films that have appeared (or at least those that are still obtainable), highlighting the dominant themes and changing discursive emphases that can be seen in depictions of Nightingale on screen. Two common threads will emerge. First, it will be shown that most of the films, particularly the earlier ones, incline towards a simplistic narrative of Nightingale's life focused almost exclusively on the Crimean War, often with significant distortions of the historical reality. Second, racial identity will emerge as a consistent element—whether because Nightingale was being celebrated as an exemplar of the supposed virtues of the white race, or condemned as racist towards Mary Seacole, a British woman of Jamaican origin also present in the Crimea. The essay will conclude by arguing that Nightingale's current reputation is caught between the impulses to celebrate and to condemn, both of which have been developed by the corpus of films about her.

In recent decades, a gap has opened between academic work on Nightingale, which has tended to focus on her nursing reforms in the broader context of changes in gender roles and women's work in Victorian Britain (for example Vicinus, 1985; Poovey, 1988; Summers, 2000; Penner, 2010) and the popular legend, which remains firmly focused on her Crimean War adventures. Historians have attributed the durability of the legend to the idea that Nightingale's Crimean War work inaugurated a new stage in the relationship between civilian populations and national militaries. Between 1854 and 1914, civilians became ever more closely engaged in national war efforts and concerned about soldiers' welfare (Crossland, 2018; Hutchinson, 1996). With the emergence of steam ships and international telegraph cables, noncombatants could follow wars in more-or-less real time via the press. The phenomenon of celebrity may be understood as a co-production between the celebrated individual and a social collective that assigns significance to their actions; Nightingale caught the imagination as one of the first people to embody and direct the new popular concern for soldiers' wellbeing. In fighting the British army's inertia and bureaucracy on behalf of the suffering troops, cheered on by the press and public, she represented "a living, breathing watershed in the history of military medicine" (Crossland, 2018: 15–16). Furthermore, this development was not confined to Britain. By the 1860s, Nightingale had become an international symbol of the new charitable, caring mood towards sick and wounded soldiers and the drive to improve their medical and nursing care. In the American Civil War, Nightingale inspired Dorothea Dix's Women's Nursing Bureau and the United States Sanitary Commission, while in *A Memory of Solferino* (1862), the book that sparked the creation of the International Red Cross, Henry Dunant cited Nightingale as an example of the new spirit of "sublime self-sacrifice" and "passionate devotion to suffering humanity" (Dunant, 1939: 120).

Dunant in fact rather misunderstood Nightingale, believing that she had primarily been leading a short-term philanthropic mission rather than a concerted effort to bring about systemic improvements in army medical and nursing care. Significantly, Dunant erroneously believed that Nightingale's nursing party had been made up of "ladies" (i.e., gentlewomen) who were "zealous and valiant" but unpaid (Dunant, 193: 120–121). These misperceptions proved persistent. In an era when citizens increasingly dreamed of joining military or humanitarian ventures, but non-royal female role models were rare, they made Nightingale's example seem relatively easy to emulate—in a way that, say, her prodigious education, or determined acquisition of nursing experience in several countries over a substantial period, might not. Rather than seeing Nightingale as an outlier, the idea of Nightingale as primarily an earnest philanthropist framed her success as arising out of contemporary values: caring feminine domesticity mixed with patriotism, decorum, common sense and civility—and, on some readings, Joan of Arc–style self-martyring religiosity. Such ideas fed into the production of the cultural iconography, which, in turn, reinforced these concepts further.

Early films thus tended to ignore Nightingale's impatience with and discouragement of well-intentioned but ill-prepared gentlewomen volunteers, instead celebrating such characters. The earliest surviving depiction of Nightingale on screen occurs in *Victoria Cross* (1912). This fifteen-minute silent film centers on the Charge of the Light Brigade, and the efforts of one of the Brigade's officers to win the heart of Ellen, a colonel's daughter.

Moved by the soldiers' suffering, Ellen decides to become a nurse. She is interviewed by Nightingale, played by Julia Swayne Gordon as a kindly figure, who agrees to take her despite her lack of experience. *The White Angel* (1936, discussed in more detail below), similarly inverts Nightingale's policy on nurse selection, leading to the following exchange:

> APPLICANT 1: I've worked in St Thomas' [Hospital], the Middlesex, and the Charing Cross.
> NIGHTINGALE: You've been too many places for me … [rejects her]
> [To next applicant]: What nursing have you done?
> APPLICANT 2: None. But I could soon learn. I've worked hard all my life, and I'm willing to do anything.
> NIGHTINGALE: You're the sort of person we want.

In reality, the original party of nurses that Nightingale enlisted to take to Scutari (the hospital in Constantinople/Istanbul that served as her base for most of the war), comprised sixteen experienced working-class hospital nurses alongside fourteen Anglican sisters and ten Roman Catholic nuns, all with significant prior nursing experience (Helmstadter, 2020: 49). But by misrepresenting this point, the films could speak to the cultural shift that had accompanied and fueled Nightingale's rise to fame. In the age of mass warfare, civilians were encouraged to believe that they could all do their bit, and that patriotic and humanitarian enthusiasm (and, in the case of nurses, "natural" feminine instincts) would overcome technical challenges. A now-lost half-hour biopic feature that appeared during the First World War, *Florence Nightingale* (1915), incorrectly labeled Nightingale as the founder of the Red Cross, suggesting that the film aimed to encourage women to join the Red Cross's wartime nursing efforts (Kalisch, 1983: 271). The suggestion that a good heart was the overriding qualification for nursing made it seem more accessible—at the expense of misrepresenting Nightingale's emphasis on the importance of training and experience.

Meanwhile the idea of Nightingale as first and foremost an international humanitarian philanthropist rather than a specifically British military figure—notwithstanding that much of her work was in fact conducted on behalf of the British army—helped to broaden her international appeal. Racial theorists such as the American phrenologist/physiognomist Samuel R. Wells, in his 1866 book *New Physiognomy*, held her up as an ideal human specimen. Having first distinguished the "Caucasian race"—characterized by "Causality, Mirthfulness, Ideality, and Conscientiousness"—from (among others) the "Ethiopian race" which he labeled "slow and indolent … superstitious, excitable, impulsive," Wells highlighted Nightingale's physiognomy as an ideal type representing "esthetical and refined" cultivation (Wells, 1894: 382, 390, 536). "Bright, intellectual, and spiritual," her "high moral principles" evident from her facial features, Nightingale was contrasted with "Bridget McBruiser," a lower-class stereotype considered "vindictive," "earthy," and ruled by "animal passions" (Wells, 1894: 537–538). In the context of the new system of racial segregation emerging in the USA after 1865, Nightingale was thus proposed as a pinnacle of White Anglo-Saxon Protestant racial stock.

Such ideas need to be considered as a background factor to on-screen representations of Nightingale, perhaps most obviously that in the first "talkie" biopic, *The White Angel* (1936), produced in the USA by Warner Bros. The studio conceived of the film as a cash-in follow-up to director William Dieterle's surprise hit, *The Story of Louis Pasteur* (1935), in the context of an industry-wide preference for "wholesome, middlebrow" films that satisfied the requirements of the conservative (Catholic-influenced) 1934 Motion Picture Production Code (the "Hays" Code) (Brown, 2013, 16). Hampered by a restricted budget and the Code's injunction against depicting violence (and therefore Crimean War battle scenes), Dieterle at least began with the apparent advantage of having Kay Francis, one of Hollywood's biggest female stars, lined up for the leading role. Francis had had a string of hits with Warner Bros between 1932 and 1936, playing "rich, sophisticated, big city women, attired in expensive clothes and jewelry, who often succumbed to the temptations of adultery" (Bostridge, 2009: 538). In *Mary Stevens, M.D.* (1933) Francis had played a successful female doctor, albeit one who becomes suicidal after having an illegitimate baby with an alcoholic colleague. However, she appeared miscast as Nightingale, whom she tried to play as a streetwise, cool-headed society lady, seemingly itching for lines she could deliver with her trademark sardonic humor. This was out of kilter with the historical Nightingale—and with Mordaunt Shairp's screenplay, which hammed up the sentimental aspects of Nightingale's story while rewriting significant aspects of it to add bathos. For example, Nightingale's love interest, Charles (loosely representing Nightingale's historical suitor Richard Monckton Milnes) turns up unbidden at Scutari offering to help—but soon declares that "nursing is woman's work," volunteers instead for the trenches, and ends up dying in a field hospital under Nightingale's gaze. Similarly, Nightingale's May 1855 trip from Scutari to the Crimea is transposed to mid-winter, leading to a scene in which—the army medics having refused her entry to the hospitals—she sits freezing in the snow, until eventually rescued by a drummer boy with an unexplained American accent (Francis and the rest of the cast at least attempted English accents). Perhaps in a further nod to 1930s American values, the film provides Nightingale's father with an entirely invented role as a reforming hospital inspector, thus making him into an active, respectable figure rather than an indolent gentleman of leisure—at the cost of making Nightingale's nursing vocation appear to be derived from his work rather than her own study and reflection. *The White Angel* also ends with Nightingale anachronistically reading the "Nightingale Pledge"—a modified version of the Hippocratic Oath intended for American nurses, written in 1893 in the USA and nothing to do with Nightingale.

Reviewing the film, British novelist Graham Greene wrote that while Francis had done "her best to sober down this sentimental version" of Nightingale, she had been "defeated by the scenario writers" (Greene, 1980: 121). At times, Francis appears to be struggling to bring herself to play the script straight—an interpretation which would seem to chime with a note in her diary from early 1936: "Read my new script—dear God!" (Rossman and Kear, 2006: 91). The film's producer, Hal Wallis, felt that the fault lay with Dieterle, who "should have gotten more emotion" from Francis: "In scene after scene, reacting to the sight of the injured, or clashing with an official who refused to see things her way, she looked completely blank. We weren't too happy with the picture" (Rossman and Kear, 2006: 92). Francis said in 1938 that she "shuddered" when she thought of the film (Rossman and Kear, 2006: 92). *The New York Times* nonetheless described it as "worthwhile," though its reviewer was unconvinced by Francis's attempts to portray Nightingale's inner conviction: "When she tells her opponents they cannot stop her work you cannot escape the feeling she is speaking less out of sublime faith than certain knowledge gleaned from a twentieth century encyclopedia" (Nugent, 1936).

None of the reviews commented on the film's title—seemingly indicating that the assertions it made, which to a modern sensibility appear ripe for analysis, did not seem controversial at the time. The idea of Nightingale as an "angel" was present from the earliest phase of her commemoration. It was a trope that immediately feminized her, placing her within the nineteenth-century domestic framework of the "angel in the house," emphasizing domestic, maternal qualities over intellectual ones (Patmore, 1863). Simultaneously, it pre-emptively asserted Nightingale's quasi-divinity, framing her work as an apotheosis of Christian charity while avoiding a more nuanced discussion of the role that faith played in her actions. As for "white," this was clearly consciously chosen as a motif for the film. Francis frequently appears in white clothes, often including a white headscarf or headband to create a halo effect, whereas the film's villains—the obstructionist British army doctors and bureaucrats—always wear black. The shifting of Nightingale's Crimea visit to winter allows the screen to be filled with white snow at a climactic moment, while in Scutari, Nightingale's nurses are carefully shown installing bright white bedsheets as a central part of putting the hospital in order. Much of this was conventional: the use of white clothing or lighting to indicate Christian virtue or moral goodness was already a cinematic staple, while in a medical context white was associated with laboratory science, hygiene and sterility. However, in the context of a racially-segregated culture, in which Nightingale had been proposed as an ideal physiognomical specimen, a racial reading of the title is also justifiable. Scholars of the classic Hollywood period have shown how the films of this era consistently associated "whiteness with order, rationality, rigidity" and how studios such as Warner Bros "systematized the popularization of American whiteness" (Dyer, 1988: 48; Bernardi, 2001: xv). Use of white color motifs, white lighting, and Christian iconography contributed to this process, reinforcing the cultural equation of racial whiteness with virtue—even in the absence of the overt contrasts with a non-white racial other made in contemporary films such as Warner Bros' *Jezebel* (1938) or *Gone with the Wind* (1939) (Dyer, 1997).

The *White Angel*'s identification of Nightingale as a white, Christian heroine, along with its American clothes, sets and accents, also served what was presumably considered a commercially-necessary purpose, of downplaying her Englishness and accentuating her relatability and accessibility to an interwar U.S. audience. Such a move was not necessary for the 1951 British film *The Lady with a Lamp*, starring Anna Neagle and directed by her husband Herbert Wilcox, which could afford instead to accentuate her English identity. In 1951, Neagle and Wilcox were a prolific and prominent cinematic double act, having been making films together for nearly twenty years. Rising to fame in the 1930s with a mixture of musicals, biopics, and romantic comedies, they had their two biggest successes with *The Courtneys of Curzon Street* (1947) and *Spring in Park Lane* (1948), which are still in the all-time top twenty U.K. films by cinema admissions (British Film Institute, 2012). Neagle was named Best British Box-Office Star by the *Motion Picture Herald* in 1941, 1947, and 1952. "There are better actresses than she," wrote critic Leonard Wallace in 1951, "there are more devastating personalities; but there is no one else who can touch the hearts of the ordinary [British] cinemagoer as she can" (in Dolan and Street, 2009: 36). Their fame was sufficient for crowds of fans to attend the location filming of *The Lady with a Lamp*. Local newspaper *The Matlock Mercury* made a splash of Neagle and Wilcox's stay in Nightingale's childhood bedroom during filming at Lea Hurst, the Nightingales' Derbyshire home (*Matlock Mercury*, 1951).

Having been overtly sexualized for early films such as *Nell Gwyn* (1934), Neagle had gradually morphed into a "stately icon," an embodiment of English feminine respectability and "infused with a regal aura" (Harper, 2000: 54; Dolan and Street, 2009: 37). Compared to Francis, Neagle's customary screen persona was thus less in tension with the demands of the Nightingale role. Neagle also had a better script to work with. Warren Chetham-Strode's screenplay acknowledged the influence of the stage play with the same title by Reginald Berkeley, a British Liberal MP turned Hollywood screenwriter (Berkeley, 1929). However, Chetham-Strode mostly ignored Berkeley's pedestrian dialogue and retained only a few key elements, especially the suggestion of a flirtatious relationship between Nightingale and the politician Sidney Herbert—who as Secretary-at-War had commissioned Nightingale's Crimean War venture, and subsequently worked with her on various reforms. This enabled Wilcox to carve out a substantial part for Michael Wilding, Neagle's co-star in the big Wilcox-Neagle 1940s hits, in something approaching his usual role as Neagle's love interest.

The film begins in the run-up to the Crimean War. In a ball scene at Broadlands, the home of the Nightingales' politician neighbor Lord Palmerston, Nightingale dances with Richard Monckton Milnes and fairly summarily dismisses his marriage proposal. She is then approached by a young working-class man, George, a gardener on the Nightingales' Embley estate, whose mother is ill. Nightingale accompanies him to his cottage, where, in a scene channeling her 1860 text *Notes on Nursing*, she makes a show of opening the windows ("God's good fresh air is what you need, and plenty of it") and tells George to scrub everything thoroughly. This is followed by an Embley dinner scene, at which Nightingale, supported by Herbert, clashes with her mother and Palmerston over women's work and the value of female army nursing. After a further confrontation with her anxious sister Parthenope ("But why must you be so different? *Why* must you go on blowing a trumpet for humanity?") Nightingale goes to see Herbert who, in a scene of mild physical intimacy between the two, suggests that she take on the management of the Establishment for Gentlewomen During Illness in London's Harley Street (which Nightingale indeed ran for a year from 1853, though not at Herbert's instigation). The film soon advances to the Crimean War, switching between Nightingale's struggles in Scutari and Herbert's battles to secure her government support at home. Nightingale has showdowns with representatives of the army's bureaucratic intransigence, notably Dr. Menzies, who initially refuses to let her nurses treat the soldiers, and an obstructive army purveyor. Eventually prevailing, Nightingale imposes order and calm in the hospital, setting up the inevitable scene of her doing her ward rounds with her lamp. She is shown doing quite a lot of hands-on nursing, including of George, the Embley gardener, who dies as a soldier in her care. In London, meanwhile, Herbert's best efforts are not enough to prevent the fall of the government, with Herbert declaring to his wife that he is "sick and tired of this endless battle." This provides the set up for the final part of the film, derived from Lytton Strachey's *Eminent*

Victorians, in which Nightingale's constant exhortations in the service of her post-war reform projects are shown as contributing to an overworked Herbert's early death (Strachey, 1918). The film however ultimately ends on a celebratory note, with a visit to the elderly Nightingale's home in 1908 by two public officials to present her with the Order of Merit. "How little people know about Miss Nightingale who only know about the lamp," one official says in a discussion with Nightingale's housekeeper—despite the film having done little to illustrate any other aspects of her legacy, and indeed closing with a recital of the "lady with a lamp" passage from Longfellow's *Santa Filomena*.

Much more historically accurate than *The White Angel*, *The Lady with a Lamp* nonetheless was far from a documentary and can be seen as carrying certain political connotations, especially when set within the context of the Wilcox-Neagle corpus. Scholarship on Neagle has emphasized her "English rose" image and her relationship to what Josephine Dolan and Sarah Street have called "the mesh of a racialized imperial hegemonic Englishness" (Dolan and Street, 2009: 37–39). Neagle had partly established her reputation with a series of biopics of famous/heroic British women, including Queen Victoria (*Victoria the Great*, 1937; *Sixty Glorious Years*, 1938), *Nurse Edith Cavell* (1939), and the Second World War heroines Amy Johnson (*They Flew Alone*, 1942), and (French-born) Odette Sanson (*Odette*, 1950). *Odette* and *They Flew Alone* both raised the issue of the relationship between femininity and wartime heroism. Neagle played Johnson, an aviator, as a woman whose patriotism, and refusal to be constrained by conventional conceptions of femininity, carried her into military occupations without thereby masculinizing her. The same dynamic was at play in her depiction of Nightingale, whose feminist belief in women's ability to work (which the film faithfully represents) coexisted with Neagle's decision to play her as "intensely feminine," manifest in her demure relationship with Wilding's Herbert and her patriotic-maternal attitude to the suffering soldiers (Kalisch, 1983: 273). In one scene, perhaps included with an eye on its audience's experiences of Second World War grief, Nightingale visits the Scutari grave of the Coldstream Guards, saying "goodbye, my children, I can do no more for you who have suffered and died in your country's service … you have not sacrificed your lives for little or no purpose, because I for one shall never forget." Dolan and Street also emphasize the political undertones of Neagle's voice: gentle enough to be considered feminine, sufficiently "establishment" to narrate the 1947 Royal Wedding for Pathé news, yet sufficiently un-aristocratic as to help make upper-class characters like Queen Victoria and Nightingale seem relatable to a broad English public (Dolan and Street, 2009: 40–41).

The Lady with a Lamp was commercially successful—not on the scale of the late-1940s Wilcox-Neagle films, but enough to place it among the largest-grossing British films of 1951 (Thumim, 1991: 258). The cultural authority that Neagle brought to the role perhaps encouraged a sense that hers was a definitive performance, discouraging other filmmakers from tackling Nightingale; there has not been a cinema biopic since. Nightingale has however been portrayed several times in made-for-TV movies since the 1960s. The earliest of these, *The Holy Terror* (1965, dir. James Lee), made for the American *Hallmark Hall of Fame* series, appears to be lost. According to Beatrice and Philip Kalisch, Julie Harris, in an Emmy-nominated performance, played Nightingale as a "driven fanatic" who hounds and bullies people into supporting her reforms (Kalisch, 1983: 275–276). A more conventional American depiction appeared in a 133-minute film for NBC, *Florence Nightingale* (1985), starring Jaclyn Smith of *Charlie's Angels* fame. Directed by Daryl Duke, the film reprises many elements of the cinematic releases, while adding extra elements of Nightingale's backstory such as her training at Kaiserswerth, Germany, and her family's friendship with the Massachusetts physician and abolitionist Samuel Gridley Howe. Smith's impressive range of facial and emotional expression in the title role stands out in comparison with Neagle and Francis's more detached performances. Otherwise, this version is most notable for the expanded part afforded to future James Bond actor Timothy Dalton as Richard Monckton Milnes, who doubles as the film's narrator. Placing Milnes at the center of the story necessitates a distorting compression of the historical events, such that Nightingale's final rejection of Milnes appears to occur in 1853–54 rather than 1849. The decision to make Milnes central feels inherently conservative, in the sense that exaggerating the importance of the love interest, as almost all of the films do, makes her choice to forego romance into a crucial part of her heroic self-sacrifice—as if asserting that love was an indispensable component of true happiness. The NBC version further adds in a trope of feminine jealousy by inventing a "bad nurse" character who, racked by envy and class antagonism towards Nightingale, causes multiple problems before finally cutting Nightingale's hair off out of spite during her Crimean illness.

A different take on Nightingale is offered by the 2008 BBC TV drama, also called simply *Florence Nightingale*, starring Laura Fraser and written and directed by Norman Stone. Unusually, the first half of this film focuses not on Nightingale's family/romantic life before the Crimean War, but on her troubled mental state in the months after it, when she went through the British army medical figures with the statistician William Farr and realized that the hospital with the highest mortality had been hers, Scutari. This realization is shown as crushing to Nightingale, provoking a spiritual crisis which she ultimately resolves with her father's help. This storyline was clearly derived from Hugh Small's 1998 book *Florence Nightingale: Avenging Angel*, and controversy ensued when Small complained about the BBC's failure to acknowledge this, instead trailing its version as an "untold story" (Wavell, 2008; Small, 1998). Other interesting facets of this film, which was co-produced by an interfaith production company, include the way it juxtaposes Nightingale's soaring public reputation—depicted through scenes of music hall performances—with her private crisis of faith. Fraser's Nightingale reacts to this with fourth wall breaking commentaries to camera explaining her emotional torment—such that my wife, who patiently sat through all these films with me, labeled this version "*Fleabag* Florence" in reference to Phoebe Waller-Bridge's similar technique in her BBC comedy series.

By the twenty-first century, the issue of Nightingale's racial identity had taken on a different dimension, owing to the rediscovery of the story of Mary Seacole, the mixed-race Jamaican woman who travelled to the Crimea during the war. Though widely celebrated in her own lifetime, Seacole essentially dropped out of British historical consciousness following her death in 1881, until rediscovered a century later by Ziggi Alexander and Audrey Dewjee, who republished Seacole's memoir, *Wonderful Adventures of Mrs. Seacole in Many Lands*, in 1984 (Alexander and Dewjee, 1982; Seacole 2005). Seacole's fascinating life story, the resourcefulness and larger-than-life generosity that are evident in her memoir, and the underdog aspect of her historical neglect, held strong public appeal at a time when Britain was beginning to become aware of its neglect of Black history and the absence of Black figures in the curriculum (a critique which has become all the sharper in recent years and with the emergence of the Black Lives Matter movement). To some nurses, the Seacole story also provided an opportunity to remind the public about the existence of, and discrimination against, Black nurses—and thereby to help move British nursing on from the stereotype of the Nightingale-inspired "white girl who lives in a nurses' home" who "has 'Doctor and Nurse' romances on her bookshelves" and "will never strike" (Crawford, 1992, 58). By 2004, Seacole's re-found prominence was such that an internet poll named her the greatest ever Black Briton (Taylor, 2004). *Wonderful Adventures* was reprinted as a Penguin Classic in 2005, and since 2007 Seacole has featured on the British school curriculum alongside Nightingale—surviving an attempt by Conservative Education Secretary Michael Gove to remove her in 2013 thanks to a popular campaign to retain Seacole.

Seacole and Nightingale were not big parts of each other's lives. Prior to the Crimean War, Seacole had lived for most of her life in Jamaica as a businesswoman—running hotels, stores, restaurants and making investments—and folk healer. She had treated cholera patients in Jamaica in 1850, and again in Panama between 1851 and 1854, both times in an unofficial capacity alongside her business activities. In 1854 she travelled to England to attend to her interests in mining stocks. Upon reading newspaper coverage of the Crimean War, she "shared in the general enthusiasm" to improve conditions for the soldiers, and sought to help in some capacity (Seacole, 2005: 67, 70). She was however turned down both by the army, and by (Sidney's wife) Elizabeth Herbert on behalf of Nightingale's nursing mission. Seacole suspected that racial prejudice contributed to these refusals—though she would likely have been refused as a nurse regardless, for lacking formal hospital experience (Seacole, 2005: 73–74). She decided to travel to the Crimea anyway, along with her business partner and two servants, where she set up the "British Hotel," a general store and restaurant. Seacole's ability to procure all kinds of items from anchors to handkerchiefs, and to supply food and first aid to soldiers, "brewing tea for all who wanted it," made her well-known and respected as someone who "did not spare herself if she could do any good to the suffering soldiers" (Reid 1911: 14). Seacole and Nightingale met only once, briefly, when Seacole passed through Scutari *en route* for the Crimea, and Nightingale found her a bed for the night. Nightingale comes across as friendly in Seacole's memoir: "What do you want, Mrs. Seacole—anything that we can do for you? If it lies in my power, I shall be very happy" (Seacole, 2005: 82). Nightingale contributed to a fund created in 1857 to support Seacole, who lost money in the war and subsequently settled in Britain (Bostridge, 2009: 274, 590).

Since the 1980s however, Seacole and Nightingale have become inextricably intertwined in popular commemoration, often as rivals or enemies. Despite the divergence in their historical experiences, the temptation to contextualize Seacole's re-emerging story and its previous neglect by characterizing her as "another Nightingale" or a "Black Nightingale" proved irresistible. Some commentators went further, implicating Nightingale in Britain's century-long failure to commemorate Seacole; Salman Rushdie wrote of Seacole as "another magic-lamping Lady" who "being dark, could scarce be seen for the flame of Florence's candle" (Rushdie, 1988: 292). A 2010 sketch for the children's BBC series *Horrible Histories* showed Seacole and Nightingale squabbling over who merited the most recognition, with Nightingale at one point saying that "the nursing corps was for British girls—you're from Jamaica!" Taking on the role of Nightingale's defender, Lynn McDonald has documented how various texts celebrating Seacole embellished her story, or erroneously credited her with Nightingale's reforming achievements (McDonald, 2014). McDonald's Nightingale Society led an unsuccessful campaign to prevent Seacole's statue being located at St Thomas' Hospital, the site of the Nightingale Training School for nurses and the Nightingale Museum but a place unconnected to Seacole. It did however get the BBC to remove the *Horrible Histories* episode from its website, on the grounds that it unfairly portrayed Nightingale as racist (BBC News, 2014).

A major contribution to the idea of Nightingale as Seacole's enemy was made by the 2005 Channel 4 (UK) TV docu-drama *Mary Seacole: The Real Angel of the Crimea*. Written and directed by Sonali Fernando and starring Angela Bruce, the film helped cement Seacole's status as a major historical figure—and, with its subtitle, claimed her as superior to Nightingale, who became the villain of the piece. Somewhat oddly (and inaccurately), the film presents Nightingale as having only a managerial and administrative role in the war, as opposed to Seacole's "hands-on care." It makes prominent use of a private 1870 letter from Nightingale to her brother-in-law, in which Nightingale wrote of having sought to prevent Seacole associating with her nurses during the Crimean War, and accused Seacole of having kept "something not very unlike ... a 'bad house'" [i.e., where prostitutes were available] and being the source of "much drunkenness and improper conduct." In the film, Michelle Bunyan plays Nightingale as icy and aloof. Her encounter with Seacole at Scutari is filmed from the point of view of a seated Seacole, such that the upright Nightingale appears to be looking down snootily at both Seacole and the audience. The affable exchange from Seacole's memoir is turned into a hostile confrontation, as Bunyan's Nightingale sneers, "what do you *want*, Mrs. Seacole?" This scene appears to have influenced subsequent representations of the Nightingale-Seacole relationship, such as that in a 2011 book by the then-Mayor of London Boris Johnson, who wrote of Nightingale looking "down her beaky nose" at Seacole (Johnson, 2011: 272) (The publication deadline for this book came too early to incorporate the *Seacole* feature film due for release in 2021, directed by Charlie Stratton and starring Gugu Mbatha-Raw.) Whereas *The White Angel* claimed Nightingale as a symbol of racial virtue, *The Real Angel of the Crimea* portrayed her as an embodiment of Victorian racism.

A consistent feature of the Nightingale filmography, whether sympathetic or hostile, has thus been a lack of nuance and the assertion of simplistic—or even moralistic and didactic—narratives. An interesting exception to this, in terms of highlighting complexity and nuance, is *Miss Nightingale* (1974), a British TV film directed by David Reid for the ITV channel and adapted from John Bowen's successful stage play. The film follows a 1970s undergraduate student, "Sally," who has been asked to write an essay on Nightingale. Having initially concluded that Nightingale was "dull," a discussion with her supervisor prompts Sally to throw herself into researching Nightingale's personality. The film then stages various episodes from Nightingale's life as Sally encounters them in her research. This device allows *Miss Nightingale* to approach its subject in a non-linear way, jumping between different periods of her life to illustrate different aspects of her work or personality, using Sally as a conduit to fill in gaps in exposition. It enables more aspects of Nightingale's life to be covered, such as her daydreaming, or her sister Parthenope's nervous breakdown, which do not feature in other productions. The device also frees the film from committing itself to a single interpretation of Nightingale, giving her a kind of right of reply—for example, staging a scene in which Nightingale works Sidney Herbert to death, but following it with a monologue from Nightingale giving her side of that story. Sally's conversations with other 1970s characters are used to debate contemporary theories about Nightingale, such as when she meets a psychology lecturer to hear (and ultimately reject) his cod-psychoanalytic theories about Nightingale being a "hysterical obsessive" and "defined by violence." The film refuses to end on a note of triumph or certainty, with Sally saying "you can admire [Nightingale], you can dislike her, you can feel sorry for her, but you can't ever know her. She escapes you."

Historical drama is always subject to tension between accuracy and entertainment, and films that set out to challenge audience preconceptions or portray complex historical debates are a risky route to commercial success. While *Miss Nightingale* successfully indicates a complexity to Nightingale's character that simplified/romanticized depictions had missed, it remains a fairly obscure work. In retrospect, it nonetheless appears significant as the first postmodern Nightingale production—in the sense that it tries to break down and question the older myths rather than, or at least as well as, reproducing them. The BBC 2008 *Florence Nightingale* can also be considered in this category, in that it makes Nightingale's reputation into a kind of character in its own right via music hall scenes charting the progress of her fame. So, too, can *The Real Angel of the Crimea*, insofar as it tries to force a rethink of Nightingale as a symbol of moral virtue by showing her transgressing the new moral code of anti-racism, and proposes Seacole as an alternative candidate for the previously unassailable position in British cultural memory that Nightingale has occupied. In recent decades, there certainly seems to be an unwillingness to play Nightingale "straight" in the sense of reproducing the unproblematized narratives that dominated for the century after the Crimean War. Each new representation seeks a new angle or a new way to undercut conventional expectations; the British sketch show *Big Train* even tried her out in 2002 as a hard-drinking potty mouth.

From the perspective of Britain in the early 2020s, it feels as if

Nightingale's reputation is caught between two stools: on the one hand, the persistence of a celebratory, laudatory, patriotic tendency with its roots in the 1850s; on the other, a postmodern desire to undercut metanarratives of Nightingale's heroic virtue, a tendency that is caught up with the long-term trend away from Nightingale's vocational vision of nursing towards an academic model, as well as with contemporary sensibilities on questions of race and empire and the drive to commemorate Seacole. In other words, there are both still plenty of people who want to keep celebrating Nightingale as a "white angel," and many others who see it as vital to dismantle that idea as an imperialist myth that hampers today's diverse nursing profession. As this essay has shown, film has played a large role in developing and reflecting both of these trends—yet this dichotomy may also go some way to accounting for the relative paucity of screen depictions of her. With no commonly accepted version of Nightingale that can easily be reached for, no agreement on what Nightingale *means*, she is a hard character to get right.

Films and Television Productions Referenced

Florence Nightingale (1915) British & Colonial Kinematograph Company.
Florence Nightingale (1985) Cypress Point Productions.
Florence Nightingale (2008) BBC.
The Holy Terror (1965) Compass Productions.
Horrible Histories (2010. Episode 206) Lion TV.
The Lady with a Lamp (1951) Herbert Wilcox Productions.
Mary Seacole: The Real Angel of the Crimea. (2005) Channel 4.
Miss Nightingale (1974) Southern Television.
Victoria Cross (1912) Vitagraph Company of America.
The White Angel (1936) Warner Bros.

References

Alexander, Z., and Dewjee, A. (1982) *Mary Seacole: Jamaican National Heroine and "Doctress" in the Crimean War.* London: Brent Library Service.
BBC News, Entertainment & Arts (2014) BBC Rapped Over Horrible Histories Florence Nightingale Sketch. Available at https://www.bbc.co.uk/news/entertainment-arts-29426242 [accessed 29 Oct. 2020].
Berkeley, R. (1929) *The Lady with a Lamp: A Play.* London: Gollancz.
Bernardi, D. (ed.) (2001) *Classic Hollywood, Classic Whiteness.* Minneapolis: University of Minnesota Press.
Bostridge, M. (2009) *Florence Nightingale: The Woman and Her Legend.* London: Penguin.
British Film Institute (2012) The Ultimate Chart: 1–100. http://old.bfi.org.uk/features/ultimatefilm/chart/complete.php [accessed 27 Oct. 2020].
Brown, N. (2013) "A New Movie-Going Public": 1930s Hollywood and the Emergence of the "Family" Film. *Historical Journal of Film, Radio and Television* 33, 1: 1–23.
Cook, E. (1913) *The Life of Florence Nightingale.* 2 vols. London: Macmillan.
Crawford, P. (1992) The Other Lady with the Lamp. *Nursing Times* 88, 11: 56–8.

Crawford, P., Greenwood, A., Bates, R., and Memel, J. (2020) *Florence Nightingale at Home.* London: Palgrave Macmillan.

Crossland, J. (2018) *War, Law and Humanity: The Campaign to Control Warfare, 1853–1914.* London: Bloomsbury.

Dolan, J., and Street, S. (2009) "Twenty Million People Can't be Wrong": Anna Neagle and Popular British Stardom. In: Bell, M., and Williams, M. (eds.) *British Women's Cinema.* London: Routledge, pp. 34–48.

Dunant, H. (1939) *A Memory of Solferino* (1862) Trans. the American Red Cross Geneva: International Committee of the Red Cross.

Dyer, R. (1988) White. *Screen* 29, 4: 44–65

Dyer, R. (1997) *White.* London: Routledge.

Fox-Leonard, B. (2015) The 50 Greatest Britons Revealed. *Daily Mirror* 22 Sep. 2015. Available at https://www.mirror.co.uk/news/uk-news/50-greatest-britons-revealed-wills-6495706 [accessed 26 Oct. 2020].

Gill, G. (2004) *Nightingales: The Story of Florence Nightingale and Her Family.* London: Hodder & Stoughton.

Greene, G. (1980) *The Pleasure-Dome: Graham Greene, the Collected Film Criticism, 1935–40.* Oxford: Oxford University Press.

Harper, S. (2000) *Mad, Bad and Dangerous to Know: Women in British Cinema.* London: Continuum.

Helmstadter, C. (2020) *Beyond Nightingale: Nursing on the Crimean War Battlefields.* Manchester: Manchester University Press.

Hutchinson, J. (1996) *Champions of Charity: War and the Rise of the Red Cross.* Boulder: Westview Press.

Johnson, B. (2011) *Johnson's Life of London: The People Who Made the City That Made the World.* London: Harper.

Kalisch, B.J., and Kalisch, P. A (1983) Heroine Out of Focus: Media Images of Florence Nightingale. *Nursing & Health Care* 4: 181–187, 270–278.

Longfellow, H.W. (1857) Santa Filomena: A Poem. *The Atlantic*, Nov. 1857. Available at https://www.theatlantic.com/magazine/archive/1857/11/santa-filomena/531180/ [accessed 27 Oct. 2020].

Macdonald, I.W. (2013) *Screenwriting Poetics and the Screen Idea.* Basingstoke: Palgrave. *Matlock Mercury*, 7 July 1951.

McDonald, L. (ed.) (2001–2012) *The Collected Works of Florence Nightingale.* 16 vols. Waterloo, ON: Wilfried Laurier University Press.

McDonald, L. (2014) *Mary Seacole: The Making of the Myth.* Toronto: Iguana Press.

Nugent, F. (1936) THE SCREEN: A Worshipful Biography of Florence Nightingale Is "The White Angel," at the Strand. *The New York Times,* 25 June 1936.

O'Malley, I. (1931) *Florence Nightingale 1820–1856: A Study of Her Life Down to the End of the Crimean War.* London: Thornton Butterworth.

Patmore, C. (1863) *The Angel in the House.* London: Macmillan.

Penner, L. (2010) *Victorian Medicine and Social Reform: Florence Nightingale Among the Novelists.* New York: Palgrave.

Poovey, M. (1988) *Uneven Developments: The Ideological Work of Gender in Mid-Victorian England.* Chicago: University of Chicago Press.

Reid, D.A. (1911) *Memories of the Crimean War, January 1855 to June 1856.* London: St Catherine Press.

Rossman, J., and Kear, L. (2006) *Kay Francis: A Passionate Life and Career.* Jefferson, NC: McFarland.

Rushdie, S. (1988) *The Satanic Verses.* New York: Viking.

Seacole, M. (2005) *Wonderful Adventures of Mrs. Seacole in Many Lands* (1857). London: Penguin.

Small, H. (1998) *Florence Nightingale: Avenging Angel.* London: Constable.

Smith, F.B. (1982) *Florence Nightingale: Reputation and Power.* London: Croom Helm.

Summers, A. (2000) *Angels and Citizens: British Women as Military Nurses, 1854–1914.* 2nd ed. Newbury: Threshold.

Taylor, M. (2004) Nurse Is Greatest Black Briton. *The Guardian*, 10 Feb. 2004. Available at https://www.theguardian.com/uk/2004/feb/10/britishidentity.artsandhumanities [accessed 27 Oct. 2020].

Thumin, J. (1991) The "Popular," Cash and Culture in the Postwar British Cinema Industry. *Screen* 32, 3: 245–271.

Vicinus, M. (1985) *Independent Women: Work and Community for Single Women, 1850–1920.* Chicago: University of Chicago Press.

Wavell, S. (2008) BBC Drama About Florence Nightingale Sparks Controversy. *The Sunday Times*, 1 June 2008. Available at https://www.thetimes.co.uk/article/bbc-drama-about-florence-nightingale-sparks-controversy-f8mmh0m5gdx [accessed 26 Oct. 2020].

Wells, S.R. (1894) *New Physiognomy* (1866). New York: Fowler & Wells.

Woodham-Smith, C. (1950) *Florence Nightingale 1820–1910*. London: Constable.

"Women bow"

The Shifting Power Dynamics Between Nurses and Doctors in Tenko

Mark Aldridge

Introduction

The BBC television drama *Tenko* (1981–85) focused on the stories of women placed in a female prisoner of war camp in Singapore during the Second World War. Across the course of thirty episodes, and a reunion television film, the series followed a group of women from different walks of life who were interred together and sought to find ways to survive in a world that was markedly different to the society that they had come from. In the first series of ten episodes, three of the main characters had medical backgrounds, including Dr. Beatrice Mason, and two nurses who were under her supervision in the outside world, Kate Norris and Nellie Keene. In this essay, I will explore the ways in which *Tenko* portrayed these two nurses, paying particular attention to how the series expressed changing power dynamics and a new idea of social order once the characters were in the camp, compared to the outside world. Concentrating on the first series, which shows the contrast most dramatically, I will first outline the important background context of the series' creation, before providing a textual reading of key episodes and moments. I will then draw on existing scholarship and other material relating to both *Tenko* and female ensemble dramas in general in order to highlight the distinctive approaches made by the series' writers and production team.

The origins of *Tenko* are particularly important, as they demonstrated that real-life experiences of nurses in particular would be a key component of the program's influences and identity. The series was created by Lavinia Warner, who had worked as a researcher for a 1978 episode of *This*

Is Your Life that celebrated the achievements of Dame Margot Turner, who had risen to the rank of Brigadier as a British military nurse. When in a more junior position in 1941, Turner had been posted to Singapore and was there when the Japanese invaded. Despite attempting to evacuate, the ship in which she was travelling sank following an air attack, and after escaping first by swimming and then on a life raft (on which she was to be the only survivor), she was eventually found and captured by Japanese forces who interred her in a camp on Bank Island, off Sumatra, where she would stay for three and a half years. Warner found this story fascinating and admired the fortitude of both Turner and those who had been in the camp alongside her. Consequently, Warner was inspired to tell their stories in more depth, which first resulted in a 1979 BBC documentary *Women in Captivity*. A memorable section saw Margot Turner reunited with fellow nurse (and captive) Betty Jeffrey, who stated that:

> I often make people laugh when I say I like women, I like nursing women, but never again do I want to be locked up with a thousand other women, never, I want to be locked up with some men next time! Because women can be unreasonable, they can be very very brave, very very tenacious, if it hadn't been for their tenacity their bravery their sheer guts to win, but to live with a lot of women, they all had minds of their own, and for some reason or another you can't regiment women like men. And I think they had a tremendous amount of guts, I really do, to do what they did, and to be able to survive, because we had no men to help us. It was only our strength, it wasn't anybody else's [*Women in Captivity*, BBC 1979].

As this recollection showed, for Jeffrey being imprisoned alongside women was an impactful part of the experience, rather than a secondary consideration—hers was not just a story of imprisonment, but of living in a world where she co-existed only with women, and this would come to be an important part of *Tenko*. The stories told by the camps' survivors helped to convince Warner that there was dramatic potential in the series, and with Turner and Jeffrey having been nurses it was perhaps obvious that such characters would have a central role to play in the series. Nevertheless, despite the influence that her experiences would have on the program, when Margot Turner was asked if *Tenko* was authentic, she replied that "No, I don't think it was. They had too many clothes for a start.... But then one is apt to judge a thing by your own circumstances and your own camp" (Imperial War Museum interview, quoted by Starns, 2010: 171).

However, *Tenko* was not designed to take a strict documentary-drama approach to its topic, even though it was based on real experiences. It was not intended to tell a single person's story, nor to closely depict specific events, but instead to give an overall impression of a largely untold history that had been largely neglected, possibly because it was one that was concerned almost entirely with women. In her exploration of female ensemble dramas, Ros Jennings, drawing on Alison Landsberg's writings on "prosthetic memory," discusses both *Tenko* and *Call the Midwife* (BBC, 2012–present), suggesting that they perform "as technologies of prosthetic memory which immerse viewers into a 'larger history' (Landsberg 2004: 2) of both the historic periods in view and also a rich 'herstory' of women who have been marginalized by dominant historical accounts" (Jennings, 2017: 182). In *Tenko*, women's stories were not sidelined, and were instead given prominence, even though the more general popular historical retelling of the war had paid them little attention. By contrast, the gender of the program's key characters and creatives would be important to its development, and would allow the stories of two female nurses to be elevated to a position in drama where they might otherwise be neglected in favor of more male-dominated environments. Perhaps more significantly, the series would also tell a story that depicted the realities of women's experiences in a way that had previously been considered to be too unpalatable for television drama.

In the first two episodes of *Tenko*, which deal with the Japanese invasion of Singapore and life before the characters' imprisonment, the two nurses Kate and Nellie are initially shown to have important but inherently subservient positions in their roles at the hospital, where they work under Dr. Beatrice Mason (an example of the series showing women in a position of authority). Jennings points out that these opening episodes "highlight the initial tensions and divisions of class, nationality, race, education and sexuality that exist between the central characters before they are then forcibly confined and grouped together as prisoners" (Jennings, 2017: 185). They do this by establishing the complex power-relations between characters, in which public expectations can be contrasted with private thoughts. For example, in the first episode, the nurses describe Dr. Mason as a "battle-ax" and "wicked witch of the west" in private while fastidiously following her orders on the hospital ward. There are already hints that the superficial attitudes are not necessarily all that they seem, however, when the nurses' request to change shifts for social reasons is granted by the doctor, albeit begrudgingly, showing that her brusquely professional exterior is at least partly for show. The series does not pay much attention to the relative unusualness of a female doctor at this time (although camp records show that there were indeed female doctors imprisoned alongside Margot Turner), but the audience can surely draw an inference from the fact that they will understand that Dr. Mason will have had extra struggles to contend with in order to reach her position of authority, and that this may explain her no-nonsense attitude. She is certainly someone who has worked hard to ensure that she commands respect, and perhaps does not wish to show any weakness that could be ascribed to her gender, such as taking on a motherly role for the younger nurses.

These early appearances of the nurses show the duality of their lives, with the formalized work environment in which they are required to follow instructions contrasting with their relaxed and liberated personal lives. In the following months and years their professional skills will become an important and valued part of life in the prison camps, but prior to this they are shown to be less important in the British community than the military wives and socialites who attend dinner dances with regularity, whereas for the nurses this is a special occasion, and they revel in its glamor. The strongest character of the two is certainly Kate, an Australian who is brimming with confidence and is not shy when it comes to making her voice heard. In his comprehensive book that covers the history of the series, Andy Priestner reproduces the original character outline for twenty-five-year-old Kate, who we are told, had decided to become a nurse in order to travel the world, and that "she did not start out very dedicated to her profession." Once she reached Singapore she started work under Dr. Mason, but (in what became a recurring character theme) this "was not a happy working relationship as the doctor found her to be too independent and free with her opinions. The arrival of another nurse, Nellie Keene, ameliorated the situation somewhat and the pair became friends as well as colleagues" (Priestner, 2012: 67).

While Nellie seems uninterested in lasting relationships, Kate enjoys dating the British man Tom Redburn (Daniel Hill), and lives a somewhat carefree life outside of the hospital. She is also sexually liberated, as she works with Tom to hire a hotel room where they can sleep together for the first time. Just as Dr. Mason is to-the-point in her professional life, so Kate is in her personal life, and so when Tom proposes after they have had sex she unromantically but pragmatically replies, "Okay, sport, let's give it a go." Minutes later, an explosion signals military action from the Japanese, and the consequent medical emergency means that Kate must quickly revert to being under the command of Dr. Mason, a position that she accepts. In the series' second episode, Dr. Mason tells the nurses to evacuate Singapore, demonstrating that despite her clinical manner she clearly cares for her nurses' wellbeing, even at the expense of the local patients. Dr. Mason's initial plan is to remain at the hospital ("She's going to stay behind and play the hero," says Nellie) but all three characters will find themselves in a prisoner of war camp by the next episode, at which point the pre-existing boundaries between professional roles and personal lives will start to break down.

These first two episodes of *Tenko* are anomalies in the series, as they are the only two to be written by a man, Paul Wheeler (all the others were written by Jill Hyem or Anne Valery), and the explanation for this mirrors the gender presumptions that occasionally occur in *Tenko*. Julia Hallam (2013) and Ros Jennings have both drawn attention to the fact that female creatives in the television industry have been influential in the creation of female focused dramas; as Jennings puts it, such programs often "evolved as vehicles for female writers and producers who, on entering a previously male-dominated television industry, took opportunities when they arose to make both the representation of women and their own industry presence more meaningful" (Jennings, 2017: 182). However, while the core team of Warner as creator, with Hyem and Valery as lead writers, was entirely female, this was not the whole picture. As Hyem herself pointed out in a 1987 article:

> … the two producers, five directors and the original script editor appointed to the series were all male, as were the designers, the composer and the person in charge of publicity. It is also worth noting that a man was commissioned to write the first two episodes before the women reached the camp. These dealt with the fall of Singapore. It was not thought that a woman writer could "handle the military side," in spite of the fact that Anne Valery had been in the army at this period and that anyway events were meant to be seen through the eyes of the women [Hyem, 1987: 153].

Even with these gendered assumptions in the wider production team, the creation of such a female focused series which would eschew glamor in favor of the miserable (but dramatic) reality of life in the camps was not seen as a recipe for success among the male-dominated "powers-that-be." Hyem recalls that the general feeling was that "No-one'll want to know about an all-woman cast looking their worst," and that the series was "such a depressing subject, they'll switch off in droves" (Hyem, 2017: 153). In the event, the series was a commercial and critical success, with reviewers drawing attention to the realism of the camp environment as one of the program's biggest attractions (Priestner, 2012: 221).

An early indication of the ways in which the (perceived) class and backgrounds of characters would come to be important points of drama in the series, at least initially, occurs when many of the show's regular characters board a ship to evacuate Singapore. Kate and Nellie comfortably assert themselves and fit in with the overcrowded surroundings, as they appear to draw on their nursing backgrounds that allow them to cope and keep calm in a crisis. When society lady Rose Millar expectantly asks them to separate so that she can be more comfortable by sharing the cabin with her lover she is given short shrift by a dismissive Kate. Great play would be made of the fact that Rose's socialite background did not make her suitable for life in the camp, as she misses the excess and glamor that she had become accustomed to in Singapore—while the nurses understand that they will need to adapt to their new lives. They also understand their own strengths and skills—when the ship is attacked and sunk, Nellie is seen to tend to one of the survivors on the beach where they have been washed up, shortly before they are captured and moved to the camp. Jennings has highlighted the way that these differing experiences and attitudes of women placed together in a single environment can resonate as a universal theme, perhaps particularly with female audiences, as she points out that "tensions and divisions continue to permeate the women's relationships in the camps," and that "their differing worldviews … are then explored throughout the series in ways that resonated with the experience of female audiences" (Jennings, 2017: 185).

The creation of these interactions, friendships and divisions in the camp that would not have occurred in the characters' previous lives is rooted in the truth of the situation. In her book about the real-life camps, *Women Beyond the Wire*, series creator Lavinia Warner quotes one unnamed prisoner as saying that "One learnt to live with and understand people better. The old order of politeness broke down and one got to the bare bones of living" (Warner in Warner and Sandilands, 1983: 5). This is a crucial aspect of the series, which soon establishes that pre-existing values and expectations quickly lose their currency in times of crisis, which has a leveling effect on society.

The removal of the prisoners from the men in their lives—whether friends, relatives or lovers—creates an entirely new structure for the relationships between the women as, apart from the guards almost all of their time is spent as a single-sex unit, where their character interactions do not need to rely on day-to-day lives lived alongside men in the way that most dramas demand. Jilly Hyem was acutely aware that female characters often seemed to only operate in relation to men on television, often either as allies or enemies of a central male protagonist, rather than as independent entities. She wrote that "There is a tendency among men to dismiss women characters who are not young and attractive as 'unappealing' or 'uninteresting.' Unless, that is, they fulfil the usual stereotype of nagging wife or mother-in-law" (Hyem, 1987: 154). The series needed to create its own idea of relationships and character types, and the placement of nurses and a doctor within this new order automatically gave them significance and importance—for the first time, in the case of the nurses, who had been used to being ordered around as staff, rather than praised and consulted as trained professionals. Thus, things that had been considered important outside of the camp—such as wealth, connections, and ancestry—no longer had any value, and characters such as Rose and Marion Jefferson, wife of a British colonel who had risen to the top end of society's hierarchy, now found that they would no longer be treated in the way that they had been accustomed to. More than this, they would be mixing with people whose lives would never normally intersect with theirs.

Despite its attempts to break away from the established order, *Tenko* does foreground its middle-class characters by assigning them important roles, either within the new camp hierarchy or in terms of story development. However, Anne Valery was very aware that history tends to preserve the voices and stories of those who have the opportunity and means to tell it, as she told a contemporary documentary about the writing of the program:

> There was one danger here in that all the books one was able to read by women were obviously written by middle class women, it was nurses, doctors, families…. But one realised, out of the corner of your eye from things you read, that there were other women in the camp, there were tarts, there were whores, there were people who'd been in Shanghai who'd been washed up, there were cockneys, and they hadn't had a voice, so one had to invent the voice for them [*General Studies: TV Writer*, 1982].

For Valery, then, nurses were seen as middle-class, even if the characters may not have felt that themselves, and other characters such as Blanche Simmons (Louise Jameson), a cockney sex worker, help to challenge the pretentions of some of the previously more privileged characters, although she stands out precisely because the middle-class characters are given more of a voice. However, despite that fact that the established order is seemingly destroyed, as all characters are placed in the same difficult situation, writers Valery and Hyem then placed Marion as the voice of the prisoners who will liaise with the camp's commandant, the complex Captain Yamauchi. Marion's background as a wife of a man of high rank in the military had previously required her to do little more than issue instructions to her servants each day, and yet the privileges of her earlier life gave her some weight within the camp. "In real life I was sure that there must have been irritation," said Hyem (*General Studies: TV Writer*, 1982). Nevertheless, whatever the characters' backgrounds, Warner saw a similarity in the types of women who would then survive the camp. She felt that there was "a confidence and a strength and a predisposition to the same kind of humour, understated and wry" (Warner in Warner and Sandilands, 1983: 4). Such understatement and humor would allow what would seem to be a superficially gloomy series to feature characters who could make the most of their situation, and provide entertainment as well as interest.

Given the appalling conditions of the camp, illness inevitably follows, and so the role of the nurses becomes important for the camp. The assumption that they would continue their outside paid roles in this new free-for-all environment initially goes unchallenged by Kate and Nellie, but it soon becomes clear that the power structures that had limited their autonomy in their professional lives have now been somewhat dissipated.

In the third episode, the first to take place inside the camp, Dr. Mason pointedly refers to Kate and Nellie as "*my* nurses" (emphasis mine), which immediately irritates them. So does the doctor's decision to volunteer Nellie for work without consultation, referring to her by her surname—"we're not being paid to work with her any more," they grumble to each other. Despite being characters who had spent some time together before the camp, even imprisonment is not enough to allow Dr. Mason to dissolve the barriers between professional distance and personal friendship. At this point, Kate's character in particular is not driven by her nursing background, as instead it is her confident attitude that marks her out, as she demands to know about food and drink and refers to one of the guards, Sato, as "Satan." When one of the prisoners appears to be pregnant, she offers a decidedly un-medical response—"Oh boy!"

In the following three episodes, irritations continue to rise, although they generally simmer under the surface as characters accept that offering medical support is the top priority. Dr. Mason continues to maintain the pretense of a hospital environment in a hut being used as a sick bay, as she firmly orders the nurses as she considers necessary, but this sows the seeds of division, with Kate and Nellie both making it clear that they are unhappy. For Dr. Mason, the preservation of order as she understands it is essential, and she complains to Marion that she is losing authority over "her" nurses. However, it is clear that Dr. Mason is clinging to these pre-existing structures of authority and order because she is so concerned by the reality of the situation, particularly in the case of an unwell baby, who subsequently dies, and then an outbreak of malaria. In a telling judgment about their feelings about the apparent authority figures in the camp, Nellie (who even dons a makeshift nurse's hat) later remarks that the Marion is "out of her depth" in her role as ostensible leader of the prisoners. Kate responds "Aren't we all?," tacitly acknowledging that simple survival is the priority.

By the sixth episode the differences between Kate and Dr. Mason finally boil over as Dr. Mason tries to enforce relatively minor points of order in a traditional hospital environment, including nurses not talking over a patient. This leads to an argument in which Kate argues that she is not Dr. Mason's nurse, she is *a* nurse. Kate cannot see why the new relationships between prisoners needs to mirror the pre-existing expectations adhered to outside of the camp, including the ways that she and Dr. Mason interact. However, Dr. Mason struggles to see beyond the old power relations that offer her stability, and perhaps even comfort in an impossibly difficult new environment. Both are sympathetic to the patients, but each feels devalued in a different way—Dr. Mason because she perceives there to be a rebellion from her nurses, and Kate because she feels that she and Nellie are not given the voice and autonomy that they deserve. The argument is a tempestuous one, far beyond any minor disagreement that may occur on a traditional hospital ward. This stand-off between the two characters is indicative of the fact that the disruption of the previous social hierarchies is welcomed by those who had less power, and angrily reacted against by those who did, including the likes of the wealthy Dutch woman Dominica Van Meyer, who snootily and selfishly refuses to see herself as operating on the same level as most of her campmates. For a while, Dr. Mason can't see how to continue in the face of such disruption. "I never realized how protected I was before," she says. "Hospital routine. Everything to hand."

As Jennings points out, the "usual order" is upset by *Tenko* because of the way that different backgrounds are not only juxtaposed, but that the characters are forced to co-operate in a way that would be unthinkable outside of the camp. Instead, rather than a typical emphasis on youthful femininity so prevalent in popular dramas, the program offers "a more diverse range of age groups and female identities: celibate, lesbian, single mother, leader, doctor, housewife, secretary, nurse, teacher and, indeed, combinations and intersectionalities of all of these that form a more diverse female imaginary for the construction of possible identities along the whole life course." In *Tenko*, such matters are more significant than just questions of friendship—as Jennings says, such co-operation is a "necessity for survival and the day-to-day realities of disease, starvation and physical punishment mean that frailty, so often culturally associated with older age, is understood to strike in a remarkably egalitarian way at any age" (Jennings, 2017: 187). Indeed, those who had led privileged but sheltered lives are just as much at risk of death or disaster as any other character, perhaps even more so. The way that the series strikes against traditional depictions of femininity may have been a cause for concern amongst some of the senior (male) management at the BBC, but in *Tenko* it proves to be an essential component of its leveling out of characters so that they face the same dangers and problems, even if their coping mechanisms differ.

These "unfeminine" conditions (which included the cast growing their body hair and donning an array of wigs and unkempt hairstyles) marked out the program as something different, offering women coping in situations little acknowledged or understood elsewhere, either directly or through similar scenarios being depicted. Hyem recalls that maintaining this was difficult when the series went into production, as "we found that music and lighting would often be used to soften or romanticise scenes which we had intended to be stark" (Hyem, 1987: 156). Even with a series telling the story of such appalling circumstances, the BBC production struggled to grapple with the idea of presenting women in a realistic way—although the actors themselves had mutually agreed to lose gradually weight for the camp scenes, a task that resulted in the short-lived installation of scales in the rehearsal room (Priestner, 2012: 153).

Cat Mahoney points out that despite the distinctiveness of certain aspects of the story told in the program (particularly in terms of gender), there are elements of the series that feel both familiar and yet are presented in a new way. As Mahoney argues: "The setting of *Tenko* within a female prisoner-of-war camp is conducive to more recognizable wartime narratives. This removes it from the domestic and elevates it beyond the dichotomy of the masculine front line and the feminine home front" (2015). Although there had been earlier screen depictions of women in prisoner of war camps, such as in *Two Thousand Women* (1944), it was generally male prisoners whose stories had been told most frequently, and the serialized format of *Tenko* allowed individual stories to be told with more depth. Vicky Ball has drawn attention to the way that the series "offered some insights into those marginalized aspects of women's history" (2013: 246), and points out that, along with other programs of its type, "the female ensemble drama moves to centre stage that which is celebrated only periodically in British soap opera: women's relationships with other women outside of their familial roles as wives and mothers" (2013: 246). These relationships may be questions of respect and diplomacy, as well as relationships of all types—including, as *Tenko* demonstrated, friendships and rivalries alongside occasional romance. Ball goes on to say that "the female ensemble drama constructs alternative lifestyles for women based upon meaningful social relationships with other women. In so doing, it undermines the heteronormative ideologies that have governed the normative feminine life course" (2013: 246). In *Tenko*, the breakdown of this heteronormativity is never more apparent than in a storyline that sees nurse Nellie Keene form a romantic attachment with fellow campmate Sally Markham shortly after Sally loses her unborn baby.

Such a relationship between the two characters is a striking contrast to the rigidly structured order imposed in the professional world of the hospital that Nellie had been familiar with, and is perhaps the first season's most explicit acknowledgment that it was not only the environment that had changed for the characters, but also a different sense of freedom to express themselves in ways that may have been frowned upon outside of the camp. However, the series' producer was unhappy with the inclusion of a lesbian storyline, demonstrating that there seemed to be a somewhat vague set of boundaries of what would be considered acceptable in a mainstream television series, even one based on such traumatic events that would surely be more troubling than a dash of homosexuality. Nevertheless, Jill Hyem, who wrote the episode that focused on the relationship, recalled the difficult journey that the story had to take in order to reach the screen:

> I wanted to write a story about a relationship between two of the younger women. This was not such an unlikely occurrence in a camp with several hundred of them; indeed, ex-prisoners had told us of women who were "special friends." The idea was rejected out of hand. I was told that if we introduced such a subject it would be "turn-off time" and that the characters concerned would lose audience sympathy. I argued my case. Anne Valery and Lavinia Warner supported me. The producer remained adamant. I said that if the series was going to dodge such issues I would sooner not work on it. A compromise was reached. I was told that I could write my story provided I did not use the word "lesbian." It was probably one of the best episodes I wrote [Hyem, 1987: 156–7].

These two characters come from middle class backgrounds that are conventional for television dramas of the period—Sally is married, and had previously lived a comfortable lifestyle in the English Home Counties, while Nellie had only shown superficial interest in men while demonstrating diligence in her nursing career. That the storyline was given to them, rather than one of the more overtly sexually promiscuous characters, says something of the subtlety with which the series wished to talk about their relationship, which is shown to be one of affection and dependence, even while comments from other characters make it clear that their relationship is a physical one (albeit off screen). Sally's rejection of heteronormativity is made explicit when she reveals that she is relieved to have lost her unborn child; "at least I've got you," she had earlier said to Nellie, while she also reveals that the child will be named after Nellie if it's a girl. Dr. Mason attempts to use what power she has to break up the attachment between the women, but Nellie stands her ground in a way that would have been unthinkable pre-camp. "You can't order me here, we're not at the hospital now you know," she tells Mason. Soon, Nellie and Sally are giggling like schoolgirls and are shown to be closer physically (although a kiss is only implied). Others in the camp notice and prejudices from life outside the camp make their way into the new surroundings as graffiti describes the characters as perverts. Nevertheless, they publicly dance together and flirt, while Nellie shows flashes of jealousy when others take an interest in Sally. Most camp mates are not concerned about the burgeoning romance—"at least they care about each other," says Blanche.

True to her character, Dr. Mason's biggest concern about the relationship is the extent to which it distracts Nellie from her nursing. "I think you could go a long way in the profession," she says. "I think you're in danger of losing your direction…. When we were in Singapore I always used to think of you as one of my more reliable nurses but now…. It seems to be playing second fiddle to your extra mural interests. People are talking about you and Sally." For Dr. Mason, Nellie is a nurse, "first and foremost." "No

I'm not," Nellie retorts. "First and foremost I'm a person." This exchange highlights the differences between the outlooks and attitudes of the doctor and nurses, as the new camp environment allows Nellie to break free of the expectations of her as a person, formed in a heteronormative society and a strictly formalized professional world. Imprisoned in the camp, she now has new freedom that defines her beyond heterosexual relationships and a nursing career. However, when Sally abruptly ends the relationship, Nellie throws herself back into her role as a nurse, becoming "all work and no play," as Kate puts it. Having perhaps finally seen Kate and Nellie as people rather than nurses, Dr. Mason starts to call them by their first names, a small but definite shift in the relationship in the direction of friendship, and a sign that even characters who cling to the previously established hierarchies most strongly will eventually loosen their grip.

Nellie Keene does not return to the series after the first season, as she is moved to another camp where she dies—a typical fate for *Tenko* characters. However, Kate continues to work at the side of Dr. Mason and comes into her own when the camp has to contend with another doctor at their new camp, who seems more interested in experimentation than caring. Over time Dr. Mason's eyesight starts to fail, meaning that Kate takes over most of her duties that require intricate medical and physical skills. This gives her confidence to train to be a doctor once the camps are liberated by the Allies, although by the time of the final *Tenko* episode (a reunion special set in 1950) we learn that she is considering leaving her studies because she feels that she already knows more than most, due to her experiences in the camp, and she ends up staying in Singapore to undertake important community work, a sign that her character's growth is more than just a development of her medical career.

Tenko allowed its characters to find new directions in their lives, and not always in expected ways, with Nellie and Kate serving as particularly good examples of this. Freed from the formal structures and expectations of the hierarchical hospital, each found their characters developing in ways that would likely have not occurred if they had stayed within established social order. As is so often the case for the series, such personal growth has links to the reality on which the program was based. As Warner and Sandilands put it in their history of life in the camps:

> These many years afterwards it is possible to see these events not only as a conventional story of hardship, but as a singular experiment: a "laboratory" in which there was a great deal to be learned about women. Long before it became fashionable to examine women for their strengths rather than their weaknesses, to ask what they are able to accomplish rather than underlining what they cannot, here was a case history with all its elements neatly laid out [Warner and Sandilands, 1983: 15].

For *Tenko*, its own take on the "case history" of women in prisoner of war camps allowed characters from throughout society to become an important part of the newly established camp life, and the nurses had significant roles to play. However, the series also considered them as characters in their own right, rather than as one-dimensional caregivers supporting those who society would generally expect to be more prominent or even important. *Tenko* made some effort to show that not only were the women in the camp fully formed characters in their own rights, away from traditional gender expectations (particularly those seen in drama), but that backgrounds and careers were not the entirety of their lives. Nellie and Kate were nurses, but their lives and stories were much more than simply their jobs.

Films and Television Productions Referenced

Drama Connections: Tenko (2005) BBC One.
General Studies: TV Writer (1982) BBC One.
Tenko (1981–85) BBC.
Women in Captivity (1979) BBC One.

References

Ball, V. (2013) Forgotten Sisters: The British Female Ensemble Drama. *Screen* 54, 2: 244–248.
Felton, M. (2009) *The Real Tenko*. Barnsley: Pen & Sword Books.
Hallam, J. (2013) Drama Queens: Making Television Drama for Women 1990–2009. *Screen* 54, 2: 256–261.
Hyem, J. (1987) Entering the Arena: Writing for Television. In: Baehr, H., and Dyer, G. (eds.) *Boxed In: Women and Television*. London: Pandora Press. 151–163.
Jennings, R. (2017) Ageing Across Space and Time: Exploring Concepts of Ageing and Identity in the Female Ensemble Dramas *Tenko* and *Call the Midwife*. *Journal of British Cinema and Television* 14, 2: 179–195.
Landsberg, A. (2004) *Prosthetic Memory: The Transformation of American Rememberance in the Age of Mass Culture*. New York: Columbia University Press.
Mahoney, C. (2015) "Not bad for a few ordinary girls in a tin hut!": Reimagining Women's Social Experience of the Second World War Through Female Ensemble Drama. *Frames Cinema Journal* 7.
Masters, A. (1981) *Tenko*. Slough: Hollen Street Press.
Priestner, A. (2012) *Remembering Tenko*. Cambridge: Classic TV Press.
Smyth, J. (1970) *The Will to Live*. London: Cassell.
Starns, P. (2010) *Surviving Tenko*. Stroud: The History Press.
Valery, A. (1986) *Tenko Reunion*. London: Severn House Publishers.
Warner, L., and Sandilands, J. (1983) *Women Beyond the Wire*. London: Hamlyn.

The Death of Judy Hill

*Arctic Nurses, Northern Bush Pilots
and the Crash of '72*

Travis Hay

Introduction

The Arctic nurse and the northern bush pilot are two enduring figures of the social history of post-war Canadian medicine. Part folk tale and part historical reality, these two profoundly gendered constructs are associated with so-called "mercy flights," or medical evacuation flights chartered in response to an emergency situation in a northern community. Most often, a mercy flight transports a First Nation or Inuk patient whose home community lacks access to emergency, surgical, palliative, obstetric, or other forms of healthcare. Due to these treacherous service gaps, Indigenous peoples who live on-reserve in the provincial and territorial north of Canada have historically had to rely upon bush pilots and Arctic nurses to access a wide range of emergency and other medical services. This colonial double standard within the structure of Canadian healthcare created the historical conditions of possibility for cultural productions and folk tales that celebrate the bush pilot and the Arctic nurse as an intrepid duo.

"The legend of the bush pilot," as *Maclean's* magazine describes it, is that of the "pioneer and knight-errant of the frontier, the guy who can fly anywhere by the seat of his pants" (Philips 1973). Masculine, brave, and daring, the northern bush pilot is often pictured roguishly as a "high-wire cowboy of the Arctic" who flies off into the "midnight sun" whenever an Arctic nurse deems his services necessary (*Edmonton Journal*, July 27, 1977: 27). In 1941, for example, in *Captain of the Clouds*, Hollywood film star James Cagney portrayed a Canadian protagonist who plies his skills as a northern bush pilot for the Royal Canadian Air Force in the Second World

War. The bush pilot, however, only arrives when he is called for by the Arctic nurse, who is seen to carry considerably more power, autonomy, and responsibility than her southern counterpart. Canadian newspapers have variously described the Arctic nurse as an adventurous woman "hooked on the frontier," "canoeing through icebergs," and keeping a "cool head" as she relies on an astute combination of training and experience to determine "the urgency of summoning an evacuation plane at the cost of anywhere between $600 and $4,000" (*Star-Phoenix,* August 3, 1966: 13; Kelly, 1970). Portrayed as hardened by their travel through northern lands and sanctified for their delivery of health services to Indigenous peoples, the Arctic nurse and northern bush pilot were, for several decades, celebrated colonial characters in a Romantic national narrative about the provision of modern healthcare on the frontiers of the Canadian north.

In 1972, this national mythology collided with the grim realities of healthcare gaps and crises of care in the Canadian north. On November 8, 1972, an under-trained northern bush pilot named Marten Hartwell crashed a mercy flight *en route* to Yellowknife in the Northwest Territories. An Arctic nurse named Judy Hill was killed instantly. The crash also caused the death of a young Inuk mother named Neemee Nulliayok as well as her unborn child. The fourth and final passenger on the plane was Nulliayok's 14-year-old nephew David Kootook, whose abdominal pains had been wrongly diagnosed as appendicitis. Hartwell, who had received his flight training in Hitler's Luftewaffe, shattered his knees and ankles in the crash. Heroically, the young David built the pair a shelter and shared emergency rations as they awaited the arrival of what was to become the most expensive search and rescue mission in Canadian history. Kootook passed away 19 days after the crash due to starvation. As Canadians learned during an inquest into the death of Hill, Nulliayok, and Kootook in March of 1973, Hartwell had cannibalized Hill and harvested 38 lbs. of flesh from her body prior to being rescued as the sole survivor on December 9 (Philips, 1973: 1). Though the story had already garnered both national and international media attention, the death of Judy Hill and the grisly fate she had suffered put Arctic nurses, northern bush pilots, and mercy flights into sharp global focus.

In this essay, I use Canadian newspaper coverage to recount this major media moment and to investigate its legacy on northern nursing and healthcare services. Though two novelists have approached this rather sensationalistic narrative, little scholarly attention has been paid to it (McDougall, 1977; Tadman, 1991). My critical review of the coverage will be divided into four chronologically arranged sections: the background to the ill-fated mercy flight; the controversial search and rescue mission (which was called off, criticized, and called back on again); the funeral scandal, wherein the politics of public mourning exalted Judy Hill while conveniently forgetting the Inuuk victims; and, finally, the inquest and the cannibalism revelation, which put the story back on the front-page in March of 1973. At each successive stage, the story became more and more sensational and thus more and more popular in Canadian newspapers. In the broad sense, this essay will use Canadian newspaper coverage to retrace the contours of the successive revelations made about the tragic series of events. My argument is that Canadian newspaper coverage shone a spotlight on the grisly elements of the crash as well as the working conditions of Arctic nurses and northern bush pilots. Spotlights, of course, serve the double purpose of concealing what they do not illuminate. As we shall see, the public grieving and memorializing of Judith Hill obscured what had happened to the Inuuk victims of the crash, who received a very different kind of treatment. Ultimately, the larger national meaning that was made out of Hill's death was not related to the dire need of reforming northern healthcare provision systems (the poor administration of which had, in effect, caused her death). Rather, the crash was contained within a colonial politic of recognition wherein Neemee Nulliayok, David Kootook, and the community of Spence Bay sat in the shadows of the somewhat salacious spotlight that was shone on the grisly fate of the Arctic nurse. Thus, in titling this essay in a way that privileges "The Death of Judy Hill," I seek to name, identify, and critique the colonial lens through which much newspaper coverage cast this series of events. As I highlight in the following section, it is important to clearly underscore these dynamics of power and race, lest such sensational narratives of northern bush pilots, arctic nurses, and mercy flights be presented as harrowing folk-tales rather than the very real and painful histories that they are.

Historiographies of Indian and Northern Health Services

Though Canada has a common reputation of enjoying a "universal" healthcare system, this is a mythology that erases the experiences of Indigenous communities who have been historically subject to the genocide of federal Indian policies and segregated systems of healthcare. I am speaking here not only of the biological and cultural genocide of the residential and day schooling system, but of a long series of particularly violent policies that targeted Inuit communities beginning in 1939 (Starblanket, 2015). Though not originally considered "Indian" under the legislative force of Canada's *Indian Act* of 1876, a Supreme Court decision in this year defined "Eskimos" as "Indians" within the framework of federal policy. Inuit communities immediately began facing administratively intensive forms of colonial governance. This period in Canadian federal Indian policy saw the rise of what was termed the "Eskimo disk list system," wherein community members were assigned a numbered disk as a personal settler state identifier. As Derek Smith argued, "the Eskimo Disk List System indicates how the assignment of unique personal identification numbers through that list forged a direct state-to-individual link that rendered ineffective and irrelevant for most state purposes virtually all traditional Eskimo structures of social solidarity, including the family" (1993: 43). Writ large onto northern Indian policy, then, was an attempt to atomize, individuate, and govern each individual "Eskimo" with state-centered techniques of surveillance and control. This era also initiated the horrific practice of forced Inuit relocations. Discussed at length in Peter Kulchyski and Frank Tester's *Tammarrniit (Mistakes)*, these relocations have been criticized for their cruel logics of Canadian Arctic sovereignty, wherein the Inuit were used as "human flagpoles" in a federal government attempt to assert Crown sovereignty over High Arctic locations (1994).

The post-war period also saw the emergence of what the federal government called Indian and Northern Health Services. Prior to this period, healthcare in Inuit communities was left largely to travelling doctors, Indigenous practices, fur trade outpost provisions, and the active role of Christian institutions present in the Canadian north. As Myra Rutherdale explains, American soldiers present in the Arctic during the Second World War noted that "many Inuit suffered ill-health. Their complaints, inspired partly by the increase of tuberculosis, placed pressure on the federal government to compensate for their apparent neglect. Instead of the handful of federally funded doctors who periodically travelled across the north, a new Indian and Northern Health Services (INHS) branch was established. By 1963, the branch had a staff of 2,500 people, including nurses, doctors, dentists, and administrators" (2008: 57). In a 2012 article, Leslie McBain focused on the role of outpost nurses in the provision of healthcare in northern Saskatchewan. Though McBain noted that "nurses were considered key players in the plan" to achieve healthcare coverage in the Canadian north, she explained that "the level of financial support and commitment necessary for the nurses to achieve such goals were simply not forthcoming" (2012: 310). In a paper that focuses on the disproportionate amount of public grieving visited upon an Arctic nurse compared to Indigenous people, it is important to underscore at this juncture that Judy Hill and other northern nurses did not receive sufficient infrastructure support when attempting to provide healthcare coverage in the territorial and provincial norths of Canada. Though Hill was exalted in death, she was not supported professionally in life and was in fact endangered by the colonial gaps in healthcare she worked to close.

It was during these same decades (1930–1970) that Canada's racially segregated Indian Hospital System was established (Drees, 2016; Lux, 2016). Again, this was partly in response to fears related to the rise in tuberculosis in Indigenous communities across the country. So-called Indian hospitals were located in more southerly and urban locations to which First Nations and Inuit patients were expected to fly on medical evacuation flights organized and funded by INHS. This is the colonial structure or system that laid the conditions of historical possibility for cultural productions that depicted northern bush pilots as well as Arctic nurses as heroes that brought modern medicine to the colonial frontier. As Indigenous health historian Mary Jane Logan McCallum has warned, decontextualized and sanitized depictions of the provision of healthcare to northern Indigenous communities has been a primary discourse in which Canadian colonization in the north has been rendered a benevolent process (2005). The death of Judy Hill and its coverage in Canadian newspapers offers an example of this cultural process in action, and it is to this story that we now turn.

Background to the Mercy Flight

Judith Hill was born in Devon, England at the end of the Second World War. After training in London hospitals, the young nurse migrated to northern Canada in 1969 (*Vancouver Sun* December 11, 1972: 11). This was an era in the history of Canadian nursing in which graduates had no mandated training in midwifery, an essential skill in the profession of northern nursing. Because British nurses such as Hill had training in this area of healthcare provision, they were not uncommon in the Arctic. Indeed, less than one year into Hill's posting at Spence Bay (now called Taloyoak), she was asked to provide care to Neemee Nulliayok, a young mother and residential school survivor who was two years younger than Hill and expecting another child (Busch, 2013). By November of 1972, Nulliayok was 8-months pregnant and experiencing significant late-stage labor complications. Her nephew, David Kootook, suffered from severe stomach pains that had been misdiagnosed at the Spence Bay Nursing Station as appendicitis and were later determined to have been caused by a stomach ulcer (Slinger, 1973). On the morning of the 8th, Hill accompanied Nulliayok and her nephew David Kootook on a mercy flight from Spence Bay to Cambridge Bay. They flew on a Twin Otter airplane piloted by Ed Logozar, a northern bush pilot who worked for a flight charter company called Gateway Aviation Ltd (Philips, 1973).

Also in Cambridge Bay (and also flying for Gateway Aviation Ltd.) was Marten Hartwell (né Leopold Herrmann). Born in Germany in 1925,

Hartwell flew a glider plane as a member of the Hitler Youth at age 15; energized by the experience, he quit school and travelled to Bavaria where he received basic pilot training in the Luftwaffe (Lees, 1978). Like many Nazi soldiers, Hartwell was allowed by the Allied powers to return to civilian life following the war. In April of 1967, he moved to Canada to pursue his dream of working as a northern bush pilot. Significantly, Hartwell's training did not provide him with an "instrument rating," a particular accreditation given to pilots after they receive training in more advanced navigational techniques that assist them in flying safely when the ground cannot be used as a reference point (Philips, 2013). Accordingly, by afternoon on the 8th of November 1972, Hartwell had diverted his Beechcraft 18 aircraft to Cambridge Bay due to poor weather and visibility conditions (*Times Colonist* December 9, 1971: 1). It was here that Hartwell met Judy Hill, who urgently needed a pilot to bring her, Nulliayok, and Kootook to Yellowknife.

Canadian newspapers later suggested that Hartwell was influenced in his decision to accept the dangerous assignment by "the legend of the bush pilot" and the attendant pressures to accept any assignment no matter the danger (Philips, 2013). As one reporter in the *Globe and Mail* insisted, "had he refused and the woman died, the whole social displeasure of that community would have descended upon him for not taking the kind of the seat-of-the-pants risk that has become a foundation of the myth of the North" (Slinger, 1973: 5). Other reporters depicted the poorly trained Hartwell as having been "bulldozed into taking a flight for which he was not technically licensed and which he must have known he had no business to attempt" (*Times Colonist* 9 December 1971, p. 1). This was, perhaps, an overestimation of the power of this particular folk tale given that Hartwell enjoyed a $.08/per mile bonus, which was the most significant portion of his pay (Philips, 2013). In any case, and for whatever reason, Hartwell, Hill, Nulliayok, and Kootook departed from Cambridge Bay at roughly 5:00 p.m. on November 8, 1972. The flight to Yellowknife ought to have lasted approximately three hours.

The On Again/Off Again Search and Rescue Mission

The plane was first reported missing in a series of Canadian newspapers on the 10th of November. Though the *Edmonton Journal* found "Northern Mercy Plane Missing" a headline fit for the front-page; it was the only newspaper to have led with the story (Hume, 1972). Over the next several days, pictures of Judy Hill appeared in several Canadian newspapers alongside troubling reports of what had likely happened. These photographs depicted the tall and blonde-haired Hill providing care to a man described as an "Eskimo in Alberta"; the picture, it was often noted, had been released by her concerned parents (*Vancouver Sun* November 16, 1972: 1). Interestingly, Hartwell's identity as a German-born former Luftewaffe pilot was not reported upon as a lurid detail or deserving of any headline treatment. Neemee Nulliayok and David Kootook were far less likely to be named than Hill or Hartwell in this early coverage. When the Inuuk victims were named, their names were often misspelled as "Mullrayok" "Mulliayok," and "Klootook" (*Red Deer Advocate* November 20, 1972: 10; *Leader-Post* November 20, 1972: 8). Given the history of the Eskimo Disk List system and failed attempts of the federal government to understand Inuit familial names, the habitual misspelling of Kootook and Nulliayok's names is consistent with Canadian colonial disregard for Inuit culture. It is also useful to note here that references to "Martin" as opposed to "Marten" Hartwell made by journalists were later corrected. For example, on the 2nd of March 1973, the *Globe and Mail* ran a short piece correcting the matter, which explained that "a call to the offices of his lawyer in Edmonton yesterday verified that Mr. Hartwell spells his name Marten" (4). This same article reported that Hartwell "came from Germany ... and changed his name from Leopold Herrmann some time after he arrived in Canada" (4). Thus, whereas Canadian newspapers took care to correct the second name of a former Nazi, this same respect was not extended to the Inuuk victims of the crash.

Ten days into the search, a false spotting of the downed plane put the story on several front-pages (*Ottawa Citizen* November 21, 1972: 1; *Edmonton Journal* November 20, 1972: 1; *Calgary Herald* November 21, 1972: 1). On November 27, the head of the search and rescue mission, Colonel W.M. Houser, called the entire mission off due to its exorbitant expense as well as what he saw as a low likelihood of retrieving survivors (*Edmonton Journal* November 29, 1972: 44). On November 28, newspapers ran an interview with a woman who claimed to be Hartwell's fiancée. Though this was rather shocking news to his wife and child back in Germany, Hartwell had in fact eloped with a young 23-year-old graduate student from the University of Alberta named Susan Haley (*Leader-Post* December 1, 1972). Haley made headlines when she claimed that she would not give up hope that Hartwell would be rescued. Nor did she.

Susan Haley contacted her father and asked for his help. Dr. K. David C. Haley, the Chair of the Department of Mathematics at Acadia University in Nova Scotia, obliged. On the 29th of November, Dr. Haley published in the *Globe and Mail* a scathing critique of the cancelled search and rescue mission under the title of "Have We Abandoned a Lost Plane?" (1972: 7). Haley lambasted what he depicted as a sub-par and half-hearted effort on part of the Canadian Department of Defense. He expressed particular outrage that the search had been called after only three weeks and insisted that "to date, there have only been three days of reasonable weather for searching." Haley insisted to his audience of fellow Canadians that the calling of the search raised questions that "probe at the roots of the entire moral structure of our society." Though he was clearly very close in the personal sense to the issue, Haley's objections were not entirely unfounded. As Haley explained, "the Hercules is a cargo plane which affords nearly zero visibility of the ground. Indeed, the spotters on this plane in order to see the ground must be strapped to the end of the load ramp which is partly let down from the tail." Though he did not reference it directly, Haley was probably able to describe this logistic reality so accurately as it had been depicted on the front-page of the *Edmonton Journal* on November 16.

Haley affirmed the likelihood of survival given that the plane carried 100 gallons of gasoline, 10 sleeping bags, as well as "emergency rations for 10 people for six days each." He also lamented that local Inuit communities with high levels of land knowledge were not provided with snow-mobiles and paid to conduct ground searches for the lost plane. In somewhat dramatic fashion, Haley concluded his plea by citing the abandoned search and rescue mission as pitiable in comparison to a grander tradition of Arctic exploration and Victorian-era efforts to rescue lost ships and their beleaguered crews and captains:

> Let me describe another great search in another generation of Canadian history. Sir John Franklin was last heard from in 1845. The story of his many expeditions that went in search of him is a saga in itself. In 1853, eight years later, the British Government announced that hope for Franklin must be abandoned and proposed to give up the search. The public outcry was so great that the Government was forced to outfit further expeditions and continue. In 1859 the fate of Franklin was finally revealed. This was a search of 14 years. Our search and Rescue people began proposing to give up this search for people who risked their lives on a mission of mercy, after 14 days! The search has now been given up entirely. If the human race, if our Canadian society is not all about this, what is it all about?

Haley's letter thus drew upon a deep wellspring of Canadian social feeling that saw the lost Arctic explorer as a Romantic image worthy of national interest and action. His letter protested that the calling off of the search was a gesture counter to the essence of Canadian identity, the human spirit, and the moral foundations of civil society. Though only Franklin was named, Haley harkened to a Canadian cultural tradition that uplifts, celebrates, and to some extent mythologizes British exploration of Indigenous lands as generative of Canadian identity and nationhood. For example, there are no shortage of Canadian cultural productions and place-names that honor figures such as John Cabot, Henry Hudson, James Cook,

Alexander McKenzie, David Thompson, and John Franklin of the named Expedition. Readers might also note a kind of anachronistic irony in Haley having cited the Franklin Expedition, which has since become heavily associated with cannibalism. Indeed, Canadian archaeological research conducted in the 1980s confirmed for Canadians what local Inuit informants first told the explorer John Rae in 1854: that crewmembers of the Franklin Expedition had succumbed to cannibalism and died a grisly death in the unforgiving Arctic landscape (Beattie and Geiger, 1987). Thus, while the comparison was more appropriate than Haley could possibly have understood at the time, the rhetorical force of his letter and his depiction of Hill and Hartwell as mercy flight martyrs had considerable impact.

On the 30th of November at 4:00 p.m. the search and rescue mission was reinitiated after the Canadian public echoed Haley's outrage. This on again/off again nature of the search and rescue mission only heightened the intrigue of the increasingly dramatic story; however, what is important to note at this juncture is the extent to which newspaper coverage and discourse entered into this historical event as a constitutive element and active agent that shaped an ongoing reality. Indeed, as the late Stuart Hall wrote, "representation is not outside the event, not after the event, but within the event itself; it is constitutive of it" (Hall, 1997: 8).

Hartwell was rescued in a Vanguard helicopter by Canadian search and rescue personnel on Saturday, December 9 (*The Vancouver Sun* December 9, 1972: 1). Only western Canadian newspapers were able to report upon this development in a timely fashion due simply to the speed of the news cycle production. On the following Monday, however, newspapers across Canada led with the story on the front-page. What took center stage in this immediate burst of coverage was the heroism of David Kootook. Examples of front-page headlines include "Eskimo Youth Credited with Pilot's Survival," "Eskimo Boy, 14, proved hero right to the end," and "Eskimo Youth Emerges Hero" (*Leader-Post* December 11, 1972: 1; *Edmonton Journal* December 11, 1972: 1; *Star-Phoenix* December 11, 1972: 1; *Red Deer Advocate* December 11, 1972: 1). In this way, the normative narrative of an Indigenous person requiring the rescue of a northern bush pilot was inverted: Hartwell had only survived because Kootook had taken care of him. Because they had yet to be disclosed to the public, no discussions of cannibalism were had in this initial coverage of the rescue.

The parents of Judy Hill, despite being in Britain, appeared often in Canadian newspaper coverage that reported upon the confirmed death of their daughter. Hill's father was quoted in multiple sources explaining that his family was "comforted" to learn that Judy likely died instantly and that they had not been hopeful for her survival. "Judy would have been the one to give her life," reasoned her father, "because she would have been tending to the Eskimo patients and possibly was not strapped in" (*Ottawa Journal* December 11, 1972: 25). Newspapers also reached out to Dr. Haley for his comments on the discovery of Hartwell. "I hope that what will come out of this," pleaded Haley, "is a complete re-examination of the whole search and rescue mission for downed planes" (*Red-Deer Advocate* December 11, 1972: 1), Haley also saw fit to thank those who joined him in having "bombarded the national government to the point where they resumed the search." Few (if any) reached out to the Nulliayok or Kootook family. In fact, the community of Spence Bay learned of Neemee's and David's death over the CBC Radio broadcast (Busch, 2013). The double standards hardly stopped there.

The Funeral Scandal

Judy Hill's ornate funeral was held on the 18th of December at St. Paul's Anglican Church in Edmonton, Alberta. The funeral was highly publicized and well-covered. The arrival of Hill's mother in Edmonton was even newsworthy (*Edmonton Journal* December 18, 1972: 10). Archdeacon Albert Thain officiated at the funeral, noting that Hill was a well-known member of his congregation and a "personal friend" (*Vancouver Sun* December 20, 1972: 3). Archdeacon Thain told newspapers that the church was "full for her service" (*Edmonton Journal* December 18, 1972: 10). Health Minister Marc LaLonde praised Hill's "self-less devotion to her duty" as an Arctic nurse—a group of women he termed a "special breed" who make life and death choices "to refer patients onwards to doctors sometimes hundreds of miles away" (*Edmonton Journal* December 11, 1972: 5). "Nurses like Miss Hill in their isolated Arctic nursing stations," he insisted, "are the backbone of the Northern Health Service" (*Whitehorse Daily Star* December 20, 1972: 14). In this and other passages, Judy Hill was clearly positioned as a saintly and heroic woman who had died tragically in the line of duty.

As was reported in several Canadians newspapers, both Neemee Nulliayok and David Kootook were buried in Edmonton with no members of their family or community present (*Edmonton Journal* December 20, 1972: 1; *Montreal Gazette* December 21, 1972: 14; *Calgary Herald* December 21, 1972: 5). Archdeacon Thain, who had officiated at Hill's funeral, was selected to conduct the funeral for Nulliayok and Kootook for no other reason than "his acquaintance with Judy Hill" (*Edmonton Journal* December 20, 1972: 10). The sole members in attendance at this impersonal service were Ted Horton and Norman Burgess, who were unknown to the victims and were simply representatives of the Northwest Territorial government (*Edmonton Journal* December 18, 1972: 1). When controversy arose and such double standards were criticized by Inuk lawyer and City of

Edmonton Alderman David Ward, a member of the territorial government defended the sequence of events that led to the sparsely attended and somewhat secret funeral when they told *The Gazette* that "it would have been impossible for their immediate family to attend the funeral 'even if they could have afforded the air fare'" (*Edmonton Journal* December 21, 1972: 14). Ward took issue with this differential treatment paid to the Inuuk victims. "No one asked for money," he explained, "just a little respect. This boy gave his life in one of the most noble causes of keeping another person alive. It has me very angry" (*Calgary Herald* December 21, 1972: 14). Thus, while David Kootook was celebrated in the broad sense for his heroism, he did not receive a hero's treatment. Nor did Neemee Nulliayok or her unborn child receive much recognition or respect. All were buried in an unmarked grave with government officials claiming that they were worried a Christian burial may have been an insult to the Inuit families (*Edmonton Journal* October 9, 1974).

Horton and Burgess—the two government representatives at the Inuuk victims' funeral—claimed that a local detachment of the Royal Canadian Mounted Police had forwarded the family's consent for the funeral proceedings from Spence Bay (*Edmonton Journal* December 20, 1972: 10); however, in subsequent decades, Neemee Nulliayok's surviving daughter Denise was forced to work with lawyers as well as a series of airlines in order to organize the respectful return of her mother's remains to her home community (*Windsor Star* July 15, 2017: D3). Of course, had government officials attended to the family and community of the Nulliayoks with respect, Denise's arduous journey to recover her mother would not have been necessary in the first place. Other examples of such blatant disregard for the humanity of the Inuuk victims abound. For example, in 1974, the city council of Edmonton reaffirmed this disrespect when a motion was raised to provide David with a headstone, which was then voted down (*Star-Phoenix* May 9, 1992: 13). Shockingly, when the issue reemerged in 1992 and David Kootook was nominated for a Governor General's award, he was denied on the basis that he had not willingly risked his life (*Times-Colonist* May 10, 1992: 5). Though Kootook eventually received the award he was due in July of 1994, the stark difference in treatment between Judy Hill and the Inuuk victims of the crash speaks volumes about the colonial double standards that shaped the Canadian response to this tragic sequence of events.

The Inquest and the Cannibalism Revelation

The funerals were followed by an inquest into the crash and the deaths of Hill, Kootook, and Nulliayok. The six-person jury was assembled in

Yellowknife with a start date of February 19, 1973 (*Edmonton Journal* January 6, 1973: 4). Public interest in this particular inquest was extremely high for many reasons, not the least of which was Hartwell's general refusal to speak to the press. For example, a full-page cover story in *The Windsor Star* carried the headline "Bush Pilot Won't Talk About Arctic Horrors" (December 11, 1972: 1). Newspapers also reported that the coroner who had investigated the deaths had ordered a "clamp down" on investigations in the matter until their scope was properly determined (*Calgary Herald* December 13, 1972: 2). In the preliminary hearings for this inquest, the lawyer representing Hill's estate, family, and interests (Philip Ketchum of the city of Edmonton) made a highly publicized request that the proceedings be closed to the public. Ketchum speculated on whether or not opening up the inquest to the media was productive or prudent and suggested that "there may be some things that can be left to those people who are to decide on the matter, which when published to the world at large may produce no good at all" (*Red Deer Advocate* February 27, 1973: 1).

The perceived caginess of the inquest proceedings piqued the interest of a Canadian news media network that had only just finished covering the horrific tale of Uruguayan Air Force Flight 571, which had crashed in the Andes Mountains in Argentina and driven several of the survivors to cannibalism. In fact, Canadian newspaper headlines were reporting on the gruesome details of Flight 571 while the search and rescue mission for the mercy flight was ongoing. This storm of coverage began on the 27th of December; for example, the *Victoria Sun* reported "Cannibalism Rumours Confirmed" (3); a headline from the *Edmonton Journal* read "Cannibalism Report Causes Despair" (14); and the *Calgary Herald* "Officials Confirm: Plane Crash Survivors Had Eaten Human Flesh" (December 28, 1972: 13). Thus, when Canadian journalists heard that preliminary hearings for the inquest contained misgivings related to public disclosures of information, they were likely primed by the popularity of Flight 571 to expect a revelation of cannibalism.

The revelation of Hartwell's cannibalism came on February 27, 1973, when a ruling by Justice William Morrow determined that sensitive details would be discussed in open court (*Edmonton Journal* March 1, 1973: 49). It was at this point that a public statement from Hartwell was released that contained the following passage:

> There has been so much talk and rumour about the events surrounding my crash and rescue in the Northwest Territories that I want to make a statement about it…. After David Kootook died, I realized that I too would soon be dead because I was too weak and injured to move around. I tried and failed to get lichens to keep alive. There was no way out but to eat human flesh and this I did. It distresses me and probably others to talk more about this but I do want to

stress that it was only I who did this and that only after David Kootook's death [*Globe and Mail* March 2, 1973: 4].

By the 1st of March, Hartwell's consumption of Hill's flesh was emblazoned across the front-page of Canadian newspapers. Representative examples of full-page cover headlines include "Hartwell Says He Ate Human Flesh" (Hume, 1973) and "Hartwell Ate Human Flesh to Save His Life" (*Windsor Star* March 1, 1973: 1). In this way, the Canadian press was given its own sensationalist version of the Flight 571 narrative; however, the connection between the two crashes was not made explicit in any coverage that I encountered.

Though Hartwell had issued his statement through his lawyer J.C. Cavanagh, he refused to answer a subpoena to appear and testify at the actual inquest proceedings (*Edmonton Journal* March 1, 1973: 48). The issue at hand was that provincial inquests in Canada are not criminal trials but a public inquiry in which a jury is meant to produce recommendations to prevent similar deaths in the future; thus, the coroner who presided over the inquest had no legal authority to mandate Hartwell's appearance at the proceedings nor did he stand to face severe consequences for his non-compliance. Hartwell's failure to show did not only "rile the jury," according to the *Edmonton Journal*, but it also compromised the integrity of the proceedings in the eyes of public counsel (March 1, 1973: 48). For example, *The Vancouver Sun* reported that Crown counsel W.J. Trainor made special inquiries into the fact that Kootook "was exceptionally emaciated," that his weight had dropped from 110 to 75 lbs., and that this was comparably a far more acute period of starvation than Hartwell, whose weight at rescue was 144 lbs. compared to a normal weight of 176 lbs. (Still, 1973: 1). Trainor argued that "it is possible that Hartwell was in the process of eating human flesh before David Kootook died" and posed the question: "how was it that one of the two survivors died with this tremendous weight loss and one lived?" (Still, 1973: 1). Trainor also reportedly pressured the coroner on the fact that Hartwell's statement had made reference to Neemee Nulliayok surviving the initial impact and even walking around the crash site in the hours preceding her death; however, pathological reports on the extent of her injuries make clear that this would have been impossible (*Vancouver Sun* March 1, 1973: 1).

Hartwell's failure to appear was therefore seen by many within and beyond the courtroom as a potential foreclosure of justice for the Inuuk victims of the crash. Indeed, Hartwell's absence was especially upsetting to lawyer James Karwsick, who had been retained by Inuit Tapirisat (an umbrella political organization representing Inuit communities) to represent the Nulliayok and Kootook families. When Hartwell's solitary statement was accepted by the court as admissible and it was confirmed that he would not appear at any point throughout the inquest, Karswick withdrew from the proceedings entirely, which carried on without him (*Vancouver Sun* March 1, 1973: 1). As I have noted elsewhere, this is a common tactic of critique of protest practiced by Indigenous peoples when they are poorly served by inquests into deaths in their communities and feel that justice cannot result from the proceedings (Hay, 2018).

The inquest ultimately found the under-trained Hartwell at fault for the crash (*Ottawa Citizen* July 4, 1973: 43). Though he was not himself criminally responsible for what had happened, Hartwell's employer— Gateway Aviation Ltd.—later lost a series of civil suits related to their failure to impose their own standards regarding Hartwell's lack of instrument-rating (*Ottawa Citizen* February 4, 1974: 14). One of these civil suits, settled with the estate of Judy Hill, was used by her parents to establish the Judy Hill Memorial Scholarship, which provided "education grants to enable nurses to improve their education for service in the Canadian Arctic, and to exchange with nurses from England" (*Red Deer Advocate* December 7, 1973: 2). Reports on this particular fund often pictured Judy Hill in a white nursing outfit, smiling lovingly into the eyes of a small baby swaddled in her arms and wearing the signature nurses cap named and theorized in other chapters (*Red Deer Advocate* December 7, 1973: 2; *Edmonton Journal* December 7, 1973: 3; *Calgary Herald* December 8, 1973: 30). This saintly image was a powerful one that Canadian nurses cited when they began demanding danger pay for mercy flights made in the course of duty in the months following the inquest (*Ottawa Citizen* May 18, 1973: 4). The death of Judy Hill, therefore, had both an immediate and a lasting impact on the occupation of Arctic nursing as well as northern bush piloting.

In what is an almost unbelievable final chapter of the story, the less-than-reputable pilot Marten Hartwell crashed his plane *again* on October 6, 1987 (*Vancouver Sun* October 9, 1987: 9). Hartwell awaited rescue for two days when he was spotted by an RCMP officer near Fort Norman in the Northwest Territories. No newspaper coverage speculated on whether or not this pattern of disappearance was coincidental or indicative of instability.

Conclusion

The crash of 1972 has left a complex colonial legacy in Canada. For a brief period, the story burned bright on front-page headlines and brought the working realities of Arctic nurses and bush pilots into sharp global focus. In 1973, Canadian folk singer Stompin' Tom Connors released a song about the incident. Connors made no mention of Hartwell's decision to eat Hill's flesh and to some extent sanitized the story by mythologizing it as a kind of northern Canadian folk-tale; however, as the Canadian newspaper coverage of this tragic story demonstrates, the crash and its aftermath made incredibly real, vivid, and immediate the realities of healthcare gaps in Inuit communities and the human cost of Indian and Northern Health Services. Of course, not all victims of the crash were treated equally: whereas Judy Hill was publicly mourned in a fashion consistent with her colonial subject position as a white English nurse, David Kootook and Neemee Nulliayok were treated with the racist logics of colonial rule, wherein the lives of colonized Indigenous peoples are seen as less grievable and, ultimately, less valuable than the lives of colonists. The coverage of the crash and the response of Canadians to the dramatic series of events ultimately reproduced the same colonial double standards that made the mercy flight necessary in the first place. The colonial and racist logic here is not surprising given that this was an era of active residential schools and Indian hospitals, but the colonial politic of recognition was the starkest characteristic of the context and content of Canadian newspaper coverage. Though Judy Hill and David Kootook were both celebrated as heroes, only one of them received a hero's treatment.

References

Newspapers and Periodicals

Edmonton Journal
The Gazette
The Globe and Mail
Vancouver Sun
Victoria Daily Ties

Other Sources

Beattie, O., and Geiger, J. (1987) *Frozen in Time: The Fate of the Franklin Expedition.* London: Bloomsbury Publishing.

Busch. L. (2013) The Story No One Told. *Northern News Service*, 6 February. Available at: https://archive.nnsl.com/2013-02/feb18_13st.html [accessed: 20 October 2020].

Drees, L.M. (2013) *Healing Histories: Stories from Canada's Indian Hospitals.* Edmonton: University of Alberta Press.

Hall, S. (1997) *Representations: Cultural Representations and Signifying Practices.* London: Sage Publishing.

Hay, T. (2018) Foreclosing Accountability: The Limited Scope of the Seven Youth Inquest in Thunder Bay, Ontario. *Canadian Review of Social Policy* 78, 1: 1–32.

Kulchyski, P., and Tester, J. (1994) *Tammarniit (Mistakes): Inuit Relocation in the Eastern Arctic, 1939-1963.* Vancouver: UBC Press.

Lux, M. (2016) *Separate Beds: A History of Indian Hospitals in Canada, 1920s-1980s*. Vancouver: UBC Press.

McBain, L. (2012) "Pulling up their sleeves and getting on with it": Providing Healthcare in a Northern Remote Region. *The Canadian Bulletin of Medical History* 29, 2: 309–328.

McCallym, M.J.L. (2005) The Last Frontier: Isolation and Aboriginal Health. *The Canadian Bulletin of Medical History* 22, 1: 103–120.

McDougall, J. (1977) *Angel of the Snow: The Story of Judy Hill*. Zurich: Muller Publishing.

Philips, A. (1973) The Ordeal of Marten Hartwell. *Maclean's* July 1, 17.

Rutherdale, M. (2008) Cleansers, Cautious Caregivers, and Optimistic Adventurers: A Proposed Typology of Arctic Canadian Nurses, 1945–1970. In Elliot, J., Stuart, M., and Toman, C. (eds.) *Place and Practice in Canadian Nursing History*. Vancouver: UBC Press, pp. 53–69.

Smith, D. (1993) The Emergence of the "Eskimo Status": An Examination of the Eskimo Disk List System and its Social Consequences, 1925–1970. In Dyck, N., and Waldram, J. (eds.). *Anthropology, Public Policy, and Native Peoples in Canada*, Montreal: McGill-Queen's University Press, Montreal, pp. 41–74.

Starblanket, T. (2015) *Suffer the Little Children: Genocide, Indigenous Nations, and the Canadian State*, Atlanta: Clarity Press.

Tadman, P. (1991) *The Survivor*. Boulder: Gorman and Gorman.

A "Complex Personal Problem"

Reactions to Voluntary Sterilization in 1960s Media

Caitlin Fendley

Introduction

The Doctors and the Nurses (1962–1965), later called *The Nurses* (1965–1967), was a CBS medical drama turned daytime soap opera set in a New York hospital, centered on the dynamics of two nurses—one young and one senior.[1] Letters arrived at CBS and local television stations after their first broadcast of an episode entitled *The Rainbow Ride* on January 16, 1964. (My description and use of the episode comes from analyzing an audio recorded version since no video archive copy could be located.) It told the story of a young, white, married nurse seeking a tubal ligation after becoming pregnant for the sixth time while her husband struggled to financially support their family. The episode begins in the hospital with the main protagonist, Dory Spencer, who is both a patient and nurse there, waiting for the arrival of her physician, Dr. Ted Steffen. She is pregnant with her sixth child, is just days away from giving birth, and wants to discuss undergoing a tubal ligation afterwards. Steffen offers a defensive rebuttal, "Do you know what it means to be sterilized?" and from there, the episode follows Dory's struggles to convince many people of her need to have the procedure done, including her physician, her husband, the nurses, and the hospital's Sterilization Committee.

Though she is eventually approved for the surgery, she is first subjected to an overdramatic and often judgmental analysis of tubal ligation, as many physicians objected to performing the procedure for non-medical reasons. Not only was requesting sterilization for family planning as opposed to medical purposes portrayed as unnecessary, but the episode emphasized how "unnatural" it was for Dory to want the surgery. Given the contentious nature of this procedure in the early 1960s, the episode generated controversy among viewers. On the one hand, sterilization was portrayed in a negative fashion, with the doctors and nurses acting in an immature and unprofessional way towards the overburdened mother. Yet the episode had breached a taboo subject on television while highlighting the many social and medical objections and approvals of the procedure.

This essay analyzes the reactions to this episode following its first airing, using letters sent to CBS, mainly from doctors and other medical professionals, as well as members of non-profits like the Human Betterment Association for Voluntary Sterilization (HBAVS). It also explores the wider debates surrounding voluntary female sterilization in the 1960s, considering some of the medical and social factors that influenced its status prior to its increased acceptance and popularity into the 1970s. These debates also help illuminate how the plot and dialogue of the episode accurately portrayed the experiences of American women seeking sterilization throughout the decade. I argue that although the episode was not ultimately supportive of tubal ligation, it effectively captured the wide range of ideas and attitudes people held about it in the 1960s. Its mixed reception offered a window into understanding the complexities of sterilization in postwar America. This included: its status as a medical, family planning, eugenic, and/or socioeconomic tool; gendered attitudes towards women, their bodies, and their roles as mothers (and who is "fit" to fulfill these roles); and how the popularity of media facilitated increased public awareness of these ideas. Further, despite the debate the episode generated, Dory's story accurately reflected the obstacles and experiences that many women *like* Dory experienced at the time. This essay is part of a wider effort to contextualize voluntary sterilization, both as part of the eugenics movement and women's liberation and health movements, and as its own distinct part of reproductive healthcare history.

Eugenics, Sterilization and Reproductive Healthcare in the Sixties

The 1960s was a time of sexual liberation, new and transformative contraceptives, and feminist and reproductive rights movements (Watkins 1998: 2). The contraceptive pill, Enovid, approved in 1960, and later, the "redesign and redistribution" of intrauterine device (IUD) in 1964, revolutionized women's personal, sexual, and work lives by giving them greater control over if, and when, to have children (Kluchin, 2009: 49; Tone & Watkins, 2007: 106; Marks, 2001: xvii–xviii). But obstacles to women's reproductive care continued during this period of transition. Most notably, abortion was still illegal in every state throughout the country.[2] Many poor, black, indigenous women and other women of color were subjected to forced sterilization abuses (Kline, 2001; Kluchin, 2009; Schoen, 2005; Stern, 2016). At the same time, many women sought and were denied *voluntary* permanent sterilization. Thus, while new hormonal contraceptive technologies allowed women greater reproductive choices, restrictions persisted due to continued medical, legal, and social resistance to female sexual autonomy.

Until recently, histories of reproductive health rights and technologies focused more on non-permanent forms of pregnancy prevention, such as the contraceptive pill (Watkins 1998; Marks 2001; Tone 2001; May 2010) and abortion (Reagan 1997; Schoen, 2015; Ziegler, 2015), rather than voluntary sterilization. These national and global histories of voluntary sterilization have showcased the work of organizations and their members to promote, educate, and provide sterilization referrals. They have also highlighted the shift from sterilization as a key tool of eugenics, to one of "charity" for poor people, to a popular form of contraception (e.g., Dowbiggin, 2008; Kluchin, 2009).

The history of eugenics further complicates the history of sterilization. Coined in 1883 by British statistician Francis Galton, the term *eugenics,* or "good in birth" focused in scientific and public spheres on improving the human gene pool through encouraging the "fit" to reproduce more (positive eugenics) and discouraging or forcing the "unfit" to reproduce less, or never (Kline, 2001, p. 13). Eugenicists believed that genetics determined poverty, criminal behavior, and ill-health (Kluchin, 2009: 1). The term "neo-eugenics" reflects continued efforts to prevent certain "unfit" individuals from reproducing (Kluchin, 2009).

By the late-nineteenth century, eugenicists focused on segregating the "feebleminded" from society by forcing them into institutions. By the turn of the twentieth century, sterilization, rather than segregation, became an increasingly popular and efficient eugenic technique in the United States— with many other countries soon following—to ensure that the "unfit" would be permanently prevented from "infecting" future generations with their "faulty" genes (Lombardo, 2011).[3] But by the 1930s, several factors, including an increased emphasis on the "nurture" component of human behavior and new understandings of genetics, forced eugenicists to think of and use sterilization in new ways. Essentially, sterilization was promoted to ensure that all unfit individuals were prevented from reproducing, regardless of their genetics. While this focus on negative eugenics persisted into the postwar years, positive eugenics also gained traction in the 1930s and 1940s to promote greater reproduction and pronatalism among the "fit," with a focus on women's responsibility to uphold white motherhood and stable marriage and family life (Kline, 2009: 3; 105–106; 125; Stern, 2016: 177). Concerns about the white race and society centered on ideas about what historian Wendy Kline calls "reproductive morality," which "promoted marriage and motherhood as a central goal of womanhood," and the need for "prospective parents to consider their progeny's potential impact on the race" (126–127). Thus, a woman's right to reproduce (or not) was not a private matter between her and her sexual partner, but one scrutinized by eugenicists/neo-eugenicists, physicians, and the public.

Meanwhile, restrictions on sterilization for "fit" women, including hospital policies which prevented middle-class white women from becoming sterilized for non-medical reasons, reflected the reinforcement of neo-eugenic pronatalist attitudes. Advocates for voluntary sterilization in the United States focused on trying to convince physicians to "liberalize" their attitudes towards sterilization and accept it as an effective birth control method to help ensure greater access to the procedure. They emphasized its ability to reduce poverty and decrease the number of individuals on public welfare assistance, as well as to control the growing population in the U.S. and abroad (Dowbiggin, 2008: 8; 9; Kluchin, 2009).

The varied reactions to Dory's decision to pursue sterilization on the show serves to highlight and confirm the 1960s as a transitionary period for sterilization surgery. Though the eugenics movement lost much of its popular support after the Second World War—once, among other factors, the true horrors of Nazi Germany's eugenic sterilization program came to light—the racist and classist beliefs which bolstered eugenic causes never really went away (Kline, 2001, p. 106). Postwar neo-eugenics thrived and the forced sterilization of vulnerable groups, such as indigenous and poor black women, continued in the United States and globally, often under the guise of voluntary sterilization efforts (Kluchin, 2009: 10; 11). But by the late 1960s and into the 1970s, sterilization had also established itself as an acceptable and dependable form of *voluntary* contraception due to many factors, including the successful media campaigns and referral services of groups like the HBAVS (renamed the Association for Voluntary Sterilization [AVS] in 1965), increased concerns over non-permanent contraception such as the Pill, and advances in sterilization surgical techniques (Kluchin, 2009: 50).

Those women who opted to be sterilized did so for various reasons, including the desire to control pregnancy and limit family size (Schoen, 2005). Many others chose sterilization because of poor health, which would make pregnancy difficult or dangerous, poverty and financial concerns, and anxieties about the side effects of hormonal contraceptives. Women also had to balance the risk of getting pregnant over the risk of experiencing side effects due to the Pill (Watkins, 1998: 79). For example, in 1969 women's health activist, Barbara Seaman, published her *The Doctor's Case Against the Pill,* which exposed dangers and concerns about the contraceptive pill.

Many women, she said, were not properly informed about these dangers due to the "paternalistic" nature of the doctor-patient relationship (O'Donnell, 2019: 551). While the medical technology existed to ensure that women had some birth control options, it would not really be until the 1970s that they were able to exercise their reproductive healthcare choices more fully. Historians of women's health and medicine (Morgen, 2002; Kline, 2010; Nelson, 2015) have shown how, into the late 1960s and beyond, women's health activists transformed their own healthcare through collective and grassroots action. This included gaining more knowledge about their bodies, demanding greater power and control over their bodies and healthcare outcomes, and providing health services and education to other women.

Dory Spencer: Nurse, Mother, and Patient

Various concerns about female permanent sterilization were raised throughout "The Rainbow Ride" by Dory, her physician, the nurses, and the Sterilization Committee.[4] The episode focuses more on fleshing out why *others* felt uneasy about Dory's sterilization, and how it affected their mental states, their views on contraception, and their reputations, rather than illuminating why Dory felt this was the best decision for her. Audiences learn more about the medical profession's views of sterilization, which emphasize its drawbacks, but very little about the patient's. While Dory is approved for the surgery, she is provided with little agency or voice throughout the episode, reflecting the wider medical and social constraints placed on female patients seeking sterilization and greater family planning options.

A significant portion of the episode follows Dr. Steffen grappling with the decision to approve Dory's request because he feels the surgery goes "against nature" to solve a "socioeconomic problem." He receives religious and psychiatric counseling, and questions Dory endlessly about all the problems and regrets she might face: what if she gets divorced? What if Hap, her husband, dies? What if her children die? He even mentions that he knew a woman who regretted her own sterilization, and that it was possible Dory might as well, since in any of these scenarios she may want more children. While it is understandable that a physician would want to ensure their patient has fully thought through their decision, his reluctance to sterilize Dory also reflects the continued reinforcement of pronatalist and neo-eugenic attitudes which sought to preserve the reproductive capabilities of "fit" women like Dory.

The hospital nurses are also generally against her decision to be sterilized, stating that they feel "uncomfortable" and "funny" about the idea.

One of them even refused to help prep for the surgery because, as a nurse otherwise "liberal about medical necessity," she did not feel right about the procedure. This preceded the signing into law of a 1973 federal policy that included a conscience clause which allowed medical professionals working at federally funded hospitals to refuse to provide sterilization surgery, as well as abortions (Haugeberg, 2018: 435). Thus, her refusal was more likely intended to highlight the moral and social objections to sterilization surgery, rather than her right, as a nurse, to medically object to it. Near the end of the episode, the main senior nurse of the show, Liz Thorpe, belittles Dory's decisions and makes it known to her how the student nurses feel about them. Being a nurse-patient in this context, who also works at the hospital, likely gave Dory a more in-depth understanding of the internal gossip. It also gave the medical staff room to openly lecture her more harshly. However, her established relationship with the hospital workers gave her more agency and power to openly discuss the reasons she desired the surgery, though she never got very far. And, as a white woman, she would generally have more agency to make reproductive decisions, though this also meant receiving more pushback when trying to end her own fertility. Otherwise, it is unlikely that a female patient would have "talked back" to her male physician given the highly paternalistic nature of the doctor-patient relationship in this context.

Conflicts between a medical professional's personal beliefs and medical authority are most evident in women's reproductive healthcare.[5] The conversation that takes place between Dory and Thorpe reflects how personal ideas about sterilization, and by extension, motherhood and childbearing, interfered with providing quality medical care and choice for patients. "Dory Spencer: Wife, mother, nurse. The fulfilled triple threat lady of the hour, and the envy of all the other nurses," Thorpe begins, explaining that the student nurses were positive they could "have it all": a family and a career, with "enough love" left over for nursing, as evidenced by Dory's life, but now "they're not so sure anymore." Thorpe agreed and seemed to take Dory's decision as a personal attack. It also threatened Dory's otherwise glowing medical credentials: "Dory, you're an intelligent woman, with medical training; 16 years of being a nurse. And the only way to control the size of your family is through permanent sterilization?" (One letter writer to CBS likewise was appalled that Dory, a "well educated person," would need to resort to permanent contraception to prevent pregnancy) (Carson et al., 1964). She envied Dory as well, having never had a baby herself since her husband died before they could have children, and said that it was "hard for me to imagine killing that chance to have children." Thus, this dialogue implies that the nurses are projecting their own insecurities on to Dory, viewing her as the "gold standard" woman who could successfully juggle a family with children, a career, and family planning responsibilities (episode *The Rainbow Ride*, 1964).

By contrast, Dory argues for bodily autonomy and personal responsibility. She already has enough children and wants the choice to make the best decision for her and her family. Near the end of the episode, however, it becomes clear that she has other reasons as well, and the episode takes a decidedly harsh and morally judgmental tone (episode *The Rainbow Ride*, 1964). For example, there is an indication that Hap is struggling to provide for Dory and their children. Though he is required to sign a spousal consent form before she can receive the surgery, a standard requirement at the time, he seems unsure about what sterilization even is, and Dory is too apprehensive to talk about it (Kluchin, 2009). The need for her husband's signature, despite his ignorance of the procedure, reflects the restrictive and patriarchal obstacles many women faced when seeking sterilization. It reinforces the idea that women's husbands should ultimately determine what they do with their bodies.

After a short argument at the hospital, Hap leaves, and Dory calls in a nurse. She is close to having the baby, so she needs that form signed; Nurse Thorpe reveals that Hap signed it before he left. Quite suddenly after hearing that, Dory says she feels "funny," and later it is revealed that her newly delivered baby has died. Dory states that this was God's way of punishing her for wanting to be sterilized. She ends up calling off the tubal ligation surgery; she no longer feels she needs it, and her subsequent conversations with Hap confirm for her a new life is on the horizon where everything will change, and he will be able to provide for their children (episode *The Rainbow Ride*, 1964).

While the purpose of this drama was more to entertain than educate the public on sterilization, its importance lies in how it portrayed the surgery to those who viewed the episode and how it fits into the wider social and medical context of sterilization surgery during the 1960s.

Reactions to The Rainbow Ride

In a letter to members of the HBAVS, Executive Director John R. Rague wrote that "voluntary sterilization will be presented as an integral part of a dramatic theme on a nation-wide television program—for the first time." He invited members to watch the episode, to "commend" the producers if they favorably portrayed the procedure, "clarify and defend" if not, and then share the letter with the HBAVS (Rague, 1964a). This call to action was part of a wider effort by the HBAVS to bring greater awareness to voluntary sterilization as a solution to many social and medical problems. They did this by emphasizing the use of permanent sterilization "as a medical solution to the contemporary social problems of poverty, illegitimacy, and overpopulation," to attempt to convince doctors and the public of the "social good" that came from it (Kluchin, 2009: 32). The HBAVS went through a transformation from actively supporting eugenics as a means of sterilizing those deemed "unfit" to reproduce, to encouraging the procedure as a safe and sure family planning method. This meant not only actively rebranding their image, and by extension, that of sterilization, but emphasizing how the procedure would help solve societal problems. Their promotion of sterilization during the 1960s, among other factors, helped pave the way for its rising popularity into the 1970s.

An examination of the letters sent by viewers of *The Rainbow Ride* reveal the range of attitudes people, including physicians and reproductive rights activists, held toward sterilization in the 1960s. Situated between the tail-end of the eugenics movement and the beginnings of the women's health and sterilization movements, this decade showcases the dynamic attitudes to permanent sterilization. Some viewers felt that painting sterilization as a controversial subject "in this day and age" was immoral and wrong-hearted, referring to the changing attitudes towards women's reproductive rights, and the increased emphasis on access to family planning (McGaughty, 1964). There were also growing concerns about overpopulation, and sterilization was viewed as one key strategy to curb the population. However, others commended the episode for the public exposure it provided to the procedure. One letter described it as a "remarkably helpful program" that "handled this sensitive subject both objectively and entertainingly" (Anderson, 1964). It also emphasized the need for television to both educate and entertain, revealing different ideas about what television should provide for its viewers.

A letter from a woman named Mrs. Hanloy Quock (1964) congratulated Herbert Brodkin, Executive Producer of the show, and his staff "for breaking through this 'hush-hush' subject in a factual and open manner," noting that such dramas would help educate people about the role sterilization should play in curbing population growth. Another letter remarked that sterilization had been "taboo for too long" and its coverage was "essential to provide the desired individual freedom of thought and action in our society" (Unke & Unke, 1964). While many reactions were negative, or neutral at best, what the positively-written letters revealed was that these changing ideas about sterilization—as a key family planning tool, and a solution to socioeconomic and population-related problems—were already emerging socially and in other media formats but were not yet properly addressed on television (VanEssendelft, 1978: 14).

Viewers also reacted negatively to the show, emphasizing the dramatic nature of the program, the judgmental attitude of the physicians and nurses, and the misunderstanding of voluntary sterilization itself. Rague used his personal experience as a physician to argue against the idea of sterilization as being stigmatized or rejected by medical professionals, as it was portrayed on the show. He stated that the episode "incorrectly implied to the public that difficulty and even disgrace would face any individual who presents himself to a physician or enters a hospital for such a procedure" (Rague, 1964b). Other physicians who wrote in agreed that the overdramatic responses to Dory's sterilization did not accurately reflect real-life hospital settings (Mitchell, 1964; Easley, 1964). While some physicians still discussed sterilization in the context of "human betterment," they also increasingly promoted its contraceptive benefits; not only was it a safe and effective form of birth control, but it could positively contribute to mental health by, among other things, reducing the anxiety associated with unwanted pregnancy (see Laidlaw, 1964; Blacker, 1964). Regardless, though, many women were denied the procedure and stigmatized for wanting to permanently control their fertility.

Permanent sterilization was forced on many women and denied to many others. Historian Rebecca Kluchin (2009), for example, shows how women struggled to voluntarily secure sterilization throughout the 1950s to the 1970s, though by the latter decade such access increased. These struggles partly reflect the entanglement of the procedure with coercive sterilization and the eugenics movement. But for those who *wanted* to be sterilized, rejection was sufficiently accepted to warrant legal campaigns to sue physicians and hospitals on behalf of these individuals. For example, from 1971 to 1973, in a campaign called "Operation Lawsuit," the AVS, the American Civil Liberties Union (ACLU), and population activist group Zero Population Growth (ZPG) worked to overcome obstacles placed on sterilization, such as spousal requirements and "age-parity" restrictions (a number, usually 120, which multiplied a woman's age by her number of children) (Dowbiggin 2008; Kluchin, 2009). Despite this, many women would continue to struggle to access the procedure voluntarily.

Though fortunately not a common reaction, a few letter writers reinforced eugenic ideas which promoted sterilization of the "unfit" as socially desirable and a societal good. For example, one letter from Dr. Lee R. Dice (1964), Professor Emeritus of Zoology at the University of Michigan, rightly pointed out that the "possibility that sterilization might sometimes be desirable was not discussed" in *The Rainbow Ride*. However, his reasons for believing so were less than desirable. He wrote that:

> It could have been suggested that sterilization possibly might aid in solving the problem of the mentally subnormal woman who continues to have a succession of illegitimate children and thus places a severe burden on the community

welfare funds and rears her children in an extremely unfavorable environment where they may grow up to become potential juvenile delinquests [sp] or even criminals.

Proponents of eugenics and neo-eugenics argued that health and social problems, such as poverty, could be dealt with through controlling reproduction—namely, though ensuring that control over a woman's access to abortion, birth control, and sterilization, remain in the hands of the state (Schoen, 2005). Some justified this by arguing that poor, uneducated women could not be trusted to properly use birth control or make their own reproductive healthcare decisions (Schoen, 2005: 4). Promoting sterilization to aid the "mentally subnormal woman" both reinforced such attitudes and ignored the real problem: that such women were often denied access to these reproductive technologies (Schoen, 2005). It also reinforced the neo-eugenic idea that children who grew up in "unfavorable environments" to "unfit" women were more likely to become criminals and/or "burdens" to their community and the welfare state. Thus, perceptions of and access to sterilization often depended on ideas about who should and should not reproduce.

While there were a variety of responses to *The Rainbow Ride*, overall, many viewers argued that public exposure to sterilization alone helped bolster it as a legitimate form of contraception, whether that portrayal was at times dramatic and critical, perhaps even inaccurate. Some who otherwise disliked the episode admitted that, despite its dramatic and exaggerated portrayal of the procedure, the exposure itself that the episode had provided was promising. Though other factors are more widely noted for the procedure's rising popularity—such as the increased sophistication and safety profile of medical technologies, and the desire to find other, non-hormonal and permanent, forms of contraception—this dialogue of acceptance was important for helping to ensure the procedure's increased popularity and legitimacy into the 1970s (Kluchin, 2009). The episode was part of the wider media campaign formed and encouraged by the HBAVS, which used popular media to better inform and educate Americans on voluntary sterilization. No matter how poorly or positively it was represented, the HBAVS used it as a learning opportunity to bring awareness to the procedure, how difficult it often was to access, and the stigma that plagued it.

Betty Gonzales: Patient, Nurse, and Sterilization Advocate

It was the attitudes and actions of the 1960s that helped give rise to the women's rights and women's health movements, as well as the active shift away from sterilization as a procedure of the eugenics movement and forced sterility. Groups like the HBAVS not only encouraged this shift but helped to provide resources and referral services to those interested in voluntary sterilization. A woman named Betty Gonzales, who sought out HBAVS for this very reason, serves as an interesting real-life case to examine alongside the fictional Dory Spencer. Like Dory, Gonzales was a nurse who struggled to gain access to tubal ligation. She used her personal experience to help others become sterilized through her work at the HBAVS and later the AVS.

After having five children, and while pregnant with her sixth, Gonzales—a married, white woman—requested a postpartum tubal from her physician. Each of her pregnancies involved complications, including "dangerous episodes of phlebitis" and "bilateral saphenous ligations to remove varicose veins, with twenty-two scars on my legs to prove it." She recalled how after each delivery she "had to be treated with anti-coagulants and elevated legs to prevent dangerous blood clots" (Gonzales, 2014: 11).

Very pregnant with child number six, she "begged" her doctor for a tubal. But neither her doctor, nor her vascular surgeon, believed that she had "sufficient medical reasons" to receive a tubal because pregnancy did not threaten her life. She describes that as the moment when she realized that, as a woman, she did not have full control of her own body, and that the tubal would only be performed when the doctor themselves decided it was appropriate, not when *she* did (Gonzales, 2014, p. 8; 11). Like Dory, she felt that she could not truly exercise her bodily autonomy and the right to plan her family as she saw fit. Both women also had large families already and expressed financial insecurities as part of their rationale for seeking sterilization. As fairly young, educated white women, resistance to their desires to be sterilized reflected neo-eugenic ideas about reproductive fitness and promoting childbearing and pronatalism among "fit" white women by denying them a permanent way to prevent pregnancy (Kluchin, 2009: 23).

A year later Gonzales became pregnant again, but this time sought an abortion. She was unable to find a trusted abortionist to ensure a safe procedure, however, so she performed the abortion on herself. "My subsequent hemorrhage and emergency surgery finally convinced my gynecologist that I was serious about not wanting another pregnancy," she said (Gonzales, 2014: 13). Gonzales was then referred to Dr. Alan Guttmacher, obstetrician-gynecologist and member of the HBAVS, who referred her to the organization for a tubal ligation (Gonzales, 2014). After receiving the surgery, she used her own experience and work with the AVS to help educate others about tubal ligation and permanent sterilization. Her story also reveals a lot about the status of women's bodily autonomy and contraception use in the 1960s.

As a nurse, Gonzales was expected to be aptly educated about her body and family planning; after all, these are subjects she probably spoke with her own patients about regularly. But she struggled to use contraception effectively before surgery. She initially relied on a diaphragm with jelly, and later dismissed the Pill and IUD after they arrived on the market in the 1960s, concerned about what the hormones would do to her body. This also reveals just how few, truly effective and safe methods were available; even the Pill, generally recognized today as both safe and highly effective, came with a much greater risk of side effects at the time due to the significantly higher concentration of synthetic estrogen. These included weight gain, nausea, headaches, and in more serious cases, deep vein thrombosis and pulmonary embolism (Tone, 2001: 245–246). Permanent sterilization was not only highly effective, with few side effects other than that which comes with invasive surgery, but would ensure no family planning accidents in the future (depending, however, on the type of surgical technique used, failure rates of tubal ligation varied) (Seiler, 1984: 178–179).

Conclusion

Despite being a fictional character for a dramatized soap opera, Dory's brief journey to become sterilized mirrors the real-life struggles of many women at the time. By the 1970s, sterilization became a highly popular form of contraception among both males and females in the United States. For example, rates of tubal ligation surgery increased by 164 percent throughout the decade and more women under 25 sought the procedure (Lee, 1984: 1363). But even today, many American women face rejection from their physicians when requesting sterilization, reflecting both medical and cultural biases towards women as mothers. It often takes women years of doctor shopping, sharing information about "sterilization friendly" physicians, and preparing "sterilization binders" in the face of opposition (No rugrats no ragrets, 2020). Ultimately, the choice of whether to sterilize a woman remains in the hands of her physician "in the absence of state laws that mandate otherwise" (Tazkargy, 2014: 135).

While the status of women's rights in the United States is a far cry from that of the 1960s, there is a continuous struggle to provide nationwide access to not only abortion and birth control, but also permanent sterilization. The legal status and social constructs of motherhood, fertility, and pronatalism create both perceived and actual obstacles as well as stigma towards a woman who seeks sterilization, especially if she is young and does not have children. As the struggle to protect and expand women's reproductive rights continues, we should keep in mind that reproductive choice—not only the access to birth control, but the *type* of birth control—is part of this fight, as it has been for generations.

Unfortunately, while shows like *The Doctors and the Nurses* may have exposed many viewers to ideas about permanent sterilization, we continue to see few positive media portrayals of the procedure. Medical dramas of the 1950s and 1960s had already addressed many of the complex, contentious, and often emotional aspects of women's reproductive healthcare, including but not limited to: pregnancy, childbirth, motherhood, abortion, and hereditary illness, as well as birth defects, stillbirth, miscarriage, and teen pregnancy.[6] In recent years, vasectomies receive much more attention in popular culture, as do abortions, pregnancy, and non-hormonal contraceptives. Female characters seeking sterilization on television are still few and far between and they are more likely to regret or be forced into the procedure. For example, Black Widow in *Avengers: Age of Ultron*, is forcibly sterilized as part of her Red Room graduation ceremony. Yennefer, a sorceress in the series *The Witcher*, is sterilized and comes to regret her decision and seeks ways to restore her fertility. The western drama *Yellowstone* also addresses the history of forced sterilization in the United States, while shows like *The Handmaid's Tale* depicts the reverse: the forced breeding of fertile women. While it is crucial to continue to tell stories depicting America's dark history of forced sterilization, and to contextualize the real possibility of regret among women who seek sterilization, these narratives need to be balanced with inspiring and liberating examples of the procedure. The lack of such narratives reflects the continued social stigma against female sterilization and the women who seek it. Recognizing the obstacles and stigmas attached to female sterilization, from the past to present, helps us challenge the cultural biases against women who choose a permanent method of contraception, such as the endurance of pronatalism and ideas that womanhood equates motherhood (Lalonde, 2018). Doing so will help ensure that women can access the birth control of their choice without struggle or judgment.

Notes

1. One newspaper advertisement described Dory's dilemma as a "complex personal problem" ("The Nurses," 1964).

2. There were some exceptions: for example, if a woman was suspected to have contracted rubella during her pregnancy (Reagan, 2010). Throughout the 1960s, some states began to allow abortion, such as in cases of rape and incest (Reagan, 1997).

3. In 1907, Indiana became the first place in the world to pass a compulsory sterilization law (Lombardo, 2011: ix).

4. A Sterilization Committee commonly comprised 3 to 5 physicians whose task was to decide whether a hospital patient should be sterilized. Many were phased out by the early 1970s (Lippman, 1973).

5. Historically, many medical professionals have objected to providing abortions, birth control, and sterilization for female patients for personal, religious, and other reasons. For a discussion of nurses' objections to abortions, for example see Haugeberg, 2018.

6. Medical dramas which addressed one or more of these issues include *The Doctor* (1952–1953), *Medic* (1954–1956), *Marcus Welby, MD* (1969–1976), and *Dr. Kildare* (1961–1966).

FILMS AND TELEVISION PRODUCTIONS REFERENCED

The Doctors and the Nurses (1962–1965) CBS
The Handmaid's Tale (2017–present) Hulu
The Nurses (1965–1967) CBS
Yellowstone (2018–present) Paramount Network

REFERENCES

Alderman, G. (Planned Parenthood Center of Syracuse) (1964) Letter to M.L. Carson, C. Sampson, H.B. Liddiard, E.K. Zimmerman, H. Gross, and N. Fox (cc: Human Betterment Association). 30 January. Association for Voluntary Sterilization Records [AVS Records], University of Minnesota [UMN], Minneapolis.

Anderson, J.P. (1964) Letter to WTVR Channel 6 (Richmond, VA). 24 January. AVS Records, UMN, Minneapolis.

Blacker, C.P. (1964) Voluntary sterilization: its role in human betterment. *The Eugenics Review* 56, 2: 77–80.

Carson, M.L., Sampson, C., Liddiard, H.B., Zimmerman, E.K., Gross, H., and Fox, N. (1964) Letter to CBS-WSYR Radio & Television Center (Syracuse, NY). 27 January. AVS Records, UMN, Minneapolis.

Dice, L.R. (1964) Letter to WCBI-TV (Columbus, MS). 20 January. AVS Records, UMN, Minneapolis.

Dowbiggin, I. (2008) *The Sterilization Movement and Global Fertility in the Twentieth-Century.* Oxford: Oxford University Press.

Easley, E.B. (1964) Letter to Channel 2 Station WFMY-TV (Greensboro, NC). 17 January. AVS Records, UMN, Minneapolis.

Gonzales, B. (2014) *A Public Health Journey: My Quest to Provide Permanent Contraception.* Betty Gonzales.

Hansen, R. (2013) *Sterilized by the State: Eugenics, Race, and the Population Scare in Twentieth-Century North America.* Cambridge: Cambridge University Press.

Haugeberg, K. (2018) Nursing and Hospital Abortions in the United States, 1967–1973. *Journal of the History of Medicine and Allied Sciences* 73, 4: 412–436.

Kline, W. (2001) *Building a Better Race: Gender, Sexuality, and Eugenics From The Turn Of The Century to the Baby Boom.* Berkeley: University of California Press.

Kline, W. (2010) *Bodies of Knowledge: Sexuality, Reproduction, and Women's Health in The Second Wave.* Chicago: The University of Chicago Press.

Kluchin, R.M. (2009) *Fit To Be Tied: Sterilization and Reproduction Rights in America, 1950–1980.* New Brunswick: Rutgers University Press.

Laidlaw R.W., and Bass, M.S. (1964) Voluntary Sterilization as It Relates to Mental Health. *The American Journal of Psychiatry* 120, 12: 1176–1180.

Lalonde, D. (2018) Regret, Shame, and Denials of Women's Voluntary Sterilization. *Bioethics* 32, 5: 281–288.

Lee, N.C. (1984) Tubal Sterilization in Women 15–24 Years of Age: Demographic Trends in the United States, 1970–1980. *American Journal of Public Health* 74, 12: 412–436.

Lippman, M. (1973) Hospitals Liberalize Rules: A New Sterilization Technique. Asbury Park Press.

Lombardo, P.A. (ed.). (2011) *A Century of Eugenics in America: From the Indiana Experiment to the Human Genome Era.* Bloomington: Indiana University Press.

Marks, L. (2001) *Sexual Chemistry: A History of the Contraceptive Pill.* New Haven: Yale University Press.

May, E.T. (2010) *America and the Pill: A History of Promise, Peril, and Liberation.* New York: BasicBooks.

McGaughty, J.B. (1964) Letter to WTAR-TV (Boush Street, Norfolk, VA). 17 February. AVS Records, UMN, Minneapolis.

Mitchell, A.D. (1964) Letter to Mr. E.K. Hartenbower, KCMO Television. 23 January. AVS Records, UMN, Minneapolis.

Moore, J. (2020) The Fixed Childfree Subjectivity: Performing Meta-Facework About Sterilization on Reddit, *Health Communication,* https://doi.org/10.1080/10410236.2020.1773697.

Morgen, S. (2002) *Into Our Own Hands: The Women's Health Movement in the United States, 1969–1990.* New Brunswick, NJ: Rutgers University Press.

Nelson, J. (2015) *More Than Medicine: A History of the Feminist Women's Health Movement.* New York: New York University Press.

"The Nurses" (1964, Jan. 16) *Fort Worth-Star Telegram* (Fort Worth, TX).

O'Donnell, K. (2019) Our Doctors, Ourselves: Barbara Seaman and Popular Health Feminism in the 1970s *Bulletin of the History of Medicine* 93, 4: 550–576.

Quock, H. (1964) Letter to Manager of KPIX-Television Channel 5 (San Francisco, CA). 18 January. AVS Records, UMN, Minneapolis.

Rague, J.R. (1964a) Letter to "Friend" (of Human Betterment Association for Voluntary Sterilization, Inc.). 9 January. AVS Records, UMN, Minneapolis.

Rague, J.R. (1964b) Letter to H. Brodkin. 18 February. AVS Records, UMN, Minneapolis.

Reagan, L.J. (1997) *When Abortion Was a Crime: Women, Medicine, and Law in the United States, 1867–1973.* Berkeley: University of California Press.

Reagan, L.J. (2010) *Dangerous Pregnancies: Mothers, Disabilities, and Abortion in Modern America.* Berkeley: University of California Press.

Schoen, J. (2005) *Choice and Coercion: Birth Control, Sterilization, and Abortion in Public Health And Welfare.* Chapel Hill: University of North Carolina Press.

Schoen, J. (2015) *Abortion After Roe.* Chapel Hill: The University of North Carolina Press.

Sterilization Binder. *No Rugrats No Ragrets.* https://norugratsnoragrets.wixsite.com/binder [accessed 23 November, 2020].

Stern, A. (2016) *Eugenic Nation: Faults and Frontiers of Better Breeding in Modern America.* Berkeley: University of California Press.

Tazkargy, A.S. (2014) From Coercion to Coercion: Voluntary Sterilization Policies in the United States. *Law & Inequality: A Journal of Theory and Practice* 32, 1: https://scholarship.law.umn.edu/lawineq/vol32/iss1/5.

Tone, A. (2001) *Devices and Desires: A History of Contraceptives in America.* New York: Hill and Wang.

Tone, A., and Watkins, E.S. (eds.) (2007) *Medicating Modern America: Prescriptions Drugs in History.* New York: New York University Press.

Unke, W.R., and Unke, M.J. (1964) Letter to WCCO Television (Minneapolis-St. Paul). 17 January. AVS Records, UMN, Minneapolis.

VanEssendelft, W. R (1978) "A History of the Association for Voluntary Sterilization: 1935–1964," University of Minnesota Ph.D.

Watkins, E.S. (1998) *On the Pill: A Social History of Oral Contraceptives, 1950–1970.* Baltimore: The Johns Hopkins University Press.

Ziegler, M. (2015) *After Roe: The Lost History of the Abortion Debate.* Cambridge, MA: Harvard University Press.

M*A*S*H*e*d and Harassed?

Nurse Margaret "Hot Lips" Houlihan as Gendered Hate Object

Susan Hopkins

Introduction: The Meanings, Messages and Misogyny of M*A*S*H

This essay uses a close feminist textual analysis to deconstruct depictions of sexual harassment and the character of Margaret Houlihan in the film *M*A*S*H* (1970) and in *M*A*S*H* (1972–1977) the television series, season one and season two. This critical analysis identifies and explores intersecting misogynistic myths around femininity, sexuality, nursing and sexual harassment evident within the film, and to a lesser extent the early seasons of the television series. It includes close, critical analysis of both the scripted dialogue and visual content of relevant scenes from the film and television series and the gendered cultural myths and misconceptions that circulate within these texts. The fictional character of *M*A*S*H*'s Margaret Houlihan, as she appears in the original American film directed by Robert Altman and in the early period of the television comedy produced by Gene Reynolds, provides an illuminating and widely known case study for interrogating the misogynistic moral narratives, vocabularies of motive and sexist stereotypes which continue to underpin the harassment and abuse of women. Moreover, the representational universe of *M*A*S*H* is a memorable and misogynistic media (mis)representation of the role of nurses and the nurse-doctor relationship. As Smith (2001: 78) has pointed out, nurses have long been stereotyped in communications media as "bossy and overbearing," with characters such as Ratchet (see also essay in this collection by Harmes, Harmes and Harmes 2021) and Houlihan sending negative messages which may ultimately impact public perceptions, as well as nursing recruitment and retention. I argue, through close study of relevant *M*A*S*H* scenes, that the regular punishment and humiliation of the bossy and overbearing Houlihan character is presented in both the film and the television series as a kind of moral mission and disciplining backlash threat (see also Faludi, 1991; Faludi, 2020) to undermine female empowerment and legitimate male dominance in the workplace.

In both the real world and the representational world, shaming sexist humor and hostile misogynistic speech is used to degrade, dehumanize and silence women, and this patriarchy-enforcing hate speech is today increasingly amplified by social media and other new communication technologies (Lim, 2020; Manne, 2018; Sunden and Paasonen, 2018; Richardson-Self, 2017; Ford, 2016; Hopkins and Ostini, 2015). Hence, this essay particularly focuses on close and critical feminist analysis of the patriarchy-enforcing, misogynistic or woman-hating *speech* captured in extracts from the *M*A*S*H* scripts and dialogue relevant to the development of the Nurse Houlihan character. Moreover, I argue that within this speech there are certain moral judgments, moral language and "vocabularies of motive" (see Bassil-Morozow and Proctor, 2018) or defensive justifications which are still used to explain sexual harassment and other abuses of women today and which also deserve critical feminist interrogation. As Berns (2004) has pointed out, media frames and media representations of sexual violence are important because they shape public perceptions of victims and perpetrators and their motives.

While on the surface "only" a medical black comedy (the film) or even "safe" situational, slap-stick humor as family entertainment (the television series), *M*A*S*H* is actually far more politically significant than we might at first imagine, especially for the generation who grew up watching it and learning from it as text. As we shall see, *M*A*S*H* is absolutely rife with degrading pranks, sexualized humor and gendered hate speech underpinned by victim-blaming moral narratives and hostile misogyny, most of it directed toward the target or token female hate object of Margaret Houlihan. The reasons *why* chief nurse Major Margaret Houlihan is targeted, and other female nurses are not, illustrates how the language and logic of misogyny (Manne, 2018) worked and continues to work to place the responsibility for "bad" attitudes, actions and feelings upon victim-survivors rather than on (mostly male) perpetrators (see Bassil-Morozow and Proctor, 2018). Moreover, these particular popular culture texts are not only a thing of the past but continue to be widely broadcast and celebrated as 1970s and 1980s nostalgia products available for viewing on demand on the internet, on streaming television "classics" replays or for purchase in "collector's edition" DVDs. The *M*A*S*H* (1970) film, which is particularly brutal in its hostile targeting and humiliation of Houlihan, is still widely regarded as cinema art; it received an Academy Award for best adapted screenplay as well as winning what is now known as the Palme d'Or at the 1970 Cannes Film Festival. In 1996, *M*A*S*H* was included in the selection deemed by the Library of Congress as historically and culturally significant. Yet in this feminist analysis and its critical alternative reading of the moral value of these texts, I argue that *M*A*S*H* is also perhaps historically and culturally significant to a whole generation of women who grew up with it, for its deeply misogynistic treatment of Houlihan and its portrayal and legitimation of her sexual harassment. Now more than ever, it is important to look back and look again at this classic pop culture text and what it teaches us about how and why misogyny works in workplaces, as the #MeToo movement continues to expose toxic cultures of sexism and sexual harassment, even and especially in medicine today.

Almost everything we need to know about the *M*A*S*H* universe, and its attitudes toward women generally and nurses in particular, is captured in the original, three minute 1970 movie trailer for the feature film; trailers are, after all, both an introduction and advertisement for the film. The *M*A*S*H* trailer begins and ends with pranks and sexualized insults directed at the unit's chief nurse, Major Margaret Houlihan, including highlights of the infamous shower prank scene which is discussed further below. The male narrator of the film trailer firstly introduces us to, "a United States Army field hospital somewhere near the front line" and tells us, "this is the story of two indispensable military surgeons—they have the army over a barrel" with shots of the two male (anti)heroes of the film, Captain "Trapper" John McIntyre and Captain Benjamin "Hawkeye" Pierce. However, the first character dialogue spoken, less than one minute into the trailer, is a senior commanding officer commenting; "Let's check this place out and see what the nurses are like." After this "comic" overt sexualization of nurses sets the emotional tone, next comes a blatantly misogynistic scene wherein one of those "indispensable" male military surgeons, "Trapper" John, points at Nurse Houlihan declaring: "Bring me that one over there. That one. The sultry bitch with the fire in her eyes. Take her clothes off!" The narrator tells us that *M*A*S*H* is "a motion picture that raises some important moral questions—and then drops them." Perhaps ironically, I argue in this essay that the *M*A*S*H* universe, by which I mean, the original film, the television series and even its film poster iconography, does indeed raise "some important moral questions" which are still relevant today, fifty years later. They relate however to the moral philosophy of misogyny and the socio-cultural vocabularies of motive which typically underpin the sexual harassment and abuse of women, even in the contemporary #MeToo era. It is indeed important to focus on what might be called the *moral economy* of these texts, because the humor of the scenes and scripts relies on particular moral assumptions and value judgments to be made about women, their value and their place at work.

M*A*S*H, *Morality and #MeToo: Theoretical Frameworks and Historical Contexts*

*M*A*S*H* assumes that the rightful role of women, especially nurses, in the field hospital workforce, includes the enthusiastic provision of sexual services and emotional labor to men, especially doctors, to help relieve them of the stress of practicing medicine in a warzone. Women, like Margaret Houlihan, who fail to comply submissively with this expectation are judged to be failing or lacking by hetero-patriarchal standards and thus in need of correction (which typically takes the form here of sexual harassment, humiliation humor and sexualized pranks). The woman who does not comply, like the perpetually angry, assertive and resistant Margaret Houlihan character, is subjected to ever escalating hostility and punishment for not adapting to the dominant hetero-patriarchal norms. As the feminist philosopher Kate Manne (2018) explains it in *Down Girl: The Logic of Misogyny*, misogyny is not just about regarding certain disagreeable women as less than fully human, hateful objects—it is also about systematic social and cultural processes of policing and enforcing the patriarchal order, especially when and where it is challenged. I argue that popular culture too can work in this disciplining and shaming way, especially where film and television audiences are invited to identify with and take the perspective of misogynistic male characters through the setting of scenes, scripts and camera work. *M*A*S*H* has been particularly effective in teaching these patriarchy-enforcing moral lessons across generations of viewers, because it invites viewers to see sexual harassment through the perspective of the male perpetrators (as "heroic" surgeons McIntyre and Pierce), thus perpetuating the notion that sexual harassment, especially through sexist humor, is not only acceptable and excusable, but cool (rebellious), fun, flirty and even sexy. Both the film and television series construct the female characters (mostly nurses) and the way they are to be looked at, not only through a "male gaze" (see Mulvey, 1975) but through a *disciplinary* male gaze, which punishes certain moral "types" of women while rewarding and romanticizing others.

Hence, the kind of special treatment Nurse Houlihan receives from her male colleagues is not just simple sexism but blatant misogyny or "woman-hating" (see also Richardson-Self, 2017) which targets and punishes particular types of women who are deemed "bad," worthy of scorn, humiliation, hostility and hatred. This is why the political-philosophical work of feminist moral philosophy is particularly helpful in understanding the moral messages of *M*A*S*H* and why they are still so relevant today. Currently, female journalists, politicians, academics and other outspoken women are facing, as Faludi (2020: xi) recently put it, "harassment and threats on a whole new front" in a "misogynist blitzkrieg" thanks to an online epidemic of "bile-spewing swarms of trolls." While Faludi (1991 & 2020) explains this historical cultural moment in terms of political "backlash" (against female empowerment), feminist moral philosophers have also explained exactly how this hate speech is built upon misogynistic *moral* judgments between good and bad types of women—those "good girls" who deliver feminine-coded labor and services to men (mostly free of charge) while pandering to male interests, versus those "bad girls" who refuse and resist the dominant patriarchal order—like the feisty and fierce Nurse Houlihan. Feminist moral philosophers, such as Kate Manne (2018) and Louise Richardson-Self (2017), have explained how and why misogyny increasingly pushes back, hard and fast, against its most vocal critics through gendered hate speech in particular and through *victim-blaming* moral narratives in new and mainstream media. As Kate Manne (2018: 307) puts it: "One woman's misogyny is thus some men's poetic justice." Hence, for the modern misogynist, feminist activists are not just wrong, they are morally disgusting as well as less than human; they are essentially hate objects.

This is where the work of feminist theorist and public intellectual Sara Ahmed (2017: 67) is also helpful in her feminist critique of those dominant, hetero-patriarchal cultural narratives which use hate and violence as "a moral correction." Sexual banter, observes Ahmed (2017, 35) is part of a gendered and often institutionalized system of reward and punishment: "You might participate in that banter because it is costly not to participate: [or] you might become the problem, the one who is disapproving or uptight." In other words, the female character who does not play along or takes herself too seriously, like Houlihan, is painted as a kind of unlikeable killjoy which, as Ahmed (2017) points out, is equivalent to the "kiss of death" in the increasingly competitive culture industries. Yet, as part of her own steadfast refusal to participate or laugh along with such punitive patriarchal cultures and her commitment to instead speak up against misogynistic moral judgments, Ahmed (2017) has consciously embraced for herself and her followers the title and theoretical framework of "the feminist killjoy." Ahmed coined the term "feminist killjoy," firstly in her online blog to refer to the principal and practice of not pandering to the patriarchal culture, and calling it out when she feels uncomfortable, no matter the social cost she may incur (https://feministkilljoys.com/about/). As she explains on her blog (2020): "My name is Sara Ahmed, and this is my research blog.

I am a feminist killjoy. It is what I do. It is how I think. It is my philosophy and my politics…. I am writing to those for whom complaints of this kind, complaints about abuses of power, complaints about institutional violence, are companions." Ahmed's (2015) work on the cultural politics of emotion is also helpful for explaining how Othered people, especially women, are turned into hate objects. For, as Ahmed (2015) has observed, in the affective economies of hate in contemporary hetero-patriarchy, the female Other may be turned into an object of hate, where all negative feelings are projected onto her by the hostile male subject(s), when she fails to comply with patriarchal norms. To treat someone as an object is to fail to appreciate their full inner life as a human being and imagine them instead as a thing, as a means to an end (see also Manne 2018, 136). Ahmed (2015, 95) also suggests the internet has become the new and powerful means by which we watch or call upon others to witness our own performativity of hate and disgust directed toward Others perceived as wrong, contaminating or repulsive.

These cutting-edge philosophical feminist theories around woman-hating and hate objects explain how, within the *M*A*S*H* moral universe, Houlihan is constructed as both a *killjoy* and a *hate object* through the punitive, disciplining and misogynistic male gaze. This process of moral alchemy in the representational world has much to teach us about how sexual harassment and other abuses against women work today, even and especially in the (post)modern, (post)feminist age. As Kate Manne (2018) has pointed out, the kinds of scripts or cultural narratives which are still used to explain harassment and abuse of women still tend to objectify and ascribe responsibility and blame to women, while exonerating and humanizing men—a process which allows perpetrators to (sometimes literally) to get away with murder. A woman who withholds feminine-coded services of emotional labor, a woman who appears cold, selfish, anti-social or ambitious, is especially likely to lose sympathy and attract the most misogynistic hostility and anger (Manne, 2018, 296). Manne (2018: 266) also points to just how long it has taken, despite multiple credible reports and case studies, to have sexual harassment seriously addressed in our key institutions, suggesting this is a collective symptom of women learning to stay silent, to stay loyal to authority figures, to avoid attracting hate or jealousy, to be the "good" woman, rather than risk being seen as a killjoy or trouble-maker.

Helena Bassil-Morozow and Katy Proctor (2018) have recently engaged the sociological concept of "vocabularies of motive," developed by C.W. Mills, to challenge the ways in which perpetrators of sexual harassment like Harvey Weinstein typically explain and minimize their conduct and intent. Common defensive claims, excuses, rationalizations or "blame-shifting" narratives include: accusations that women are overreacting or fantasizing and seeing harassment where it isn't, misunderstanding the line between flirting and harassment, claiming "it was a different time back then" and sexual attention norms have changed over time, citing "political correctness gone mad," and the claim that women secretly enjoy the attention. While the *M*A*S*H* stories and characters are fictional, they illustrate, personify and exemplify this kind of misogynistic logic and language which perpetuates and excuses sexual harassment and other forms of sexual violence. The same threats of public humiliation, exposure of private information and malicious attacks disguised as controversial "humor" which the fictional Houlihan endured, are still experienced by real women today, only amplified by new communication technologies, especially social media (see also Hopkins & Ostini, 2015).

While sexual harassment and discrimination is illegal in Australia (under the *Sex Discrimination Act* 1984) it continues to be a major social, cultural and economic problem for women across professions, including medicine and nursing, where a particularly "toxic culture of bullying, overwork, sexism and harassment is devastating young female doctors sometimes to a fatal end" (Carlton, 2021: 62). Popular culture provides an important tool for understanding and illustrating how these gender hierarchies work in the workplace, especially in high pressure environments like medicine and especially where they are underpinned by misogynistic moral narratives about who has the *right* to be confident, powerful and assertive at work and who is told they need to be more caring, agreeable and modest! As we will see in close feminist and textual analysis of the *M*A*S*H* scripts, Houlihan is a classic pop culture lightning rod for these issues of gender politics, as she is frequently targeted, blamed or scapegoated, humiliated, questioned about her sex life, the butt of sexual jokes and comments, asked for sexual favors but most often insulted with sexual insults—in other words, sexually harassed.

With the feature film released in 1970 and the early seasons of the television series running from 1972 to 1977, *M*A*S*H* was a product of its time, reflecting back the sexist atmosphere in many workplaces in the 1970s. As Faludi (2020: x) points out, back in the 1970s and 1980s, "complaints of sexual harassment and assault were met with scoffing skepticism, even as they plagued schools, the military and workplaces nationwide." It was not until 1975 that a group of feminist activists in New York coined the term "sexual harassment" to put a name to the unwanted sexual demands, looks, comments, contact and coercion that they had experienced in the workplace, but which was not yet widely acknowledged in official discourse (Baker, 2008: 1). While widespread, sexual harassment in the workplace was treated as a kind of joke at time or trivialized as harmless flirtation until feminist activists and organizations, such as the Alliance Against Sexual Coercion, began to raise awareness of the issue in the 1970s and 1980s (Baker, 2008). As it gathered pace, sexual harassment litigation became a kind of testing ground for feminist arguments that women had an equal right to participate fully in the workplace, and the women's movement made important advancements both politically and legally (Baker, 2008). By the 1980s and 1990s however, hostile backlash narratives were also gathering momentum, expressing in media culture particularly, a kind of moral condemnation of victims, blaming women or accusing them of being deceitful or opportunistic (Faludi, 1991 & 2020). M*A*S*H pop culture parallels real world attempts to undermine the authority of individual women, and the empowerment of women as a group. The sexist stereotypes, bullying and victim-blaming narratives encountered by "Hotlips" Houlihan persist today, which is why it is so important to interrogate the powerful gender bias that's captured and legitimated in our popular culture and centered on nursing. While individual legal solutions or remedies for sexual harassment cases are of course important, it is also important to investigate the misogynistic mediated myths of wider patriarchal culture which continue to enable and trivialize the harassment and abuse of women in the guise of controversial "humor" or black comedy.

Who Is Hot Lips? The Cinematic Origin Story and Other Dehumanizations of Women in M*A*S*H

As Bassil-Morozow and Proctor (2018) have pointed out in their critical analysis of the contemporary discourses and vocabularies of (male) motives which frequently underpin sexual harassment in the workplace, colleagues should avoid name-calling or nicknames which express romantic attachment, as sexual slang can easily cross the line into dehumanizing, denigrating expression, especially where it involves projecting (male) fantasies on to women: "It all boils down to treating people as individuals, not objects." In both the M*A*S*H film and the television series, the male hero doctors frequently refer to female nurses not by their actual names, but by sexual or romantic nicknames like "sweetheart," "baby," "dish" or "darling." The most often used female nickname in the M*A*S*H universe is the label "Hot Lips," reserved for the highest ranking female of the 4077th and the unit's chief nurse, Major Margaret Houlihan. The Houlihan character is significant in these texts as the only prominent female central member of the television series cast, the only female who features on the television DVD promotional images (pictured alongside the five central male characters) as well as the only female character introduced in the early episode voiceovers ("attention all personnel...") alongside Hawkeye, Trapper, Henry, Frank and Radar. Hence, the sexualized slang and shaming pranks routinely directed at head nurse Houlihan in both the film and early television series are also performances which produce gender politics as well as slap-stick comedy, for Houlihan comes to stand in and act for all (difficult) women in the moral narratives and discourses of the show. Indeed, it is her resistance to the patriarchal order, her refusal to get along and go along with the male characters that (supposedly) makes her humiliation "funny" and deserved. Moreover, the backstory to how Houlihan came to be known as "Hot Lips" is particularly illuminating, as it demonstrates the real shaming and disciplining function of the name assigned to her by her male colleagues. As we know, discourses are all about (socio-cultural) contexts and it is clear in the *M*A*S*H* context that the term indicates not romantic attachment, but playful punishment and humiliation for a chief nurse who is seen (through the disciplining male gaze) as both too sexual and not sexual enough.

The *M*A*S*H* narrative backstory to the overtly sexualized nick-name "Hot Lips" is told first in the film, when Trapper records Frank and Margaret passionately kissing in her tent with a hidden microphone and then broadcasts it over the public address system. Unaware that the whole camp is listening to her private and passionate conversations, Margaret declares to her lover, "kiss my hot lips!" Screams and confusion follows, however, when Margaret realizes they are being recorded and publicly humiliated in this scene, which reminded me of an early analogue version of what we would now know as revenge porn. Hot lips Houlihan thus finds herself thus stuck with this sexualized and dehumanizing label through the film and into the television series that followed it, forever mocked for being a difficult woman who is both sexual and unlikeable. It sets up a misogynistic dynamic for the rest of the narrative whereby Margaret is punished for both being too sexual and not sexual enough; women who have encountered online gendered hate speech or technology facilitated violence against women will be all too familiar with how this shaming and disciplining narrative (still) works. While the name "Hot Lips" may appear on the surface to represent innocent, friendly and fun humor between characters, it is also possible to read this sexualized slang as a form of gendered hate speech, because in the text it is also used by the anti-establishment male (anti) medical heroes of the story to silence and shut down the chief nurse when they feel threatened by her. The iconic *M*A*S*H* "Hot Lips" cinematic origin story sets up a common pattern in both the film and in the early television series whereby the active sexuality of Margaret is judged very differently from the sexual aggression of male characters in the moral accountancy of the narratives. The private desire of Margaret for Frank, or any man, is mostly set up as comic and ridiculous (and deserving of punishment through public humiliation) whereas the public sexual harassment exercised by Hawkeye and Trapper is presented differently as further evidence of their virile and medical masculinity—thus once again invoking and relying upon a gendered, sexual double standard in the moral judgments implicitly invited by the text.

Next, Margaret is further humiliated and defeated in the even more infamous "shower prank scene" of the *M*A*S*H* film. The shower scene is so indicative of the sexual libertarian moral message of the film and its misogynistic underpinnings that it deserves further explanation in some detail. A group of nurses who are walking to the showers, are delayed by Trapper, Hawkeye and their gang. The reasons they are delayed, reflected in the dialogue, are clearly gendered and loaded with misogynistic moral meaning. All except Margaret are detained by the men with questions and help seeking requests for their various emotional and physical pains, such as missing their children, attending to their sore feet and various other desires for feminine coded care services. In this apparent misogynistic moral accountancy, the nurses who are constructed as "good" women stop and voluntarily and cheerfully perform the unpaid labor and traditional gendered role of attending to men's feet, nursing their wounds, healing their emotional pain and providing positive attention as requested by Hawkeye, Trapper and the gang. Only Nurse Houlihan replies that she is "not the least bit interested" in viewing photos of their children, or nursing their sore feet and with head high strides on to the shower tent alone. Houlihan's immediate and unapologetic reaction of dismissing her male colleagues of course furthers the moral narrative that she is thus deserving of the spectacular public punishment and humiliation which follows, for failing to fulfill the gender role of the "good" (nurturing, maternal and self-sacrificing) nurse. Kate Manne (2018: 267) calls this kind of gender bias and unspoken expectation for women to be more giving and attentive than men "care-mongering"—a term with connotations too of petty enforcements of order. As Chemaly (2018: 84) points out, when women at work don't do the unpaid work of emotional labor expected of them (especially in the "feminized" profession of nursing) by suppressing their own negative feelings in the service of others, they are judged harshly by men and women alike: "A 'no-nonsense' woman is 'cold,' 'bitchy' and disliked." Certainly, when Nurse Margret Houlihan refuses to moderate her authority and rank with displays of feminine submissiveness and emotional labor, the audience anticipates she will soon be punished for this gender transgression in the moral accountancy of the film. Moreover, by setting up the scene in this way, the director, writer, producer and other male authority figures behind the scenes are clearly elevating this symbolic punishment of the unruly "Hot lips" woman to a *moral* task and lesson. We are being implicitly told she is *deserving* of her own harassment because she is *wrong* and has *wronged* Hawkeye and Trapper. Moreover, significantly, we the viewer are invited and encouraged to experience the disciplining of Nurse Margaret Houlihan as pleasurable and comic. As Chemaly (2018: xx) observes, treating women's anger and pain as something to be mocked is central to the systematic exploitation of women's labor and sexuality.

Once Margaret is alone inside the shower, Trapper gives a signal, and the shower tent collapses revealing Margaret naked to the whole camp—naturally she screams in alarm and falls to the ground crawling for cover in an attempt to recover her dignity. Hawkeye and Trapper cheer and raise their martini glasses at the sight of this "entertaining" spectacle. From a critical feminist reading it is difficult to interpret this scene as anything other than a representation of a traumatic event and violent, unprovoked response to an assertive and independent woman—the fact that it is presented as slap-stick comedy suggests a sexually assaultive "male gaze" at work (see Mulvey, 1975) in the construction and reception of the scene. Moreover, the text clearly reflects and reproduces, if not actually a rape, then certainly the kind of depiction indicative of what Sarah Projansky (2001) has identified as a wider rape culture within the hetero-patriarchy. As soon as she recovers herself and a robe, Margaret strides over to the tent of commanding officer Henry Blake to complain, eventually crying in frustration and exhaustion: "This isn't a hospital! It's an insane asylum!" Expertly acted by Sally Kellerman, the screaming, the tears, the pain, the humiliation of Major Margaret Houlihan in this iconic film scene is, from a female perspective, absolutely shocking and heart-wrenching. The movie, however, runs through a misogynistic male gaze or perspective and the dominant or preferred reading presented in the arrangement of the scene is that the victim deserves her punishment. In the final humiliation, the *M*A*S*H* commanding officer does nothing to help her and instead tells her to go ahead and resign her commission if she has a problem. Again, the message is clear—by naming the problem, she becomes the problem and thus speaking up makes her even more of a target for the remainder of the cinematic story. Her complaint clearly "falls on deaf ears" and is not taken seriously by her supervisor (commanding officer). This representational scenario of sexual harassment of a nurse by doctors, and a telling moment in the media history of nurses, might have been dismissed as a thing of the past had this essay not previously provided 2021 examples of real world authority figures who also apparently "didn't want to hear it" let alone deal with it (see Curtis and Crowe, 2021). The darkly comic, misogynistic moral narrative is compounded further by the fact that Henry Blake himself has a naked woman in bed with him during this post-shower meeting scene. The meeting and the scene concludes with Henry turning to the naked, far more obliging and submissive nurse next him, offering, "more wine my dear?" The misogynistic moral message is clear, that Margaret is the killjoy and the naked, cool "good-girl" bed companion is the ideal nurse. Women are divided into categories here in the moral accountancy of the film, and those who fall on the wrong side of the good nurse/ bad nurse binary must apparently pay for it with their pride.

Both these key scenes in the cinematic origin story of the "Hot Lips" character discussed above are also picked up in the television series in numerous episodes. For example in the Season Two episode titled "Divided We Stand" Margaret complains about Hawkeye and Trapper ("they're both impossible") only to have Trapper respond: "You stay out of this Hot Lips or I'll stop selling tickets to your shower" (Followed by laugh track). Hence, the same misogynistic myths and victim-blaming narratives mobilized in the film are continued in the television series, with the suggestion that not only does Margaret deserve the sexual harassment, but that she secretly enjoys the sexualized attention.

Margaret as Sexualized Hate Object

Manne (2018, 164) makes the important point that the logic of misogyny, like other dehumanizing ideologies, relies on (supposedly) amusing "put-downs" to keep difficult women down, which is why hate speech functions to insult, intimidate and belittle, as well as hate. The hate the male doctor heroes feel for chief nurse Margaret Houlihan in the film is apparently visceral, especially where they feel both threatened and fascinated by her *at the same time.* Captain "Duke" Forrest says of Margaret: "You know I damn near puke every time I look at her." As Ahmed (2015, 94) observes: "To abject something is literally to cast something out … a form of vomiting, as an attempt to expel something whose proximity is felt to be threatening and contaminating." Ahmed (2015) goes on to explain that in the cultural politics of emotion, such intense hatred can thus reveal a perverse form of attachment, especially when the (male) subject is threatened or fearful. And in keeping with Ahmed's theory the sexual desire of Duke for Margaret is quite clear by the end of the film narrative.

On this point, it is interesting to note that while the film and early seasons of the television series are clearly woman-hating, they are equally man-loving—the relationship most celebrated is the homoerotic relationship between Trapper and Hawkeye. While Margaret is insulted in both the film and television show for supposedly being too masculine, being a man is actually also celebrated by the *male* characters in the show as the human ideal. Apparently, to not be male is to have a life not worth living, as this misogynistic philosophical appraisal from the film puts it: "If a man isn't a man anymore, what's he got left that he should be living for?"

The reason Nurse Houlihan is hated by both male and female characters is in part because she is painted as the token no-nonsense but ridiculous "kill-joy" villain of the comedy—the uptight mother figure who gets in the way of the sexual adventures and libertarian ethos of our juvenile, anti-establishment male (anti)heroes. It is significant, therefore, that Hawkeye's first dismissal of Margaret's authority is laced with sexual insult and is clearly positioned to penetrate her (supposedly) inflated sense of importance: Hawkeye to Margaret: "Under normal circumstances, you being normally what I would call a very attractive woman, I would have invited you back to share my little bed with me, and you might possibly have come. But you really put me off. I mean, you're what we call a regular army clown" (*M*A*S*H*, 1970).

The insults directed at women in the *M*A*S*H* universe are at times ageist as well as sexist forms of discrimination, typically expressed through male characters cracking offensive jokes and through demeaning nicknames (as previously mentioned). Senior nurses who are aged out of the category of sex object in the film are differently degraded by being referred to as "mother" instead of their name or rank, invoking the classic overbearing monstrous-mother caricature of psychoanalytic theory and Hollywood horror (see also Kristeva 1982, Creed 1993). Indeed, Trapper John apparently puts an older nurse back in her place in the film (and film trailer), by reminding her that he is the superior, genius surgeon under time pressure (and she is positioned as the emasculating mother getting in the way of innovation whose authority must be overthrown), declaring: "Look, *mother,* I want to go to work in one hour." Clearly this sexist and ageist language is designed to frame the nurse as excessively bossy and maternal while imagining himself as playfully young and vital. It is another example also of impossible and unequal standards required of women, who may be criticized both for being not maternal enough ("cold and uncaring"), yet also for being too maternal ("nagging," "smothering," "grumpy" "outdated" "mother-hen"). Hence, here is another example of how the female killjoy character, tasked with policing the sexual behavior of others (basically ruining their "free love" fun) is painted as a traditional conservative moralist, invented in unflattering contrast to the supposedly progressive sexual libertarian male heroes of *M*A*S*H*.

Good Nurse/Bad Nurse

Just as Margaret the hate object (that viewers love to hate), is frequently painted in unflattering opposition to Hawkeye and Trapper, nurses are pictured in moral contrast to each other in these misogynistic narratives and mythologies. As Manne (2018, 34) explained, misogynistic hatred does not necessarily target all women equally, but will selectively typically target certain *kinds* of women who are perceived as a threat to the patriarchy, or failing to live up to its sexist standards. Hence, both men and women make moralistic judgments about how women provide (or fail to provide) feminine-coded services and appearances, by dividing women into different moral types of "good" and "bad women" (Manne 2018, 296). These moral judgments then incite powerful emotional reactions. I argue that the old Western moral dichotomy of good girl (obedient virgin) vs. bad girl (unruly whore) is also presented in *M*A*S*H* as a kind of moral division between the good nurse and the bad nurse, determined and decided in part in terms of their submission (or lack of) to the heroic male characters. In this way gendered characters we love, or love to hate, are constructed in the *M*A*S*H* scripts and scenes. The strategic placement of the laugh track sound effect in the television series is also particularly significant because it reinforces the notion that we are *supposed to be* laughing *along* with the sexist insults and pranks directed at female nurses. It thus "eggs us on" to laugh at Margaret and women like her as part of the function of the disciplining male gaze. The laugh track tells us, in the moral accountancy of the show, that sexual harassment is funny, trivial, a joke—and those who complain about it deserve to be mocked as supposed killjoys.

In the episode, "Requiem for a Lightweight" from series one of *M*A*S*H* the television show (1972), Hawkeye talks Trapper into entering a boxing match in order to "win back" their favorite new nurse, Nurse Cutler, who was transferred out of the 4077th for being too "distracting" to the doctors. The opening scene of the episode, which is titled "the Semi-Nude Nurse," positions the young and naïve new arrival to the 4077th, Nurse Margie Cutler (played by Marcia Strassman) accidentally bumping into Hawkeye and Trapper, exiting the shower and wearing only a towel. Thus the shower motif, so memorable from the original film, is repeated here, however with Cutler constructed as the good-girl, submissive nurse in opposition to the aggressive killjoy character of Nurse Houlihan. Both women, as women, are still sexualized by the doctors first and foremost:

> Nurse Cutler: "Excuse me doctors I wasn't looking."
> Hawkeye [holding on to her with both hands while looking her up and down]: "I'm doing enough looking for both of us."
> [laugh track follows]

As Nurse Cutler scurries off and exits the frame, the audience sees that Hawkeye has "accidentally" pulled off her towel. Both men salute the, presumably now naked, woman as she hurries away. In the operating room the harassment continues and the good nurse character thus again obliges.

> HAWKEYE: "Nurse!"
> NURSE CUTLER: "Yes Doctor?"
> HAWKEYE: "That's yes Doctor Darling."
> NURSE CUTLER: "Yes Doctor Darling."
>   [laugh track follows]

Margaret and Frank overhear this exchange in the operating room and comment on this "disrespectful behavior." Later Nurse Houlihan comes between Hawkeye and Nurse Cutler, as they are "flirting" in the mess tent:

> MARGARET: "Nurse Cutler report to my office."
> NURSE CUTLER: "Now?"
> MARGARET: "Now."
> NURSE CUTLER: "Yes Sir. I mean yes Mam."
> HAWKEYE: "Well at least she didn't have any trouble figuring out your sex."
>   [laugh track]
> MARGARET: "My sex is none of your business."
> TRAPPER: "Just say the word."
>   [laugh track]
> MARGARET: "You stay away from my nurses. They are off limits to you. That's an order."
> HAWKEYE: "I think she's trying to tell us something."
> TRAPPER: "That's your basic hot lips."
> HAWKEYE: "I knew a girl like her in my home town. Her name was Rover."
>   [laugh track]

Scenes from the early television series extend themes previously mentioned; the comparison between women and dogs, the accusation-insult that powerful women are too masculine, the demonization of the feminist killjoy who disrupts male desires. In this same episode, Trapper and Hawkeye disregard Margaret's orders and while up-beat, optimistic music combines with a laugh track in the background, Hawkeye and Trapper are pictured competing for the attention of Nurse Cutler (the "good girl" nurse). They "zero in on the same girl" before coming up with the "solution" that they will "share her." When Hawkeye and Trapper decide to enter a boxing competition in order to "win" her back from the other unit their boxing training begins with Trapper using Frank's bag as a punching bag, prompting this exchange with Margaret:

> MARGARET: "Just a minute, isn't that Frank's bag?"
> TRAPPER: "I thought *you* were Frank's bag!"
>   [laugh track].

Trapper wins the fight by cheating, and at the conclusion of the episode commanding officer Henry Blake leads Nurse Cutler back to the men's tent as the prize. Before leaving, Henry mutters to Nurse Cutler, "Keep moving or you're dead" and the laugh track cue follows. Nurse Cutler is the good-girl nurse character, however, so she stays and panders, obliges and flatters her heroes—with wide eyed adoration she exclaims to Trapper: "It's true you fought for me! I must say I'm impressed."

The Moral Double Standard: Slut-Shaming for Hot Lips vs. Sexual Freedom for Trapper and Hawkeye

As Manne (2018, 296) points out, according to these patriarchal moral-social categories and norms, giving sexual attention to the wrong person, and in the wrong way, makes the female hate object a bitch, slut or a lesbian through the disciplining (and assaultive) hetero-patriarchal male gaze. Margaret Houlihan is portrayed and shamed as having the "wrong" kind of sexuality—part of her framing as villain includes her habit of apparently being sexually aroused by the exercise of power and power disparities, in military rank for example. Her pleasure in the prospect of punishing Hawkeye and Trapper *back* is also sexualized and mocked, as she typically mutters the catchphrase "Oh Frank," while turning to embrace and passionately kiss Burns, when the two are plotting revenge. Inevitably their schemes and plots fail and her sex life becomes another aspect of the Houlihan character that positions her as ridiculous and deserving of the humiliation and scorn which typically follows. Hence, even the television series, serves as a kind of slap-stick (misogynistic) morality tale.

Margaret is also presented as having a strong sexual appetite and being passionate to the point of being unhinged. But while Trapper and Hawkeye are positioned as anti-establishment heroes for making impromptu passionate speeches about the futility of war—their angry outbursts under pressure framed as legitimate and righteous—the passion and anger of Houlihan is framed as ridiculous, worthy only of mockery. In contrast to the treatment of Houlihan, the "indispensable" hero surgeons of *M*A*S*H* are celebrated for their "degenerate" status. Much of the (supposed) humor derives from Houlihan attempting to stop the "degenerate" excessively sexual behavior and speech of the surgeons and failing every time with Houlihan coming off not just as the overbearing emasculating killjoy, but as frustrated and ineffectual (frequently only revealing her own weakness in her failed attempts to oppose Hawkeye and Trapper and the whole male chain of command). For example, in the season two episode of the television series titled "Divided We Stand" Margaret complains of Hawkeye and Trapper, "there isn't a nurse in this camp they haven't tried to molest" and Trapper responds "except the male ones" (followed by laugh track).

In the moral universe of the early *M*A*S*H*, the ultimate moral value is freedom, especially sexual freedom (for men at least) and any woman who is gets in the way of that moral mission is perceived as a problem that must be solved either by being screwed (or otherwise disciplined and punished) through Hawkeye and Trapper's anti-establishment antics. The libertarian "make love not war" message is taken to black humor extremes in the Altman film where sex, or more sex, is presented as the answer to almost every individual or social problem. When Captain "Pole" Waldowski, for example, starts to feel suicidal, Hawkeye pressures his own girlfriend to have sex with him and thus restores his spirits, while demanding more apparently exploitative labor for the hapless exhausted nurse. In this male-oriented scene, the film presents frontline "free love" sexual sharing as liberating and life affirming for the nurse as well, and uplifting music is played as the nurse is conveniently transported out of the unit, her multiple male-oriented caring duties apparently satisfied.

Significantly, the iconic promotional image on the original *M*A*S*H* movie poster, pictures a graphic amalgamation of the rear view of an obviously naked female in high heels, with the bottom and back disappearing into a male hand forming the peace sign. The "make love not war" message of the time is obviously reflected in this poster artwork, but it comes at the expense of women. Indeed much of the film and television series references the hero surgeons together trying to catch or otherwise get nurses naked or semi-naked, and this behavior is presented not just as comic and even endearing masculine bonding, but as evidence of their anti-establishment political credentials. Their sexual promiscuity and predatory sexualization of women is conflated with their status as creative, brave, masculine rebels—a dangerous leap of logic which has been recently exposed by the Weinstein case and the #MeToo movement as abusive.

Angry Women, Masculine Ball-Breakers and Crazy Bunny-Boilers: More Blaming the Victim Through Misogynistic Moral Narratives and Justifications

As Chemaly (2018: xvii) observes, while colleagues are more likely to defer to an angry man, an angry woman elicits the opposite reaction: when women express anger or even act assertively in our culture they risk being dismissed as irrational, incompetent, hostile, even hysterical. Nurse Houlihan is not, and cannot be an "indispensable" genius surgeon and is thus not expected or permitted to express anger without being punished for it, no matter how much pressure she might be under at the frontline. As Chemaly (2018: 83) pointed out, nurses typically do emotionally demanding and exhausting work, often in stressful life-or-death situations, yet they are expected to suppress their anger and other negative feelings and remain calm and accommodating in all circumstances. Chemaly (2018: 83) cites research which suggests all this suppressed women's anger in the workplace may lead to higher rates of burnout and depression. Hence Chemaly (2018: xxi) encourages women to embrace their rage, as "the emotion that best protects us against danger and injustice," because: "Anger warns us viscerally of violation, threat and insult."

The *M*A*S*H* film in particular makes it clear how sexual harassment actually intersects with a kind of sadistic bullying, gas lighting and explicit or implicit accusation that the victim is unstable, overemotional, crazy or oversensitive:

> TRAPPER [Referring to Houlihan]: "Well, what's the matter with her today?"
> HAWKEYE: "Oh, I don't know. I think it's one of those ladies' things."
> TRAPPER: "It's not like her to act like this. She's a bitch. Look at my new
>   flannel—I think she's going to have a nervous breakdown."
> HAWKEYE: "She can't even get out of the door."

Part of the "bad" crazy and angry woman stereotype is the moral assumption that power and wanting power is conflated with masculinity and thus the woman who wants power is not just abnormal but morally wrong and in need of punishment for stepping on to male territory. Indeed, one of the insults hurled at Margaret in the television series implies that she is too masculine, for being powerful, aggressive, especially sexually aggressive, is conflated with a male role. For example in the season two episode of the television series titled "Divided We Stand (1972)" Margaret responds to sexual insults by telling Hawkeye, "you are no gentleman" and he counters with, "good thing *you* are."

The Heterosexual Male Gaze: Looking Back and Looking Forward

What makes this harassment detailed in *M*A*S*H* so seductive for both male and female viewers is the film art of presenting every situation through the male point of view or as Mulvey (1975) famously put it, through the hetero-patriarchal "male gaze." In the film especially, viewers are encouraged not only to identify with the more sympathetic characters of Hawkeye and Trapper, but to take an almost erotic pleasure from looking at and treating women through their eyes. This is evident in both the camera angles and in the script. In the film for example, Trapper comments to one of his co-workers: "It's a good thing you have a nice body, nurse, otherwise they'd get rid of you quick." We are also encouraged to sympathize with the male perspective, feeling compassion for the male heroes under pressure in a warzone—although this compassion is not extended to the female characters, at least not in the early series. Another common myth being manufactured here, which remains in cultural circulation today, is the belief that it is understandable that men behave badly when they have lost control due to stressful circumstances, that sexual harassment is a kind of normal and acceptable reaction to stress, a way of "letting off steam." This scene from *M*A*S*H* demonstrates:

> TRAPPER: "Now listen Frank. I have just completed three days' surgery without rest and now this nurse and I are going to do some nature studies." [laugh track follows] ["Cowboy" episode, *M*A*S*H* television series, 1972].

In the film trailer the narrator firstly tells us "this is the story of two indispensable military surgeons—they have the army over a barrel." Supposedly his status as genius surgeon enables and excuses Trapper John making comments under work pressures like: "give me at least one nurse who knows how to work in close without getting her tits in my way!"

This male genius under pressure motif is part of the misogynistic mythology that is still used today to excuse and legitimate abuse—it was mobilized in the Harvey Weinstein case for example. As Bassil-Morozow and Proctor (2018) have suggested, it is another aspect of the vocabulary of motive to claim, "it was [just] a different time back then." This excuse or rationalization of discriminatory behaviors has been mobilized in defense of individuals and of texts. Yet, looking forward as well as back, this study has attempted to critique these moral languages of misogyny to close these cultural loopholes and thus learn the lessons of our (media) history for the doctors and nurses of tomorrow.

Conclusion

This critical analysis of the images, language and logic of *M*A*S*H*, has presented a close case study of the iconic Margaret Houlihan character, building upon previous work by feminist philosophers such as Kate Manne (2018) in examining the cultural reproduction of misogynistic myths still dominant in our culture today. It has also built upon and extended the popular culture analysis of classic feminist texts such as Susan Faludi's (1991) work in *Backlash: The Undeclared War Against American Women* to explore how popular culture, specifically the representational mix of M*A*S*H, may reflect and reproduce political and cultural events and attitudes in the real world, at the expense of women and girls. I have followed Faludi (1991 and 2020) in exploring how popular culture texts manufactured mostly by male writers, producers, directors and other cultural figures of authority may (intentionally or unintentionally) set out with a political-moral agenda to destroy the professionally powerful, confident, assertive, and sexually assertive (post)feminist woman of the times, as a kind of cultural backlash against women and feminism. In the misogynistic moral economy, the gendered scripts and cultural narratives of the original 1970 film and in the early seasons of the television series, there can be little doubt that M*A*S*H represented a backlash against the emerging women's movement and strong, outspoken women personified by Nurse Houlihan. By belittling, infantilizing, humiliating, mocking, sexualizing and also desexualizing, Houlihan and other female characters, the male (anti)heroes of M*A*S*H act as mouthpieces for a wider culture of misogyny and violence against women—that essentially treats women as objects.

In this essay I speak back to, yet invert, the premise of the original M*A*S*H series, film and trailer in a close, critical analysis of what I *do* see as serious moral problems; I resist these misogynistic readings of moral issues and I also refuse to "drop them." Instead, through a feminist cultural studies lens, I investigate in depth, decades later, just how these texts have worked to perpetrate sexist and misogynistic ideas and attitudes about women in general and nurses in particular. It is important to note that the media representations of the Houlihan character also evolved over the series and later series were more likely to include scenes of Margaret effectively fighting back (if not always winning) in a more dramatic (liberal) feminist manner, including for example Margaret knocking out with one punch a soldier who attempts to hit on her in a bar. However, the fact that the lines between flirting and harassment are further blurred in the later seasons of M*A*S*H only serves to strengthen the relevance of the text for understanding and interpreting current events, for as Helena Bassil-Morozow and Katy Proctor (2018) have pointed out, sexual harassment is increasingly "perpetrated in the grey areas of life, not the well-defined." As we have seen, much of the humor in the M*A*S*H universe is about mocking, dehumanizing and undermining women, especially powerful and difficult women, while blurring the boundaries between seduction and abuse. In the early television series in particular the strategic placement of the laugh track makes the predatory, punitive male gaze and its misogynistic logics and motives unavoidable. For those of us who grew up in the 1970s and '80s this is the culture that made us, the soundtrack of our lives, for better or worse, as a generation raised on television in the media age. But now is our time to speak back to that culture, if we so choose, and to create new empowering cultural and social realities.

Films and Television Productions Referenced

M*A*S*H (1970) 20th Century Fox
M*A*S*H (1972–1977) 20th Century Fox

References

Ahmed, Sara (2015) *The Cultural Politics of Emotion*. New York: Routledge.

Ahmed, Sara (2017) *Living a Feminist Life*. Durham: Duke University Press.

Baker, Carrie (2008) *The Women's Movement against Sexual Harassment*. New York: Cambridge.

Bassil-Morozow, Helena, and Proctor, Katy (2018) After Weinstein: Two Women on Why We Still Need to Explain the Difference Between Flirting and Sexual Harassment. *The Conversation*. https://theconversation.com/after-weinstein-two-women-on-why-we-still-need-to-explain-the-difference-between-flirting-and-sexual-harassment-94466 [accessed January 28, 2021].

Berns, Nancy (2004) *Framing the Victim: Domestic Violence, Media and Social Problems*. New Jersey: Transaction Publishers.

Carlton, Alexandra (2021) Australian Report: On a Knife's Edge (Why Is Medicine Failing Its Future Workforce of Women). *Marie Claire*. March 307: 62–66.

Chemaly, Soraya (2018) *Rage Becomes Her: The Power of Women's Anger*. London: Simon & Schuster.

Creed, Barbara (1993) *The Monstrous-Feminine : Film, Feminism, Psychoanalysis*. London: Routledge.

Curtis, Katina, and Crowe, David (2021) "Didn't want to hear it": Liberal Staffer Says Bosses Dismissed Her Sexual Assault. *Sydney Morning Herald*. February 15, 2021, https://www.smh.com.au/politics/federal/labor-demands-answers-after-parliament-sex-assault-claim-20210215-p572l5.html.

Faludi, Susan (1991) *Backlash: The Undeclared War Against American Women*. New York: Crown.

Faludi, Susan (2020) Preface to the 2020 Edition. *Backlash: The Undeclared War Against American Women*. New York: Broadway Books.

Ford, Clementine (2016) *Fight Like a Girl*. Sydney: Allen and Unwin.

Hopkins, Susan, and Ostini, Jenny (2015) Domestic Violence and Facebook: Harassment Takes New Forms in the Social Media Age. *The Conversation*, November 30, https://theconversation.com/domestic-violence-and-facebook-harassment-takes-new-forms-in-the-social-media-age-50855.

Kadota, Yumiko (2021) *Emotional Female*. New York: Penguin Random House.

Kristeva, Julia (1982) *Powers of Horror: An Essay on Abjection*. New York: Columbia University Press.

Lim, Sun Sun (2020) Manufacturing Hate 4.0: Can Media Studies Rise to the Challenge? *Television and New Media*. 21, 6: 602–607.

Lipkin, Elline (2011) Click! Hotlips Houlihan Made Me a Feminist. *Ms*. https://msmagazine.com/2011/03/29/click-hot-lips-houlihan-made-me-a-feminist/, accessed January 29, 2021.

Manne, Kate (2018) *Down Girl: The Logic of Misogyny*. London: Penguin.

Mulvey, Laura (1975) Visual Pleasure and Narrative Cinema. *Screen* 16, 3: 6–18.

Projansky, Sarah (2001) *Watching Rape: Film and Television in Postfeminist Culture*. New York: New York University Press.

Richardson-self, Louise (2017) Woman-hating: On Misogyny, Sexism and Hate Speech. *Hypatia* 33, 2: 256–272.

Smith, A.P. (2001) Leadership Roundtable: Beyond Ratchet, Houlihan and Hathaway. *Nursing Economics* 19, 2: 78–82.

Sunden, Jenny, and Susanna Paasonen (2018) Shameless Hags and Tolerance Whores: Feminist Resistance and the Affective Circuits of Online Hate. *Feminist Media Studies* 18, 4: 643–656.

Thomas, Frank (2017) What Harvey Weinstein Tells Us About the Liberal World. *The Guardian*. https://www.theguardian.com/commentisfree/2017/oct/21/harvey-weinstein-liberal-world, accessed January 29, 2021.

Seeking the Ideal

Caps, Capes, Pins and Scrapbooks

Popular Nursing Objects of Remembrance

Jeannine Uribe

Introduction

Museums can be quiet, serene spaces with objects on walls or behind glass to protect touching from museum-goers. The objects, deemed precious and fragile, are easily marred by oil from fingers or dust from the air. Many museum objects were never meant to be enjoyed by being handled; rather they were meant to be put on a pedestal or a wall for admiration. In contrast, the Museum of Nursing History, Inc., located in St. Benilde Tower at La Salle University, Philadelphia, Pennsylvania, holds objects often stained and dented by use or being washed, sterilized, and dried and put back on the shelf for a few hours before being used many more times. As everyday and functional items, they were not designed or used with the intention that they would one day be museum pieces, following a trajectory from the quotidian to the cherished. The collection's nursing objects, worn and handled on a daily basis by nurses, tells us about the items nurses saved to represent their past. Many items have been tucked away in attics for more than 40 years and are donated by family members, who upon discovering the objects, feel they cannot imagine throwing them away, that it would be disrespectful to their loved one's memory. They recognize the objects as a legacy of their mother's contribution to nursing but also as historical objects conveying information about nursing education, practice, and professional activities. Using a material culture framework, the objects of the Museum are examined in this essay for their representation of nurses' experiences and of nursing's shifting place in society. This essay is informed by my own interactions with donors and exhibits in my role as the Museum's Collections committee chair and my own career as a nurse and a nursing academic. The experiences and insights I have gained from meeting with donors, including the owners of the items or relatives of retired and deceased nurses, provides the basis of much of the commentary and analysis in this essay, supplemented by archival and documentary sources.

The sensate appreciation for an historical object deepens an individual's understanding of the object and the historical time period when the object was used (Miller, 2017: 8). Scholars such as Knappett (2005) use material culture as a method to examine and study old but everyday objects, taking ideas from archeology and anthropology to enhance meaning and understanding of the saved items. He sees objects as interconnected to the persons who used them and worthy of study to give meaning to how things were used (Knappett, 2005).

Material culture makes history tangible and logical instead of cerebral and intellectual. Handling an item gives a different perspective on the object, allowing an individual to imagine how it felt in the hand to use it and how heavy it was. Feeling the wool of the nurse's cape, for example, provides a tactile sense of how it felt to wear it. Holding a ceramic pot used to carry boiled water to the bedside for a patient's bath gives the museum visitor a concrete view of how it was to use this object. With imagination and curiosity, the visitor connects to how the nurse lived and how the patient might have felt when the nurse brought the object into the room.

Each piece in the Museum comes with a story and is connected to a nurse. Although some objects donated to the museum are found in thrift stores or yard sales, the majority were used by nurses. Every object in the collection has a bond to a nurse or to nursing. The donations not saved by a family member who was a nurse are out of the context of a hospital setting, yet people noticed them, purchased them, and donated them knowing they belonged to a nurse. From a 1920 picture postcard of a hospital, written in pencil, telling of the sick relative's condition, to a silver cigarette box engraved with the name of a Navy nurse leader, a gift honoring her retirement from her fellow service members, these objects show a connection to nursing.

Donors who give objects to the Museum have a desire to protect and preserve nursing's history even though they are not nurses. The Museum has received many interesting items abandoned in homes or found in flea markets. Recently, a donor asked if the Museum would accept a 1912 nurse's diploma and state nurse license registration; both documents were rolled up in a paper tube with the original postage stamps and measured 11 inches by 14 inches, with hand-written calligraphy and embossed golden seals. The new homeowner found the tube in her attic during renovations and searched the internet for an appropriate repository for donation. Something about these yellowed documents kept the non-healthcare homeowner from tossing them in the trash. Seeing the date of the documents, more than 100 years old and charmingly ornate, may have been the reason for rescuing them. Or the homeowner might have respected antiquities, having purchased an old house. Perhaps, the two documents and the other objects donated to the museum are important because nursing is a trusted profession. Many people know nurses or have been patients cared for by nurses who helped them through surgery or listened to their fears during hospitalization so they recognize and respect nursing's place in society.

It is much easier to understand the familial relationship to nursing objects due to the desire to memorialize objects that one's mother used during her lifetime and in her career. This motivation represents the majority of the Museum's donations. Recently donated items come from two time periods, the Second World War era and the early 1960s, in response to demographic changes as generations age and reach retirement. Sons, daughters and grandchildren of Second World War nurses are downsizing so they are clearing out objects from their attic. Retired nurses from the 1950s and 1960s are moving into smaller living spaces and decluttering as well. They must make decisions on what to bring to their smaller homes and nursing items from their past are tentatively placed in one of three piles; worth keeping, donate to save the memories, or place in the trash. These items come out after 50 years of storage in basements, attics, and garages. White, sharply starched student aprons show brown iodine stains; caps are yellowed; and scrapbook pictures are fading. Yet even with these marks of time, nurses and families want to know if the items are worth saving. They know nursing education has changed. New technology, new systems, and different curricula are in place, but donors ask themselves if keeping items from the "old" way of nursing is important to the collective memory of the nursing profession.

Older nurses, who have come to the museum for a tour, talk about their recent experiences being a patient during a hospitalization and being cared for by nurses. Some of the nurses are complimentary of the current technology and knowledge nurses hold, while others feel nurses are not doing the expected, patient-focused, nursing activities, such as "p.m. care," which required nurses to set patients up to brush their teeth and then give each patient a backrub to prepare for sleep, which is no longer done routinely.

Retro marketing lures consumers to purchase antiques or remade items from the past. These old items draw on an emotional feeling for the old days and for old designs. Nostalgia for nursing items lies in the view of nurse's training school when young women lived and worked under apprentice-like conditions for three, long years of combined study and service in the hospital. During training, students lived together in the nurses' home and worked on the hospital floors together, learning skills and caring for patients. They were close to each other during this time and graduates of these diploma programs maintained a dedicated connection to the training school through the longstanding alumni association. Hospital schools formed their alumni association with the first graduating class and maintained the association with members of each graduating class. School mementos and yearbooks were kept in the hospital's alumni association room. Annual meetings held the nurses together by updating addresses and celebrating graduation anniversaries, job promotions, weddings, retirements, and the memories of those who died.

Diploma student nurses were inculcated with the importance of maintaining their school's history and their standardized curriculum required they studied nursing history under a nurse instructor with a required text, explaining the roots of nursing from the ancient world to the development of nursing in foreign countries. This placed the nursing history course on a par with chemistry, anatomy, and other compulsory courses. Older history texts often presented a celebratory description of nursing's past accomplishments without historical analysis; thus, many nursing history texts left out issues nursing is just coming to terms with, such as racism and sexism. These history textbooks, written by nurses, are important for their exclusion of nurses of color and of men. Thus, their nursing history education and their attachment to the post graduate alumni organization compels these nurses to keep their past, to view their saved objects with a sense of safeguarding their school and work articles for history.

As diploma graduate nurses age, however, they are not often traveling to the meetings; attendance is dwindling, leaving some nurses to keep their items and their memories for themselves. As diploma schools close, memorabilia are disposed of without a sense of historical value for the leaders or graduates of the school. In addition, some hospitals merged with larger health systems or university health systems, which displaced the school's sacred symbols and souvenirs for the branding of the new owners. By the 1980s, if applicants wanted to enter nursing they had the choice of a shorter, 2-year program in the community college setting or the 4-year bachelor's degree in the university system, which did not have the same allegiance to maintaining alumni associations nor the same communal living and training as did diploma schools.

Enthusiasm and admiration for a nurse's work leads non-family members to donate nursing objects used by their friend. If a nurse did not have children, she often had a close friend named as executor of her will. If the nurse was too ill to dispose of her nursing items before passing away, the friend inherited all of her belongings including her nursing items. The friend often sends the nurse's obituary summing up the nurse's career. One nurse, Joan Reeves, was an accomplished public health nurse with a Ph.D. who worked in several universities, including in Botswana and Korea. She worked as a visiting nurse, a nurse epidemiologist for the CDC, and as a field nurse administering the test for the polio vaccine. After her illustrious career, her friend donated three uniforms from her work as a public health nurse. The uniform was a daily part of this nurse's life. Seeing the cut of the cotton dress, the long sleeves and the attached identification pins helps us to see her working in the field and allows us to imagine seeing a public health nurse in her navy blue uniform going into a home to give the new, lifesaving polio vaccine.

When the nurse (user) is not present to tell us stories of how she used the dress, Woodward (2016) uses material culture to use the material of the object itself to understand the context of the use, to understand the meaning behind the object. Looking at the donated nursing uniform, navy blue was a standard for some public health nurse to wear. A 1932 article in *Public Health Nursing*, a journal for this nursing specialty, presented the need for public health nurses to project an image of professionalism (McDermand, 1932). Uniforms were to be "sportsmanlike," long sleeved, with wide pleats on the skirt. Navy blue was one of the suggested colors because it projected "calmness" (McDermand, 1932). The donated cotton, front-buttoned dress was soft, sturdy, and easily washed and maintained after being outside on the street and in a variety of homes. Public health nurses wanted to be recognized in the community as professionals and as helpers, as someone easy to recognize and to approach if family members had health issues.

Qualitative analysis in material culture includes using the stories connected to objects to bring depth to understanding how the objects were used by the nurses (Woodward, 2016). When a donor contacts the Museum with objects, we ask for a personal story that goes along with the objects or stories about the person who used the items. Stories enhance understanding for students who come for tours and for other visitors. The stories add a dimension to the item's place in nursing history, the location, the year, and the setting. A man donated his mother's Red Cross uniform, cap, and two pins along with training certificates, her volunteer record and a newspaper clipping. She volunteered between 1964 and 1966, traveling between Nellis Air Force Base in Nevada to Clark Air Base in the Philippines. His mother is pictured in her uniform with a nurse's style cap, known as a gray lady. The clipping reports 32 women volunteers; the wives of officers and airmen performed 300 to 500 volunteer hours to receive the "coveted caps of the Red Cross Hospital." The picture accompanying the article shows the women wearing white high heels, very impractical for nursing work. The description of the gray ladies says they were doing non-medical work to help the sick and wounded soldiers, in this case, during the Vietnam War. So, it is important to nursing history to understand the story of this picture, that the women were awarded caps and wore uniforms like nurses but were not doing nursing work because some looking at the picture would think it was about nursing.

We ask donors to tell the story and the employment history of their relatives who used the nursing items. Nurses often told stories of their work to family members and they remembered the stories. The nurses' résumés tell us many things about the women, including their movement patterns from home, to nursing school, to employment, the continuation of their education, and the awards they received for their work.

Around the 1970s, nursing students heard the term, "appliance nurse" used to refer to a nurse who returned to work to earn enough money to purchase new home appliances and then left nursing again (Brewin-Wilson, 1985). This was a derogatory term which did not account for the nurse who wanted to continue their work in nursing but lacked family support for a career. Hospitals accepted these nurses back and needed them to work however long they could. Many families portray their mothers as giving up nursing to marry and have children and then returning to work after the children grew older. These women then worked for another 20 years with some returning to school for the bachelor's degree. This was not the image of the nurse who worked to purchase domestic technology.

Caps

The nurse's cap, no longer worn by nurses in the United States, continues to carry popular media's recognition as the symbol of nursing. By the late 1980s, nurses were no longer wearing caps in school, receiving caps at graduation, or wearing them in hospital practice. What was once an instant recognition of a registered nurse lost favor with nurses, getting in the way of tubing and curtains during their work in hospitals. Up until then, student nurses received an intermediary cap with less definition than their graduation cap. In the 1924 Germantown Hospital yearbook, a graduating senior described her first-year cap as, "a queer little 'Sputum Cup' cap." Some received their official nurse's cap with a colored ribbon with the attached meaning that they had graduated. One donor recounted her school's cap ranking system. The first year of nursing was a plain white cap; second year was a vertical blue stripe; and for the third year and final year, the student placed a horizontal stripe along the outer edge. Using this system of identification, hospital workers had instant recognition of the student's level of study and capability. In a 1930 Evangelical Hospital of Chicago class yearbook, a short story dedicated to the first-year students, who wore blue uniforms, referred to the importance of understanding the cap:

> When you leave the elevator,
> Oh, beware! Of what you do,
> Look behind you! Look before you!
> Look to the right and left side, too!
> If there are any white caps near you
> Or a black band comes in view,
> Let them all get off before you,
> When you're wearing of the blue (*The Echo*, 1929).

Donors report that cap cleanliness and professional look was a student's responsibility. Students were expected to wash and starch their caps back into the required shape. One nurse donated two caps, one shaped and the other flat. She showed us how to form the three points at the back of the cap, which represented the Holy Trinity. Other nurses tell stories about washing their caps, dipping them in liquid starch and smoothing them, wet, onto their bureau mirror or refrigerator to dry overnight. In the morning, the student peeled the cap off and folded it, pinned it into shape, and went to the hospital wards. In the later 1950s, students and nurses took their caps to local dry cleaners, known for getting the caps shaped right.

Capes

The typical donated nurse's cape is hip-length, navy blue with red lining, made of 100 percent wool with a small, inside chest pocket. The school's initials are embroidered in braid on the standup collar and there are two frog closures holding the cape closed with four, plain, large black or decorative gold buttons. The nurse's initials were embroidered inside the cape or her name was embroidered in cursive inside for easy identification. One donor noted that capes were purchased by the family for the student and many nurses wore their capes to work after graduation. Like the cap, the blue cape is iconic for nurses; even a 1960s Barbie doll had a nurse's uniform with a blue cape and cap. Although the Museum no longer collects navy blue capes, unusual capes are accepted. There is a hunter green cape, which belonged to a nurse who attended a school in "the Green State of Vermont" and was the wife of a professional baseball player. Another cape donated from a graduate of Ball Hospital in Indiana had a brown exterior and a golden yellow interior. Second World War Navy capes were black wool with a velvet collar and black braiding to close the front. Those capes went below the knee. Another standout cape was black with a large, white, Maltese cross on the left side. One of the Museum's oldest capes is a 1938 navy blue wool nurses' cape from a school in Ontario, Canada. The nurse graduated and moved to work at two hospitals in New York City before moving to California.

Pins

Upon graduation, each student customarily received a nursing school pin with a distinct design representing their school and successful completion of the training program. The pin was not a brooch, or a piece of jewelry, or an accessory for dressing up. The nursing pin was worn as part of the working uniform. The pins were made of 10 karat gold and had the student's initials and year of graduation engraved on the back of the pin. Typically, they measure about one inch to 1½ inches in diameter and contain the name or the initials of the school and symbols related to the hospital, religion, or town. Latin sayings and religious values were part of some of the designs. The school's name was often prominent and found in cloisonné in the shape of a circle, an oval, or an octagon. One of the most elaborate pins of the Museum's collection is from Charity Hospital in Cleveland, 1932, a hospital run by the Sisters of Charity of St. Augustine. The pin starts with a thin, gold bar inscribed with *caritas benigna est,* Latin for *charity is love.* This thin bar has a small triangle above it with a star with nine rays emanating from it, representing the Star of Bethlehem, and a triangle below with an etched cross. Hanging from the bar by two, fine, chain links is an open wreath holding a scroll with the name of the school, the location, and the year. The wreath appears to be stamped with two different types of leaves: on the right, laurel, and on the left oak leaves. The symbolism of each pin is buried in the records of the diploma schools, but even without this understanding, the pins are objects of beauty and professionalism as well as representations of economic means and an identifiable status in society.

Student Uniforms

During hospital training, female students typically wore pink or blue checkered or striped uniforms with separate apron, collars, and cuffs with the student's name printed on each item. Before the 1950s, aprons were usually two-piece; the top with crisscross straps to attach to the bottom piece that covered the front half of the dress down to the hemline, both heavily starched and pressed. Several donated 1940s uniforms came folded and pressed by hospital laundry staff; hospitals laundered and pressed student uniforms and aprons. Occasionally, uniforms have two names stamped on each piece. Uniforms were reused frugally and kept in good repair; war-effort rationing influenced recycling fabric that was usable.

One training school's uniform from the 1960s included a navy blazer, which may have replaced the cape. Another student uniform was made of a lightweight denim fabric for the first three months of training. Students purchased identical graduation uniforms made of white cotton with an attached collar, long sleeves, and detachable buttons holding all closures together. Detachable buttons had a shank and a cotter pin to keep the buttonholes together. Buttons are often missing but replacements can be found in the Museum's donated box of different sizes of white buttons of this type.

Having the nurse's name printed on each piece of clothing was necessary because the hospitals laundered, starched, and pressed the uniforms. There are several reasons students did not have to launder their uniforms. Most likely it was because the students did not have time to hand launder their clothing, air dry it, and then press the pieces of their uniform, including long apron, collar, cuffs, and dress. The large industrial washing machines in the hospital cleaned patient gowns, sheets, blankets, and towels, so student uniforms were added and returned quickly. Students before the 1950s wore black stockings and black shoes and did not transition to white stockings until they graduated. Typically, a donation to the Museum consists of one dress, one collar, two aprons, and several cuffs because students may have owned only one uniform or may have thrown out the one that was tattered. The dress was washed weekly, and aprons were changed daily or when stains occurred during the workday. Cotton surgical and obstetric gowns, masks, and head coverings used by nurses in those specialties demonstrated concern with infection control.

Delving into the stories that accompany donated items leads to thought-provoking questions about whether the written stories sent by the families are family lore or factual. Nurses sometimes cared for important or notorious people; one uniform from the 1920s came with the statement that his grandmother had cared for Al Capone, the infamous Chicago gangster, and Gertrude Ederle, an Olympic gold medalist and the first woman to swim the English Channel in 1926. These stories could be verified with further investigation of newspaper clippings or other historical and biographical notations of the person's hospitalizations. This 1920s nurse attended Michael Reese Hospital, which was started in a Jewish neighborhood in Chicago and open to care for all people, no matter their religious denominations. The school of nursing started in 1890 and pictures show students wearing a long sleeve uniform with an organza cap and a Star of David sewn on the left sleeve to celebrate their Jewish heritage (Michael Reese Hospital, 2017).

Most of the items donated to the Museum pertain to female nurses, in line with the historic demographics of the profession but there are two male student uniforms. One nurse, one of the few male students admitted to an old Philadelphia hospital school, donated his uniform from 1969. He wore a medium blue, short-sleeve, square-shaped uniform shirt with snaps at the shoulder and without a collar, similar to Dr. Kildare from the television show. The male students wore that uniform until 1978, when the hospital closed. The other nurse was a 1971 graduate of Mount Sinai Hospital in New York. He was the only male graduate of the school. The hospital, first named The Jews' Hospital, cared for indigent Jewish people arriving at the city. The name changed to Mt. Sinai Hospital Training School for Nurses, which had opened in 1881. By the 1970s, their uniform was a blue and white plaid dress with a white apron and short sleeves and white cuffs. The donor had to wear white pants, a white, collared dress shirt with a tie made of the same material as the female student's uniform. He graduated in the last class, so he asked for a student nurse dress uniform and held on to it for 40 years. He donated his tie, the female student uniform, and his graduation invitation, program, and yearbook. He donated a 1971 hospital newsletter featuring his picture and story of being the only male student in the hospital's history.

One donated item came from an alumni association and differs from the standard student nurse uniforms collected by the Museum. It is a light-weight wool, women's basketball uniform with the number 45 crudely sewn on the back. The Hospital of the University of Pennsylvania's nursing school team wore a red and navy blue, knee-length, one-piece jumper dress with red bloomers and the school patch sewn on the front. The Philadelphia Nurses Basketball League was sponsored by the American Legion and awarded a large trophy to the winners (Award-Basketball). Nursing students were not allowed to go home very often, so schools offered a variety of activities for the students when they were off duty.

Military Uniforms

Donations of military uniforms come with stories and war mementos. One Army nurse collected a variety of crocheted doilies from her assignment in France. Another was assigned to New Caledonia and returned with a bracelet made of metal from an airplane with a bomber plane painted on it. She also collected native crafts made of island resources.

There are many parts to Second World War uniforms that varied from formal dress uniforms to field uniforms. Jackets have RN insignias and patches telling where the nurses served. Army and Navy nurse uniforms changed colors and styles several times during the war and were dependent on where the nurse was serving. One collection had a variety of pieces including slacks, shirts, and a jacket and a dress made of brown and white seersucker material used by the Army Nurse Corps. This pants uniform was used on hospital ships and planes for modesty and could be used off duty in warm climates. In 1944, the seersucker uniform replaced the white nurse's uniform for the Army and many nurses complained. However, for practical purposes, the nurses agreed the seersucker uniform was easier to pack and to wear than the traditional white (Goebel, 2011). Included in the collection was a halter top made from the same material, unquestionably against regulation, but more comfortable when off duty in hot countries. Military coats and uniforms were well made and stored well in military footlockers, which the nurses took home and used to store their World War II items. One nurse kept her combat boots, her garters, and her helmet, which has "Pinkie" painted inside. Veterans tell of needing their helmets to clean their dishes, soak their clothing, and to wash up.

Books

Nursing school textbooks are popular items to donate and some nurses have kept the complete collection of required textbooks from their training. Some nurses only kept the books they felt were most valuable to their nursing practice. One 90-year-old nurse donated three books she held onto from her student days on nursing history, nutrition, health, and a pharmacology book respectively. She wrote that she was the youngest of 13 children and the books were special because they were important to her career and they belonged to her. As one of 13 siblings, born in 1929, her nursing items were the only new things she owned, and she took care of them. The books often have the student's name inside the cover and notes written in the margins with words underlining the main concepts to learn.

Books were also given as gifts when young women left to go to nursing school and when they graduated. Several donated books are the biographies of famous nurse leaders, such as *Annie W. Goodrich: Her Journey to Yale* and *Linda Richards: First Graduate Nurse*. Dedications written inside of the covers are meant to inspire the students during their studies, or as a present for the new graduate starting her career.

Diplomas, Registration Certificates and Cards

When students graduated, they received an impressive diploma with their name in calligraphy and the handwritten signatures of the nurse superintendent, hospital administrator, and a physician. Often, diplomas arrive at the Museum in their original packaging, indicating that these diplomas were not hung on the wall for display. Family donors often explained that the diploma was found tucked in among the nurse's belongings and when the nurse did not marry or have children, the nieces and nephews inherited the belongings. The family wanted to honor their relative's nursing accomplishments but did not have a way to keep the diploma or state licensure certificate. State licensure certificates are more impressive than the diplomas; larger in size, and having a 4-inch, foil seal on the left lower corner with the state seal and date embossed in the center. The largest letters on the certificate are the name of the state and REGISTERED NURSE and includes the hand-calligraphy name of the nurse.

Occasionally, we stumble on a valuable, rare find with the signature of a nurse leader. The American Red Cross card for an American nurse has the December 19, 1912, signature of Jane A. Delano, chairman of the American Red Cross Nursing Service. Jane Delano held a variety of nursing instructor positions and served as a superintendent in the Army Nurse Corps. She left to head the American Red Cross, preparing nurses to serve in the First World War. Post war, she was on duty in France where she died after a surgical procedure (Alexander, 2019). She was buried in France, but because of her leadership position, her body was returned to the U.S. and her final interment is in Arlington Cemetery with the other nurses who died during the war.

Yearbooks and Photographs

Qualitative research methods are used in nursing. Almeida et al. (2018) propose that cultural history is a valid method for examining the content of the variety of nursing documents, such as those accepted to the Museum. Yearbooks come in a variety of sizes, types of paper, and bindings, and offer a glimpse into the female nursing students' lives and values they held. These small, often 100-pages or less, stapled or bound memorials contain pictures of nursing instructors, house medical doctors, dietary staff, interns, and community businesses who advertised in the yearbooks to help fund the printing costs. The house mother, who watched over the lifestyle of the students, and the superintendent of nurses, who supervised their training, are prominent pictures, accompanied by words of gratitude by the graduates.

The typical, 1900–1950 yearbooks celebrate the seniors with a class picture and with an individual picture. Each student was identified by her full name, her place of birth, and a nickname. In one 1929 yearbook of the Evangelical Hospital of Chicago, the graduating class had 19 students arriving from Indiana, Wisconsin, Michigan, Iowa, South Dakota, Ohio, and Minnesota, a couple from Illinois, and only three from Chicago. If the yearbook has only one picture, each senior student is wearing their all-matching, starched, white graduation uniform, pin, and cap. If there is a second picture, the student is wearing their own clothing, hairstyle, and a little makeup. Their hairstyles give clues to their individuality and their hair and eyebrows also give clues to the time period. In some schools, they all wear the same style of eyeglass frame, perhaps with the intention of creating professional similarity or to prevent vanity. When inquiries are made to the Museum to identify some information about a picture of unknown origin, yearbooks have been used to compare hairstyles, eyebrow shapes, caps, uniforms, pins, photography studios, and even glasses.

The senior students fill the rest of the yearbook with poems, a class prophecy, and the class history. These stories commemorate the lives of the students' first days, and progressive years as well as what the future may hold for each student. The pages are full of inside jokes about their experiences and remarks concerning what is most memorable about each nursing student. A phenomenon found in the group pictures of each underclass is the symmetry of the uniform lengths. Students, of a variety of heights and weights, are lined up, shoulder-to-shoulder, and all hemlines are of equal length, forming one straight hemline. This was accomplished by measuring from the floor up to a predetermined height where the skirt would end, thus, when standing, all hemlines matched. We display a framed picture of a group of approximately 30 students standing together in a horseshoe forming an impressive, level, white line of uniforms.

Loose, unlabeled photographs reveal much about the space the nurses occupied either in the hospital or in their living quarters. Black and white photographs often show the roughness of the walls and floors, the worn spots on the couch, and the machines used in surgery or in the kitchen. When one looks around the outside of the scene, one can notice other identifying items of the time, such as the style of the telephone, whether there were gas jets or electric lights overhead, and how the beds were lined up. Toys might be seen on the bed of the pediatric cases and ceramic pitchers and pans show years of use.

Conclusion

Using material culture to frame the collection of the Museum, we can divide nursing keepsakes into two categories: one of student accomplishments and the other category of the professional realm of the nurse.

Students left their homes, trained for three years on hospital floors and earned a diploma. The caps, capes, pins and student uniforms represent those accomplishments. Student nurse objects reveal the ideas of the nursing students when they were young and their earned nicknames, and predicted their futures. Textbooks document the learning of the time and yearbooks describe how the nurses lived during their training. Over time, nursing has changed, and documentation of its educational development is important for moving the profession forward. The items of the everyday student embody nursing and are appropriate for material culture research.

The second category of objects in the Museum of Nursing History represents the professional sphere of the nurse. Items are placed in the context of what was occurring in the profession at the time, namely by who wore the uniforms, who could use the tools, how these were used, and what they accomplished for patient care. Once accepted by the Museum, the object loses its sentimentality and relationship to the individual nurse and becomes a part of the history of the work of the profession of nursing. These collected items are not works of art or extraordinary items but were commonly used by nurses. The nurses did not collect assets; they saved items that were important to them. Saving nursing objects in a museum promotes these objects from simply being tools used by women to becoming representations of their stories in a profession that gave women economic power and allowed nurses to work outside of the family. These respected objects reminded the nurse of her identity when she was responsible for making clinical decisions and was independent of parental or spousal advice and admonishment, what she was before she became subsumed in the role of wife and mother.

The donations to the Museum of Nursing History are displayed as representing nursing and the (mostly all) women who shaped this profession. One can find beauty in these objects in the lines of the cape, the design and symbolism of the pin and the curve of the ceramic pitcher. These objects do not hold monetary value and are not considered fine art. Nor are they everyday objects used by an average person. These objects were used by nurses in the domain of the profession, whether in the home or in the hospital, when an individual needed a nurse's care. Holding on to these objects has allowed the nurse's family to understand a part of their mother in her world outside of the family. Donating these objects allows the world to see nurses in their profession.

References

Alexander, K.L. (2019) *Jane Arminda Delano National Women's History Museum*. [Online]. Available at: www.womenshistory.org/education-resources/biographies/jane-arminda-delano [Accessed: 13 August 2020].

Almeida, E., Silva, A., Figueiredo, J., Amorim, W., and Pellon, L. (2018) The New Cultural History as a Methodology Proposed for Research in the Nursing History Field. *Revista de Pesquisa: Cuidado é Fundamental Online* 10, 1, 130–136. Available at: file:///E:/Cultural%20History%20CHAPTER/Cultural%20history.pdf.

Award-Basketball Championship 1970–1971. [Online]. Available at: https://www.jstor.org/stable/community.21803086?tocId=100090767&tocType=collection&seq=1 [Accessed: 9 September 2020].

Bates, C. (2012) *A Cultural History of the Nurses' Uniform.* Quebec: Canadian Museum of Civilization Corporation.

Brewin-Wilson, D. (1985) How Wide Is the Generation Gap in Nursing? *RN* 9: 25–31.

The Echo (1929) Evangelical Hospital of Chicago. Available via Museum of Nursing History, Philadelphia

Goebel, K.E. (2011) Women for Victory: American Servicewomen in World War II, *History & Uniforms Series, vol. 1.* Atglen, PA: Schiffer Military History: 116–117.

Knappett, C. (2011) *Thinking Through Material Culture: An Interdisciplinary Perspective.* ProQuest Ebook Central [online] University of Pennsylvania Press, Inc. [Accessed: 22 July 2020].

McDermand, B.C. (1932) The Public Health Nurse and Her Uniform. *The American Journal of Public Health* 22, 4: 428–31.

Michael Reese Hospital (2017) *Michael Reese Hospital-Nurses, Interns, and Residents.* [Online]. Available at: https://hekint.org/2017/02/23/michael-reese-hospital-nurses-interns-and-residents [Accessed: 14 December 2020].

Miller, Peter N. (2017) *History and Its Objects: Antiquarianism and Material Culture since 1500.* New York: Cornell University Press.

Woodward, S. (2016) Object Interviews, Material Imaginings and "Unsettling" Methods: Interdisciplinary Approaches to Understanding Materials and Material Culture. *Qualitative Research* 16, 4: 359–374.

Picture Perfect?

Postcard Images of Nurses and Nursing, 1890–1920

Julia Hallam

The postcard is a fleeting art form influenced by popular ideas and fashions in visual style. Nurses and nursing have been frequent subjects on postcards for over one hundred years. No other media or art form has illustrated the nursing profession so profusely and in such variety.

—Banner 1, Pictures of Nursing travelling
exhibition, National Library of Medicine

Introduction

Between the late 1890s and the end of the First World War (1918), postcards featuring nurses were at the height of their popularity. Produced for a wide range of commercial and charitable organizations, postcards reveal how the nursing profession was represented not only in the United States, Britain and Europe, but also in what were at that time faraway places such as Japan, Russia and parts of Africa and China. Ranging from photographic portraits of individuals and groups to richly illustrative drawings and cartoons, the Zwerdling Collection in the U.S. National Library of Medicine (NLM) exemplifies, for the most part, conventional public perceptions of nursing as a female gendered profession in which a "feminine ideal" of white middle-class femininity (Hallam, 2000) predominates and the ways in which this "feminine ideal" was both enhanced (the "battle-ax," the "angel") and mocked (the "saucy," the "naughty" nurse) in popular art forms.

In 2014 I was invited to curate a touring exhibition and digital resource, *Pictures of Nursing*, from the Zwerdling Collection of 2,474 postcards dating from 1893 to the 1980s. Digitizing and cataloguing around 600 of these cards has enabled a freely available public resource of popular images of nurses to be accessible to students, social historians, health educators, nurses and the general public. Before commenting on the collection in more depth, I will briefly touch upon the development of the postcard as a visual and written form of communication, then discuss the ways in which these popular images of nurses and nursing practice can expand our understanding of the history of nursing if we are prepared to explore the "moments" caught in time that each postcard represents. The focus here is on the contrasts between the "respectable" and the "sentimental" images of nurses and nursing that are represented on the majority of these early postcards, the "saucy" images that herald the development of the "sexy" nurse stereotype and the ways in which contemporary images of the "superhero" nurse have their antecedents in images such as the heroic "battle-ax" fighting against contagious (and incurable) diseases of the time such as tuberculosis.

Throughout this discussion I will make detailed reference to the images publicly available in the NLM's digital resource housed on the National Institutes of Health website as well as drawing on Zwerdling's own book about his collection, *Postcards of Nursing: A Worldwide Tribute* (Zwerdling, 2004). Michael Zwerdling assembled his collection over many years whilst working as a hospice nurse. His book features around 600 of the postcards accompanied by extensive notes documenting the relationship of the postcards to the social and political history of the twentieth century. Drawing on arguments from my monograph *Nursing the Image* that explores how images of nurses and nursing feature in written and visual texts across a range of media forms between the 1940s and the 1970s, I will examine how these popular images of nurses are built on ideals of white middle-class femininity found in nineteenth-century interpretations of mythology in classical art and religious iconography that are re-imagined in commercial illustrations. As well as promoting health related products and services, some of these images served colonialist and nationalist aspirations, whilst others fueled women's dreams of economic independence through a career in nursing. I conclude with a brief exploration of the ways in which contemporary images of nurses circulating in public arenas such as wall murals and on social media platforms such as Facebook and Instagram share on-going similarities to the mythical and religious stereotypes found on many of these early postcards.

Postcards: An Early "Social" Media

The humble postcard plays a constitutive role in the ways in which fashions in art, illustration and photographic style along with commercial activities and prevailing social mores are interwoven with cultural and national histories and our predecessors' personal beliefs, racialized identities and gendered social behaviors. An ephemeral art form used to send quick messages, the postcard was an important form of "instant" messaging before other forms of social networking such as the telephone grew in affordability and popularity. Until the twenty-first century, the study of postcards was undertaken mainly by collectors (deltiologists) who produced the catalogues and other memorabilia that encouraged sales and exchange among the collecting community. Regarded as "ephemeral media" by cultural historians and cheap, tawdry commercial products by art and visual historians, notions of the uniqueness of an artwork being degraded by any mechanical means of reproduction held sway in the academic research and scholarly community for much of the mid-twentieth century.

Anne Kalba (2011) points out that apart from a few noteworthy exceptions, most work on forms of early modern media focuses on the reproduction of the written word with little by way of sustained attention paid to technologies designed for artistic purposes (Kalba, 2011: 441). Postcard history is driven by the desire to communicate, albeit briefly, by sending a message without having recourse to a longer letter. The creation and/or capturing of an image, the means of its reproduction and distribution, the decision to buy or pick up a card to send to someone and what to say to the recipient are all part of a complex social history that reveals much about the cultural norms and values existent at the time as well as the socio-economic patterns and behaviors of different consumer groups and individuals. For some researchers, the images on postcards extend the visual social imaginary, understood "as the set of images available to the members of a given society at a given time or, if one prefers, the visual memory of that society" (Scaglia and Bergomi, 2020 citing Vinao and Ruiz-Fumes, 2017: 33). Postcards of nurses, in this context, constitute a collective visual memory of the ways in which the profession has been envisioned and depicted, a process that continues today through the various forms of social media that have replaced them.

Postcards evolved from eighteenth-century forms of elite and upwardly mobile forms of social and commercial interaction such as visiting and trade cards. The visiting or calling card was used for various social purposes such as introductions at social gatherings ("networking") and visiting people in their homes. Scott (2004) claims that visiting cards were an essential part of social etiquette with sophisticated rules governing their use. By the early nineteenth century they were often printed on one side with the name of the visitor and presented by a domestic servant, often on a salver, to the householder on behalf of the visitor. A handwritten message could be written on the back if the acquaintance was out or not "at home" to the visitor. In parallel with the visiting card, trade cards developed to promote various products and services. Evolving print technologies enabled elaborate decoration and detail, usually on one side of the card, with some businesses commissioning highly skilled designers, artists and engravers to promote their wares (Hubbard, 2012). Reforms to the postal service in Britain in 1840, heralded by the introduction of the penny black stamp, prepaid by the sender, are generally regarded as the beginning of the postcard era in the U.K. although it took another thirty years for postcards to become a popular form of communication. In the U.S., The Postal Act of 1861 allowed cards weighing less than one ounce to be sent by mail. The Civil War delayed the development of the postcard thereafter. Meanwhile postal services in Austria-Hungary were developing a ready stamped 8.5 × 12 card with space for the address on the front and a message on the back.[1] This set a standard size for the nascent industry of manufacturing postcards throughout Europe, with Germany becoming the home of the printed color process known as chromolithography, an example of which can be seen in one of the earliest postcards in the collection: a tinted print image of a woman dressed as a nurse is used to advertise the efficacy of Johann Hoff's Malt Extract for the treatment of coughs (PoN http://resource.nlm. nih.gov/101625324). Published by a company in Vienna, Austria, this card from 1899 has space for a message on the side that advertises the product; the reverse is printed with a postage stamp outline of where to place the stamp and lines to guide the writing of an address. By 1902, new regulations permitted that one side of a postcard could be reserved for an illustration, the other split between space for a message and an address.

With the on-going development of innovations in printing technologies and processes, by the late 1890s photographic images began to be used widely on postcards; the most popular topics were rurafal and urban views sent to friends and family when people were on their travels. The development of the 3A Kodak Folding handheld camera designed for making photographic postcards in what had become, by the mid–1900s, the standard postcard format of 3.25 × 5.50 inches, led to a rapid increase in cards featuring photographic portraits. The camera became widely available in American and Britain as well as in many European countries and accounts, perhaps, for the standardization in style in the numerous portraits of nurses on postcards that appear in the collection around this time.[2]

Julia Gillen argues that the speed of change in late nineteenth and early twentieth century, Britain, Europe and North America was in many ways analogous to our own times, with developments in transportation systems, manufacturing processes and communication systems contributing to a feeling of living in an accelerating time of change. Between 1901 and 1910 in Britain, according to the Postmaster General's annual records, almost six billion cards were sent. With postal deliveries in many towns and cities numbering more than six a day, the postcard became an effective means of cheap and speedy communication. Drawing on the work of Douglas (1909), Gillen argues that by the beginning of the twentieth century, the picture postcard was considered to "epitomize the spirit of the era," and presents "a candid revelation of our pursuits and pastimes, our customs and costumes, our morals and manners" (Douglas, 1909: 377 in Gillen, 2013: 489). The ways in which this "spirit of the era" infused images of nurses and the nursing profession is illustrated in the uniforms and practices depicted in postcards from twenty different countries including Europe, North America, colonized nations in Africa and modernizing nations such as Japan.

The cards in the collection fall into two main types: photo cards, where the card consists of a photograph on one side and a divided reverse, with space for a message from the sender and the name and address of the intended recipient; and illustrated cards, where the image has been drawn/painted or otherwise created and printed, usually on one side of the card, sometimes with a decorative motif from the illustrated image on the reverse that heads or frames space for the message and an address. Photo cards of individual nurses were taken, perhaps, to provide evidence of personal achievement that could accompany job applications or to send to relatives and friends. Portraits included images of European royalty dressed as Red Cross nurses and well-known performers of the day playing nurses on stage and, from the 1920s, in films. Photo cards recorded the work of community nurses undertaking home visits; private children's nurses sitting with their infant charges; military groups and their activities; missionary work; and nurses undertaking complex medical techniques and hospital treatments. Photo cards were also used to advertise the work of medical charities such as the Red Cross and as a recruitment tool for training schools, nursing organizations, nursing agencies, hospitals and institutions.

The "captured moments" on the photo cards are often clues to a larger picture such as for example in the case of groups of nurses in uniform, the type of training an individual had undertaken, the values that the institution was instilling in its graduates, the kinds of institutions that were training nurses at that particular time, the places where training was being undertaken, the kinds of tasks that nurses were performing, and the responsibilities and duties that constituted professional identity.[3] They also reveal the ways in which nursing was regarded by those who commissioned the photographs, those who had their photographs taken and those who were writing on the cards, sometimes one and the same person (see, for example, the cards sent by nurses working at mission hospitals in places such as Nyasaland [now Malawi] and China) but often a member of the public who might have bought a card to support a fund raising event for a hospital, medical institution, charitable religious mission or the Red Cross, a prolific producer of postcards in many countries around the world.

The second type of postcard in the collection consists of a drawn or painted image, reproduced by a wide range of chromatic printing processes such as the "oilette," which was developed by Adolph Tuck to make commercially designed visuals look more like mini oil paintings.[4] A discussion of the various ways in which fashions in fine art and commercial illustration influence postcard design can be found in Chapter Two, Twentieth Century Postcard Art, of Zwerdling's book (2004: 34–107) where he focused on some of the most well-known artists and illustrators. In this article, the emphasis is on the ways in which cartoons, a very popular category of the illustrated postcard, demonstrated some particular traits in terms of the ways in which nurses were portrayed in the early twentieth century.

Saucy, Sexy and Sentimental: Cartoon Images of Nurses

In Britain, the "saucy" cartoon images created by artists such as Donald McGill in the 1930s, '40s and '50s are now valuable collectors' items. Sales of saucy postcards, often featuring seaside settings and popular stereotypes such as large ladies, long suffering husbands, vicars and nurses, reached around 16 million a year in the 1930s. The jokes relied on innuendo, often visually implied alongside verbal suggestion. In the 1950s, the Conservative government thought these postcards exemplified the deterioration of morals in British society and prosecuted Donald McGill under the Obscenity Act.[5] Saucy nurse cards invariably featured an image of a young nurse in a tight fitting uniform revealing a curvaceous figure alongside a male patient, and an older bad-tempered, overweight female dressed as a senior nurse (a sister or matron), commonly known today as a "battle-ax." A typical example from the 1940s depicts a scowling young nurse with long auburn hair wearing a tight uniform to emphasize her tiny waist and large breasts sporting high-heeled shoes that show off her shapely legs. Removing a tray from a patients' room under the watchful gaze of an older, stouter frowning Matron, she exclaims angrily "Add a black-eye to whatever he's already got"! (PoN http://resource.nlm.nih.gov/101611532).

Somewhat surprisingly, given the popularity of "battle-ax" images by the 1930s and '40s, one of the earliest popular cartoon images of a "battle-ax," the illustrations of Charles Dickens's nurse Sairey Gamp from the serial *Martin Chuzzlewit* (1842–44), rarely featured on early postcards.[6]

Only one card from the 1910s depicted a figure that looked anything like a Gamp: a child, held by the hand of a red-faced, scowling older nurse in a long cape, states a preference for another nurse nearby who is young, attractive and smiling (PoN http://resource.nlm.nih.gov/101626012). Images of young, attractive women dressed as nurses were frequently presented as objects of sexual fantasy and romantic desire. The earliest card to feature this kind of image, Medi-Kate, is from 1906; it featured a color illustration of a white Red Cross nurse pouring a liquid ("medicine") from a bottle into a glass. She wears a red striped dress that appears to be blown upwards by the wind, revealing layers of frilly petticoats and her stockings complete with garters brandishing a Red Cross symbol. The card advertised "Katy Girls series no. 8," novels written for older girls by Sarah Chauncey Woolsey that focused on a central character called Katy. Presumably the address of the card would be to a potential adult purchaser rather than the twelve-year-old girl who features in the stories (PoN http://resource.nlm. nih.gov/101611532). Early postcards often featured these "saucy" images of young attractive white women dressed in fashionable interpretations of a nurses' uniform, sometimes engaged in various forms of sexual innuendo and "play" and with their male patients. One series of cards in the collection comprised a narrative sequence with short comments in decorative graphics, creating a cheeky innuendo that paralleled the on-going visual action. In "Caught with the Goods," a woman dressed as a nurse sitting alongside her bedridden male patient laughingly resists his attempts to kiss her; they are caught in this compromising position by the patient's angry wife (PoN http://resource.nlm.nih.gov/101612369). The message on the back of this card says, "Mabel, how would you like to be this poor girl? Ha Ha." The card was unsigned, indicating that the sender was someone well known to the recipient. In a similar vein, "I'm Feeling Much Improved" is of a young man sitting in a chair in his dressing gown tying the shoelaces of young woman in a nurses' uniform sitting on the bed with her skirts lifted to show off her legs and feet. The fantasy was a more respectable version of "what the butler saw" Mutascope peep shows, popular in amusement arcades from the early 1900s, where the flip book mechanism creates a moving image of a young women removing her clothes, supposedly without knowing that she is being watched.[7] The frequency of this fantasy on early nursing post cards can be explained in part by the private health care system in the U.S. at this time. Hospitals training nurses relied on their students to care for patients; once trained, private duty nursing, where the nurse was employed by the patient or the patient's family on their behalf, was one of few employment options for professional nurses in the U.S.

Nurses were frequently depicted as sentimentalized objects of romantic attraction; before the outbreak of war they were found on Valentine and other cards that pictured the nurse as a pretty, innocent young woman, a style of depiction that emphasized good looks, childish naivety and personal attractiveness as a nurse's key attributes. An early version of this type of card from 1903 featured a child dressed as nurse, offering her doll a spoonful of medicine. An illustrated border was intertwined with the words "If you can heal a wounded heart, Pray heal mine from Cupid's dart" (PoN http://resource.nlm.nih.gov/101624066). In wartime, these attributes continued to be emphasized, with illustrations of attractive and sometimes glamorous nurses partnering their handsome soldier patient becoming increasingly common. In these illustrations, their heads were close together, the nurse a comforting presence as she supported "her" wounded soldier boyfriend, creating an intimate image of caring and adoring dependency ("If the leg is wooden, the heart is not," PoN http://resource.nlm.nih.gov/101625551).

Many of the comic cards featured male and female pairings, adopting a less realistic style that verged on caricature and exaggeration rather than saucy innuendo. Some of these images were what might be termed "cute," featuring childish images of cherubic nurses with large heads and big eyes; "Forget Me Not" by the illustrator Eugenie Richards from around 1910 is typical of the style (PoN http://resource.nlm.nih.gov/101625379). A young girl dressed as a nurse wears a white hat, a frilly underskirt visible beneath her dress; small wings sprout from her shoulders. In these cartoons, the nurses were drawn as childlike dolls, their outsized faces dominated by large, doe-like eyes and small, bow shaped lips, an image of innocence and wide eyed naivety. In a number of cartoons, nursing work was humorously interpreted as "child's play," where the female figures were always nurses, the males always either patients or doctors. In Grace Wiederseim's cartoons of the same period, the children were drawn with large heads, chubby round faces and rosy cheeks. In "His First Case" (1910), a doll lies in bed with a girl nurse standing by, her hands clasped together meekly in front of her; the boy doctor, carrying a Gladstone style bag and wearing a top hat and striped suit, is striding in with a surprised expression as he looks at his watch. The importance of the dynamic, authoritative doctor figure is emphasized by way of contrast to the static, submissive figure of the nurse (PoN http://resource.nlm.nih.gov/101611688). Nursing in these cards was visualized as "child's play," the lesser value of the female caring role accentuated by the dynamics of the graphic hierarchies played out in the drawing of the game.

Saucy and sentimental images stood in stark contrast to the portraits of women on photo cards, who, in their smart and spotless uniforms, presented themselves as serious, respectable women. Portrait photographs demonstrated the realities of these relationships: the private nurse was a paid household servant; the black nurse caring for a child replaced enslavement with servitude. In group photos of hospital staff, a doctor, often the only male who was not a patient, was frequently depicted at the center as head of a large female workforce. Group portraits also provided evidence of nursing skills: caring for patients, making dressings and bandages and preparing food, duties also shown to be carried out by members of European royalty.[8] Other cards showcased more advanced and specialized procedures and tasks such as training for the operating theatre (PoN http://resource.nlm.nih.gov/101626488). Cards depicting community nurses and district nurses were indicative of some of the professional challenges a career in nursing offered: Nurse Elizabeth McPhee, riding her motorbike through the Scottish countryside to reach patients in remote highland villages (PoN http://resource.nlm.nih.gov/101611681); and nursing's efforts to provide health care to families living in poverty. A card from 1913 advertising the free services of the Toledo District Nurse Association featured a photograph of a white nurse cradling an African American baby next to a mother nursing a young child and a toddler in a small, sparsely furnished room (PoN http://resource.nlm.nih.gov/101612116).[9]

Guardian Angels and Battle-Axes: Religious and Mythical Associations

In his introduction to his collection, Zwerdling points out that nursing's unique bond to the universal truths of human existence, birth, pain and death, gives nursing the privilege of a mythical heritage as well as a historic one, a resource "that few other professions can lay claim to" (2004: 3). Morphing between ancient archetypes of battling goddesses, religious references and modern associations of white middle-class femininity associated with Florence Nightingale's image of the "Lady of the Lamp," images of nurses as guardian angels and battle-axes are found on postcards from across the spectrum of western European nations as well as Britain and America. Designed to invoke complex emotions of female bravery, perseverance, self-sacrifice, professional pride and nationalism, they provide material evidence of the relationship between the professional "ideal" and the deep cultural roots that inform the gendering of the profession. Images of nurses in the European art traditions of the 19th and early 20th centuries were often based on ancient classical and Christian female archetypes such as healer, handmaiden, mother, angel, and guardian or warrior. In *Nursing the Image*, I argue that professional nursing is founded on Nightingale's "appropriation of the characteristics associated with 'respectable,' middle-class women circulating in mid-nineteenth-century society

in Britain" (Hallam, 2000: 11). Feminine discourse "ascribed special qualities of a moral and ethical nature (to women) which defined the domestic
realm as their principal area of expertise and responsibility; middle-class
women were expected to exercise this influence on family and friends and
to donate their leisure time to societies engaged in social and moral reform"
(Hallam, 2000: 15). The notion of "the Angel in the house" also applied
to women nursing on the nineteenth-century battlefields of Europe and
America. Nightingale, as well as being known as "the Lady with the Lamp"
was also dubbed "the Angel of the Crimea"; Clara Barton, the founder of
the American Red Cross, was popularly known as "the Angel on the Battlefield." George Barton wrote an account of the Catholic Sisterhoods in
the late civil war that he called "Angels of the Battlefield" (Barton, 1894).
These associations were drawn on and developed by postcard designers;
an Italian postcard of the First World War depicted a classical image from
a contemporary painting by Giovanni Carpanetto of a female nurse as a
guardian angel kissing the forehead of a man wrapped in a flag bearing the
red cross (PoN http://resource.nlm.nih.gov/101622089). British and American cards frequently depicted these red cross "angels" as fresh faced, attractive young women, such as in "an Angel of Mercy" (http://resource.nlm.
nih.gov/101623461) and "the Real Angel of Mons" (http://resource.nlm.
nih.gov/101611680) while European cards often featured women dressed in
nurses uniforms with wings sprouting from their shoulders that emphasized their associations with religious sisterhoods (Belgian Red Cross, PoN
http://resource.nlm.nih.gov/101625677).

There was, however, another side to Nightingale and to that of the
"angel in the house" and on the battlefield; her reforms also invoked
images of the "battle-ax," women fighting the twin evils of poverty and disease with tuberculosis in particular featuring in U.S. and European early
twentieth-century public health campaigns. Postcards were one of the ways
in which various organizations and charities tried to raise public awareness about the disease and its prevention. A number of incarnations of the
"battle-ax" featured on these cards; a Spanish card advertising the medic-
inal properties of Calcium Chloride from around 1905 drew on an ancient
image of a woman carrying a large shield and wearing a steel helmet (an
Amazon?) wielding a sword against three monsters to support their claims
for the effectiveness of its products against a range of common diseases
including Tuberculosis (PoN http://resource.nlm.nih.gov/101617049). A
postcard image from 1910 advertising life insurance depicted a female protector clothed like a goddess in a long white gown marked by the cross of
Lorraine[10]; her long red cloak shielded a child and baby from the shadowy
figure of death, her other hand holding death's arm in a firm, muscular
grip (PoN http://resource.nlm.nih.gov/101621785). An Italian image from

around the same time produced for the Genoa anti–Tuberculosis Consortium combined the head and shoulders of an ancient winged goddess with that of "the lady of the lamp," an image of nursing found internationally by this time. The art nouveau style combined the image of the goddess with that of an angel holding the lamp of knowledge or life derived from the ancient Egyptian ankh symbol (PoN http://resource.nlm.nih.gov/101623319).

The "nurse as protector" featured on numerous European cards that emphasized nursing's religious roots through the styling of the women's long white tunics and veiled headwear. In a Belgian version from 1916, the nurse's outstretched arms formed a cross that, like the first example described above, is enveloped by a cloak that embraces images of poor, suffering people wrapped in snakes. In her outstretched hand, she holds a lamp with a red cross; the cross is repeated across her breast and forehead (PoN http://resource.nlm.nih.gov/101625718). Underlying this image of strength and resilience is another, perhaps less apparent image to those not familiar with religious iconography: the female guardian wards off the serpent Satan on many fronts, preventing the theft of souls and protecting the virtuous. By invoking both ancient and modern associations of care and protection and their associations with religion and respectable femininity, these postcards reveal how deeply rooted cultural legacies of white women's role in society underpin the multi-faceted complexities of nursing's popular image at this time.

Contemporary Crises: Superheroes to the Rescue?

Battle-axes and guardian angels became popular symbols of the fight against contagious diseases and poverty in the urban ghettos and of the human price of war in North America, Europe and Britain in the early twentieth century. It is therefore no surprise to find a resurgence of similar imagery, dressed in the modern trappings of the "superhero nurse" during the global Coronovirus pandemic of 2019–2020. In England in March, when the resources to prevent deaths amongst NHS staff caring for Covid 19 patients were stretched to their limits by a lack of adequate supplies of personal protective equipment (PPE) and critical care facilities, people came out onto the streets and "clapped for our carers."[11] In May, the street artist known as Banksy created a work of graffiti art on a hospital corridor wall that spoke to the nation's admiration and thanks for its hard working nursing staff. In the illustration, a small boy has thrown his usual "boy's toys," Batman and Spiderman, into a bin and is playing instead with a female nurse doll bearing some of the signs of a superhero; her superhero mask covered by a surgical mask, she wears the traditional nurses' uniform of yesteryear, her cloak streaming out behind as she flies through the air in the hands of a small boy. Her chest proudly bears a "superhero nurse" badge on her white starched apron along with a red cross, the only color in this black and white image. Banksy has rekindled the image of nurse as a "guardian angel" for a contemporary generation reared on TV series and movie adaptations of Marvel comic book superheroes.

The development of this iconography cannot be seen apart from the ways in which these comic book superheroes permeate every aspect of popular culture; from children's play superhero costumes through computer games to films and TV series, the superhero is a distinctly modern savior, a "guardian angel" for our troubled times. In his discussion of the growing popularity of superhero fantasies during the twenty-first century, Brown draws on genre theory to discuss the ways in which superheroes confront deep-rooted contemporary fears about the nature of modern society. Although superhero films and TV series have been made since the 1940s drawing on the popularity of the Marvel comics characters, since 9/11 superheroes have become ever more dominant in North American entertainment media that is globally impactful. Hollywood in particular increasingly relies on the reliable box office success of films featuring superheroes such as *Iron Man* and *Captain America* to boost its coffers, while TV series such as *Daredevil* (Netflix, 2015–18), *Jessica Jones* (Netflix, 3 seasons, 2015–19) *Agent Carter* (ABC, 2015–16) and *Marvel's Agents of S.H.I.E.L.D.* (ABC, 2013–2020) are distributed via network, on-line and cable services. Due to the worldwide penetration of U.S. entertainment media, percolation of the superhero into all forms of popular culture has become an international phenomenon. In China, for example, although an extended version of *Iron Man 3* created in 2011 to address the Chinese audience received a mixed response, Chinese versions of the superhero are becoming increasingly popular (Zhao 2020).

As the symbol proliferates, so too does the range and variety of bodies that the superhero can, and does, inhabit. Burke and Gordon argue that the reach and power of the superhero can bring benefits to marginalized groups, for example the development of *Cleverman* (ABC Australia, 2016–17), an Indigenous superhero series set in a futuristic Australia (2020: 17). Part of the attraction of the "superhero" image is its binary and non-gendered possibilities; many of the superhero characters in the Marvel comic series are female and one of them is a nurse[12]; a new, younger gender fluid character, Kid Quick, arrived in December 2020 in a holiday themed comic book.[13] A basic on-line search using the keywords "nurse" and "superhero" in June 2020 aimed to assess how prevalent the image of the "superhero nurse" had become. Almost without exception the examples thrown up by the search engines were North American; amidst the cartoon images of many white female and male nurses, African American, South Asian and Latinx superheroes are found; masks sometimes cover the face or eyes, while hands carry syringes or stethoscopes or fly with a clenched fist to demonstrate strength. In contrast to the Banksy image, most cartoon nurses wear a superhero costume with hair length usually an indication of gender identity; a diamond shaped badge on the chest of a tightly fitting flying suit invariably indicates their RN/superhero status. In contrast, there are photographs of contemporary nurses wearing superhero nurse t-shirts or symbols on their uniforms and scrubs; some male nurses actively promote their nursing skills as "superhero" skills, as do some nursing institutions. One of the earliest on-line advertisements found using the "superhero nurse" trope is a nursing school recruitment website dated 2014, its leader page proclaiming "5 Reasons Nurses are Superheroes"[14]; other sites advertise "superhero" workforce competitions promoted by various health organizations, many of which pre-date the 2020 pandemic and the toll it has taken on health services staff.[15] For Steege and Rainbow (2017), investigating what they term the "supernurse syndrome," the qualities of Superheroes include: "extraordinary powers or abilities; a strong moral code and belief in self-sacrifice for the benefit of society; a sense of responsibility and guilt that motivates their role; a costume that projects their identity and can serve as a protective armor; an alter-ego that allows them to maintain anonymity; a weakness (e.g., Superman's Kryptonite) that makes them vulnerable to enemies and impacts their powers; and a tendency to act alone and apply their individual powers without help from a sidekick" (2017: 23).

Steege and Rainbow, like many nurses, are, rightly, skeptical about the ways in which the development of the "supernurse" draws on these attributes, arguing that it perpetuates ideas of self-sacrifice and public duty at the expense of better pay and working conditions. Similarly, McAllister et al. argue that the Banksy image has similarities to a Belgian propaganda poster from WWI "depicting a wounded soldier being lovingly tended on the battlefield by a nurse who has flown to him on her angel wings" (McAllister et al., 2020, see page x).[16] While the public "clap for their carers" in Britain and sing from their balconies in Italy, nurses are in the highest category of key workers to be killed by Covid 19, their pleas for better protective equipment and increased levels of staffing remaining unheard. Professional nurses' pay remains low compared to other graduate professions; in the social care sector, under-skilled low-paid carers deliver personal care to a growing aging population. In this context, Banksy's portrait and the many heroic images on wall murals and in cartoons and photographs that circulate on social media project idealized views of heroic nurses that are received positively by a profession suffering from a low morale generated by emotional and physical exhaustion. Rochelle Einboden argues that nurses "remain vulnerable to hero discourses because our work is entangled with our identity" (2020: 334).

The conflation of cartoon images of diversely imagined "superhero" nursing bodies with the discursive construct of the professional "supernurse" creates problems for a profession trying to achieve better pay and working conditions. Some nurses are, however, trying to raise public awareness by calling attention to the ways in which the "supernurse" discourse in the U.S. participates in installing a sense of public duty amongst nurses in the face of state irresponsibility. Drawing on the voices of young nurses demonstrating in New York City for better pay and working conditions, Einboden points out how neoliberal economics and austerity policies have led to divestment in health care in many wealthy nations, their public services privatized and ill-prepared to meet the challenges presented by a global pandemic. Amidst the ongoing crises in care, nurses' voices are increasingly calling for change: "Heroisation … opens the eyes for the need for action—among the nursing staff themselves, and hopefully, through their more proactive public appearance, also in politics and society" (Hahn, 2020).[17]

Graffiti artist Banksy's wall mural, as well as paying tribute to demoralized nursing staff at the height of the pandemic, can be read as a subtle critique of the traditional nurse as a female "superhero." Eventually the small boy who is controlling her movement will tire of her and she will be discarded, thrown in the bin with his other toys. The challenge for nursing's professional associations and institutions, as they become more publicly proactive, is to ensure that nursing's nineteenth-century discourse of idealized femininity is discarded alongside her. In countries around the world, while many mural artists continue to portray nurses as imaginary winged female "angels" and "superheroes," others are creating multivalent paintings of modern nursing's professional identity, a welcome addition to the public imaginary as nurses struggle to achieve the financial recognition they so justly deserve.

Notes

1. For a brief history of the postcard, see https://150yearsofpostcards.com/, accessed September 29, 2020.
2. For a more detailed discussion of the portraits, see Zwerdling 2004, Chapter Four.
3. Contrasting examples of groups:

a) Female and male nurses graduating with their Diploma in Nursing ca. 1910 with a statement on the back reading "hoping this will be a beautiful spat of remembrance," http://resource.nlm.nih.gov/101594341.

b) Nurses of Brewster Hospital and Nurse Training School W.H.M.S, Jacksonville, Florida, 1908, a training school for African American nurses, http://resource.nlm.nih.gov/101611713.

c) A group of male nurses from Dixmont State Hospital (for the insane), PA, c. 1910, http://resource.nlm.nih.gov/101611710.

d) A birthday greeting card featuring Dr. Aspland and hospital staff of the Anglican Hospital, Peking, China, ca. 1910, http://resource.nlm.nih.gov/101626440.

e) Trained nurses administer the Finsen Light Treatment at the London Hospital, ca. 1900, http://resource.nlm.nih.gov/101625620.

4. TuckDB postcards, History of Raphael Tuck and Sons Ltd, https://tuckdbpostcards.org/history, accessed 11 November 2020. An example of this technique dated 1917 features a child dressed as a Red Cross nurse feeding a black doll in a doll's bed; a poem printed in the top left hand corner ends with "If care and skill can save a man, A Red Cross Nurse will do it!" The card, written in Italian states "Who remembers you always always always with great affection yours forever Giulia Massagli."

5. Donald McGill Museum, Ryde, Isle of Wight, https://saucyseasidepostcards.com/?page_id=89.

6. See Anne Summers (1989) for an account of the mid-late nineteenth century vilification of the domiciliary nurse and her subsequent demise.

7. For brief information on the Mutoscope and its role the development of early 20th century erotica, see https://racingnelliebly.com/weirdscience/mutoscopes-become-butler-saw-machines, accessed 26 November 2020.

8. See, for example, Czarina Alexandra of Russia with the Princesses Tatiana and Olga nursing wounded Russians, ca. 1915, PoN, http://resource.nlm.nih.gov/101611717.

9. A range of cards featuring the work of visiting nurse associations can be accessed using the "topic" browser in the PoN digital gallery.

10. "In 1902 at the International Conference on tuberculosis held in Berlin, Dr. Gilbert Sersiron of Paris proposed that the Lorraine Cross be made the emblem of the anti TB 'crusade.'" https://web.archive.org/web/20090302074617/http://www.tbalert.org/about/cross.php, accessed 12 November 2020.

11. See, for example https://clapforourcarers.co.uk/, and https://www.theguardian.com/society/2020/may/28/clap-for-our-carers-the-very-unbritish-ritual-that-united-the-nation, accessed 18 November 2020.

12. https://superheroes.fandom.com/wiki/Night_Nurse, accessed 13 November 2020.

13. Zoya Raza-Sheik, *Gay Times*, https://apple.news/A8uGYFxpBTmua1YIN7v7C1w, accessed 27 November 2020.

14. http://findnursingschools.com/blog/5-reasons-nurses-are-superheroes/, accessed 13 November 2020.

15. https://www.hopkinsmedicine.org/news/articles/superheroes-just-another-arm-of-the-johns-hopkins-family, accessed 13 November 2020.

16. McAllister et al. are probably referring to this image, ca. 1916: PoN, http://resource.nlm.nih.gov/101625677.

17. Dr. Sabine Hahn, a Swiss psychiatric nurse specialist and Director of Nursing speaking to M. Afzali, blog of the Bernese Health Care Communication Design group, 29 June 2020.

Films and Television Productions Referenced

Agent Carter (2015–16) ABC
Captain America (2011) Paramount Pictures
Cleverman (2016–17) ABC Australia
Daredevil (2015–18) Netflix
Iron Man (2008) Paramount Pictures

Jessica Jones (2015–19) Netflix
Marvel's Agents of S.H.I.E.L.D. (2013–2020) ABC

References

Afzali, M. (2020) Superheroes in the Hospital? Hypothesis, Learning from Corona: Blog of the Bernese Research Group, Health Care Communication Design (HCCD) *Design, Healthcare and Society*, 29th June, https://hccd.hypotheses.org/1033 [Accessed: 11 November 2020].

Barton, G. (2018) *Angels of the Battlefield: A History of the Labors of the Catholic Sisterhoods in the Late Civil War*, The Project Gutenberg EBook of Angels of the Battlefield, EBook #57933 [Accessed: 11 November 2020].

Benjamin, W. (1935, 1969) The Work of Art in the Age of Mechanical Reproduction. In: H. Arendt (ed.). *Illuminations* (trans. H. Zohn). New York: Schocken Books.

Berger, J. (1972) *Ways of Seeing*. New York: Penguin Books.

Brown, J.A. (2017) *The Modern Superhero in Film and Television: Popular Genre and American Culture*. London: Routledge.

Burke, L. (2020) Introduction. Everlasting Symbols: Unmasking Superheroes and Their Shifting Symbolic Function. In: Burke, L., Gordon, I., and Ndalianis, A. (eds.). *The Superhero Syndrome: Media, Culture, and Politics*. New Brunswick, NJ: Rutgers University Press, pp. 1–24.

Einboden, R. (2020) SuperNurse? Troubling the Hero Discourse in COVID Times. *Health* 24, 4: 343–347.

Gillen J. (2013) Writing Edwardian Postcards. *Journal of Sociolinguistics* 17, 4: 488–521.

Hallam, J. (2000) *Nursing the Image: Media, Culture and Professional Identity*. London and New York: Routledge.

Hook, S.A. (2005) You've Got Mail: Hospital Postcards as a Reflection of Health Care in the Early Twentieth Century. *Journal of the Medical Library Association* 93, 3 (July): 386–393.

Hubbard, P. (2012) Trade Cards in 18th-Century Consumer Culture: Circulation, and Exchange in Commercial and Collecting spaces. *Material Culture Review* 74. https://journals.lib.unb.ca/index.php/MCR/article/view/20447 [Accessed: 29 September 2020].

Kalba, A. (2011) How Media Were Made: Chromolithography in *Belle Époque* France. *History and Technology* 27, 4, 441–453.

McAllister, M., Brien, D.L., and Dean, S. (2020) The Problem with the Superhero Narrative During COVID 19. *Contemporary Nurse*, doi: 10.1080/10376178.2020.1827964.

Moorehead, C. (1999) *Dunant's Dream War: Switzerland and the History of the Red Cross*. New York: Carroll & Graf.

Patmore, C. (1866) *The Angel in The House*. London: Macmillan.

Sachs, K. (2018) Superheroes: Just Another Arm of the Johns Hopkins Family. News and publications, *John Hopkins Medicine*, 29th October https://www.hopkinsmedicine.org/news/articles/superheroes-just-another-arm-of-the-johns-hopkins-family [Accessed: 11 November 2020].

Scaglia, E., and Bergoni, A. (2020) Education and Propaganda in the "Patriotic Postcards" Distributed by the Lombard Committee of the General Union of Italian Teachers During WWI. *History of Education & Children's Literature* 15, 1: 445–467

Scott, K. (2004) The Waddesdon Manor Trade Cards: More Than One History. *Journal of Design History* 17, 1: 91–104.

Steege, L.M., and Rainbow, J.G. (2017) Fatigue in Hospital Nurses: "Supernurse" Culture Is a Barrier to Addressing Problems: A Qualitative Interview Study. *International Journal of Nursing Studies* 67: 20–28.

Summers, A. (1989) The Mysterious Demise of Mrs Gamp and Her Detractors c.1830–1860. *Victorian Studies*, Spring, 365–386.

Viñao, A., and Martinez Ruiz-Funes, M.J. (2017) Picture Postcards as a Tool for Constructing and Reconstructing Educational Memory (Spain, 19th-20th Centuries). In: Yanes-Cabrera,

C., Meda, J., and. Viñao, A. (eds.). *School Memories. New Trends in the History of Education.* New York: Springer.

Whelan, J. (2012) When the Business of Nursing Was the Nursing Business: The Private Duty Registry System, 1900–1940. *OJIN: The Online Journal of Issues in Nursing* 17, 2, Manuscript 6 [Accessed: 11 November 2020].

Zao, S.M. (2020) Chinese Milk for Iron Men: Superhero Productions and Technological Anxiety. In: Burke, L., Gordon, I., and Ndalianis, A. (eds.). *The Superhero Syndrome: Media, Culture, and Politics.* New Brunswick, New Jersey: Rutgers University Press, Chapter 17.

Zwerdling M. (2004) *Postcards of Nursing: A Worldwide Tribute.* Philadelphia, Baltimore, New York, London, Buenos Aires, Hong Kong, Sydney, Tokyo: Lippincott, Williams and Wilkins.

Seeking Standards

*Nurses Real and Fictional
and Their Professional Standards
in British Popular Culture*

Marcus K. Harmes, Barbara Harmes
and Meredith A. Harmes

Introduction

The lost continent of British cinema, which is Julian Petley's conceptualization of a body of commercially and publicly popular films that are nonetheless on the fringes of critical and academic respectability, is now a familiar part of film studies (1986). Not all the films found in this lost continent, nor all the themes and angles they cover, have received attention and one hitherto unexplored angle is commentary on the changing profile of the nursing profession accessed via popular culture. The "lost continent" applies particularly to cinema, but other depictions of nursing in popular television equally merit analysis and will provide the source base for this essay. The two media intersect, for instance in the television specials based on the *Carry On* films (some set in hospitals), and the films made of popular television series such as *Emergency Ward 10* and *Shroud for a Nightingale*. Nurses sat and sit heavily in popular culture within this lost but popular continent of broad comedy, soap opera and crime. In 1959, the comedy *Carry On Nurse* was the best performing film at the British box office. In its wake came *Carry On Doctor, Carry On Again Doctor* and finally *Carry On Matron*, each a popular and accessible film that put hospitals, doctors, and especially nurses, in their wards at center stage, as well as *Carry On Regardless* (1961), a more episodic narrative but still with a hospital, matron, sister, and nurses. The nurses appeared organized on screen in their traditional and all-female hierarchy of matron, sister and nurse. The

124

Carry On films are not however the only instances of the nursing profession entering popular culture in post-war Britain. Among other examples, *Emergency Ward 10* introduced television viewers to the working and private lives of nurses and their interactions (sometimes romantic) with the male doctors in the titular ward and in the world of the hospital around it (Purser, 1981: 168). In place of *Emergency Ward 10* (1957–1967) came *General Hospital* (1972–1979, not to be confused with the American soap opera), while other series including *Police Surgeon* (1960) and *Owen M.D.* (1971–1973) created a consistent place for members of the nursing profession to appear on television. In later decades, *Angels* (1975–1983) and then *Casualty* (1986 to present) retained this space. Nurses in popular culture had real life counterparts, who through the 1950s, 1960s, and 1970s were experiencing change and criticism. Change came in the form of committee scrutiny of and reporting on training and education. There was also criticism expressed from various perspectives, from arguments that facilities and training were inadequate, that nurses were not intelligent enough but even criticism that they were too intelligent to compete with the male medical profession. Focusing primarily on British popular culture, this essay places the televisual and cinematic nurses against actual developments and the time frame is set by the committees, reports, commissions and public commentary on nursing across the 1950s to 1980s.

Nursing in popular culture does register in academic literature, although many works of popular culture including the *Carry On* films have attracted an equally popular type of literary interest. This essay pursues the intersection of the popular with the actual, during decades of organizational and professional development and reform. The National Health Service (NHS) came into existence in July 1948. In response many, although not all popular depictions, take place in the Nightingale wards of recognizably NHS foundations, and the fictional popular portrayal of the nursing profession keeps pace with changes to the actuality. However, this essay additionally pursues where the actual may have been influenced by, or there was a feared influence of, the distillation of nursing offered in popular culture. The key areas of Role modeling and Leadership models, training, Reputations, and Standards will be considered in pursuit of these transactional influences.

On-Screen Nursing

The type of drama featuring nurses provides an insight into perceptions of their work and roles. When the soap opera *Angels* (BBC 1975–1983, a series set in an inner city hospital) launched in 1975, advance publicity heralded it as intended to "tell the truth" about the lives of nurses, a truth inscribed in a gritty inner city reality (*Stage and Television Today* May 15, 1975: 11). Also touted as "realistic," advance publicity for the then new BBC drama likened it to *Z Cars*, a police series that had similarly sought to portray a hard bitten reality of another profession (*Stage and Television Today* May 15, 1975: 11).

The centerpiece of nursing's intersection with both popular culture and popular consciousness is arguably the *Carry On* films. Two of them, *Carry On Nurse* of 1959 and *Carry On Matron* of 1972 foreground the profession in the title. The other two hospital set-films, *Carry On Doctor* (1967) and *Carry On Again Doctor* (1969) place emphasis on the doctor rather than the nurse, but these films nonetheless carry heavy emphasis on the nursing profession, including the ranks of matron, sister and nurse, emphasizing the wards of a large NHS hospital as their natural sphere of activity, and reinforcing a strict gender divide between male medical doctors and female nurses.

The films' productions span a little more than a decade and are collectively a snapshot in time of the nursing profession, in line with the film series' general interest in institutions, as other settings included ships and business firms (Barber, 2013: 149; Landy, 2015: 77). The nurses, with the exception of the matron and the sisters, are young, single women, capped and caped in their traditional uniform. The nurses live together in a nurses' home, watched over in work and recreation by the senior nursing staff. Yet the professional and social changes over the time period of 1959 to 1972 do not pass without notice in scripting and scenarios on screen, and while the films are a snapshot in time or time capsules, they are also markers of change. *Carry On Matron* in 1972 has the same elements in place from *Carry On Nurse* in 1959, including Hattie Jacques playing the matron, the Nightingale wards of the NHS hospital, and the sisters and nurses staffing them. However the film's central plot is the theft from the hospital of the contraceptive pill, a prescient piece of writing from the scriptwriter Talbot Rothwell, pre-empting the availability of the pill from the NHS the following year and a marker of the films' awareness of social change (Hunt, 2013: 38; Gerrard, 2016: 41).

The delineation on screen of an all-female nursing profession is a study in the physicality of the profession. The role of the matron taken by the actor Hattie Jacques associated the seniority of the position with the scale of the actor. The authoritative nature of the role is noted in early critical reception of the films, as the antics in *Carry On Nurse* took place "under the watchful eye of Matron" (*Brechin Advertiser* August 18, 1959: 3). The key part that Jacques' weight played in the casting decisions made by directors is discussed critically by biographers and film and television historians, including documenting Jacques' own frustrations and dismay with her size being exploited by primarily male directors and used as a source of visual and verbal humor by writers (Merriman, 2011: 92–3). In *Carry On Doctor*, her physique is mocked as making her "Miss Bedpan 1968." Collectively, the senior ranks of nurses are a grimly formidable tier of authority against both the patients and the young nurses, with the matron at the apex. Indeed, the plot of *Carry On Doctor* culminates in an uprising in the male and female wards against the authority of matron and sister which is likened to a slave revolt. To further reinforce the exploitation of her physicality, casting decisions about the young ward nurses moved to another type of exploitation, including casting young models as the junior nurses. Thus the *Daily Mirror* announced the casting of the model and actor Laura Collins in *Carry On Matron* in terms drawing attention to her body rather than her acting talent, noting she had hitherto been seen "wrapped in winter coats on ITV commercials" (October 21, 1971: 18). Both actors, Jacques and Collins, were as such subject to the exploitation of their physicality, in order to embody a type of visual short hand of the nursing profession's most senior and junior ranks as dauntingly authoritarian and attractively available in turn. The same emphasis informs scenes in *Carry On Matron*, in which young trainee nurses are fodder for the young male doctors, while the Matron's unrequited love for the chief surgeon plays out in a scene cruelly mocking her romantic desires, and where her wish to be wooed with flowers and chocolates is met with the offer of a bar of fruit and nut. The matron and the young nurses under her charge physically and romantically embody what Darbyshire (2014) notes are among the most common stereotypes for nurses, the battle-ax and the sex symbol. Other British cultural productions of the same era made the same point. In the comedy series *The Goodies*, a comedic version of medical training, in which all the trainee doctors were men, included testing their skills in pinching nurses' bottoms and sneaking them back into the nurses' home after hours. Most nurses were the sex symbol type bar one, another oversized battle-ax matron following the visual template in the *Carry On* films.

What can be overlooked in noting the *Carry On* films' insistence on ribaldry and exploitation, especially of the Matron, is that central to Hattie Jacques' performance as the Matron is a source of medical authority who presides over a well-run hospital. In short, this Matron runs a tight ship, whether it be Long Hampton in *Carry On Again Doctor* or Finisham Maternity in *Carry On Matron*. One behind the scenes anecdote about the *Carry On* films was the director Gerald Thomas's instruction to Jacques to run her hand along the rail, looking for dust (Williams, 1993: 557–58). The small gesture added suggestive layers of depth to the character, making clear the observant Matron someone who cared for small details and overlooked nothing. The films therefore comment on and display nursing standards, most directly in *Carry On Matron*. There, the plot hatched by thieves to steal the contraceptive pills requires an inside man; the demands of farce means the inside man is a male gang member, disguised as nurse. In 1972, that entailed a transvestite disguise as a female nurse, providing an opportunity to bring cross dressing, a staple not only of the *Carry On* films' use of sexual humor and sexual taboos (Huxley, 2004: 282) but ribald British comedy generally, into the plot and onto the screen. As farcical events play out, the cross-dressing undercover criminal is advertently involved in a real medical emergency, accidentally sedates the doctor, yet successfully delivers triplet babies and is hailed for "her" medical expertise in the press and by the hospital authorities. The matron assures the nurse "I've had hundreds of capable nurses through my hands and you have that extra little something the others haven't got." While there is an obvious *double entendre* related to the cross dressing and the male physicality under the nurse's uniform, the comment is another instance where the *Carry On* films depict the Matron judging and assessing standards.

The resolution of the farce, after the robbers attempt to steal the contraceptive pills but are thwarted by the matron, nurses, doctors and the patients of the maternity ward, is the robbers' threat to reveal the successful and widely reported birth of the triplets was assisted by a man disguised as a nurse. The gang's leader threatens "if it ever got out that the nurse who delivered these babies was a fella…." It seemingly does not occur to anyone that it could be equally harmful to expose that the nurse actually had no medical training, and the plot's resolution testifies to the film's strict and enduring binary of hospital staff into male doctors and female nurses. Sue Harper and Justin Smith suggest that by the 1970s the *Carry On* films were conservative in vision (2013: 116). One aspect of that conservatism was the enduring insistence on the wholly female nursing profession, against the reality of the demographic changes in the nursing profession in the 1970s, with male nurses studying at technical colleges and becoming an evident part of the profession including in management roles (Hargreaves, 2019: 224; *The People* April 12, 1970, 18).

The *Carry On* films continued in production until 1978, but with none set in a hospital after *Carry On Matron* in 1972. They remained however prominent via repeats on television during the decade (Cull, 2015: 106), and endured therefore a means of bringing the nursing profession into popular consciousness. They therefore also remained a current and topical concern when, at the end of the decade, Dr. Hywel Davies published *Modern Medicine: A Doctor's Dissent* in 1977. Davies, an eminent cardio specialist as much as he was a notorious controversialist on a number of topics, argued his dissent against a range of aspects of modern medical practice, as it then was. A series *A Doctor in Dissent* accompanied the book and disseminated the same ideas. His text attacked his fellow doctors and other medical professionals, including pharmacists and nutritionists, but his most trenchant criticism was of the nurse, firmly conceptualized as collectively female and getting far too clever for her own good. "She should, for ordinary nursing duties, not be too intelligent or too highly educated; otherwise, she will probably cease to want to do these things." His argument resonated with some. One commentator, a nurse, found Davies' "observations on the nursing profession, and its quest for more equality with doctors, sadly true. In training nurses to keep up with the technical side of medicine, we are being led further away from the patients' basic needs." In contrast to acquiring and using knowledge and demonstrating intelligence, a good nurse would get to "know your patient, showing understanding and human warmth," while the doctor undertook the important medical tasks (*Liverpool Echo* May 3, 1977: 8). Davies's complaints, and his proposed "cure" that nurses should restrict themselves both professionally and intellectually, was a critical reaction to what he perceived as the changing nature of the nursing profession, its changing standards, and the way the interactions between doctors and nurses were changing. For example, in 1964, the Royal College of Nursing had proposed that the training of nurses needed urgent and sweeping changes, not least as "current training methods have been overtaken by a highly complex medical service," and urged a major rethink of long-standing principles to yield a cohort of better educated nurses. The Briggs Committee set up by the Department of Health in 1970 similarly proposed changes to nurses' education, including the duration of training (Dewar, 1978: 400). Stung by some of the criticisms, training establishments pointed to the educational attainments of the young women aspiring to be nurses. A class of trainee nurses at Dudley Road Hospital proudly reported their collective achievements with GCEs, O Levels and A Levels from school to a visiting reporter. Nonetheless, the sister in charge of training stressed (or perhaps reassured male doctors) that brains was not everything, because "if a girl has good practical ability and the right temperament, she also makes a very good nurse" (*Birmingham Post* October 6, 1966: 5).

Over a decade later than this comment from 1966, Davies objected to well-educated nurses in his *Dissent*. His views can be contextualized not only by the medical profession of the 1970s but also by the immediate legacy of television's distillation of how doctors and nurses appeared on screen. The soap opera *Emergency Ward 10* ended its broadcast run in 1967, a decade before Davies' book appeared in print. As will be discussed below, *Emergency Ward 10*'s production team prided itself on the medical accuracy of the series, achieved through consultation with medical professionals.

But that advice extended beyond the technical aspects of medical treatment to the portrayal of status and intellect. As Rebecca Feasey points out in her study of masculinity in television programs, both *Emergency Ward 10* and its American counterpart *Medic* (1954–56) not only used medical advisors, but also deferred to insistence from these advisors that the characters of the male doctors appear intellectually infallible and professionally competent. Set against that portrayal of male omnicompetence, the female nurses were assistants to but also evidently inferior to the godlike male doctors (2008: 67). Although these representations were intended to show the entire medical profession in the most positive light possible, and thereby reassure the general public of its skills and reliability through the reach of popular television, this reassurance was strictly gendered.

A similar emphasis on competence and the appropriate standards expected of nurses, especially those seeking promotion to sister and then matron, carried through the storylines of *Emergency Ward 10*. This soap opera, set in Oxbridge Hospital and broadcast on the ITV from 1957 to 1967, wove the standards and training of the nursing profession into its storylines. The departure of a lead character, Sister Carole Young, played by the series' star, became part of the texture of a story about the standards of nursing leadership. Passed over promotion to the position of Ward Sister, the character was informed by the Matron that "I think you are a competent Sister but immature" (*Daily Mirror* August 26, 1964: 14). Viewers had also seen the character of the Matron move through a storyline of her promotion from sister to matron, therefore showing the standards and qualities needed to make a good senior nurse in a large hospital. The series used the departure and arrival of cast members to weave stories about nursing standards and expectations and to describe what made a good nurse. In one episode, "An unfortunate nurse was fired in two minutes dead by a sweet-faced old matron." The firing allowed the series writers to bring to life on screen the examinations undertaken by nurses, and the articulation of high standards by the nursing hierarchy, as the Matron's opinion was of the nurse being "temperamentally unsuited to be a nurse," while warning the young trainee, and by extension all viewers, of the dangers that an inefficient nurse posed in a busy hospital. *Emergency Ward 10*, made by ATV and broadcast on the Independent channel ITV, is an early example of a British television soap opera, preceded only by *The Grove Family*, which commenced three years earlier on the BBC. As an early instance of soap opera on television, it nonetheless exhibits traits that have since become the norm, including a large ensemble cast and the turnover of actors, enabling a long run (Cooke, 2015: 34). These traits allowed the series to embed narratives that responded to the training, career progression and professional expectations of nurses. The scene noted above of the Matron firing a young trainee nurse had included an exchange related to the shortage of nurses in the health sector. The exchange was topical, reflecting the actual and acute shortage of nurses then available in British hospitals. The actual shortage intersected not only with television's presentation of nursing, in this case the exchange about the topic in *Emergency Ward 10*, but also with discussion of the qualities of a good nurse and the training nurses undertook. In 1964, the Royal College of Nursing concluded a three-year investigation on the training of nurses. The investigation as reported made associated criticisms of what comprised training, the way training turned off potential good students, and the result of there being too few nurses to staff the NHS (*The Press and Journal* June 18, 1964: 6).

Emergency Ward 10 aimed for verisimilitude in the enactment of the medical procedures, and also the presentation of the medical and nursing profession. One television critic bemoaned that later episodes in the program's decade-long run no longer portrayed the "bustling efficiency and sense of dedication which is all I want to believe about hospitals" (*Daily Mirror* December 1, 1964: 18). The comment is revealing of viewer expectations among the 17 million people who were watching *Emergency Ward 10* at the time. The use of an actual hospital for filming exterior shots, and the presence on set of a general practitioner, nurse and surgeon as advisors to the production team, added to the perceived authenticity and to the show's didactic purpose regarding the public understanding of medical treatment (Thumim, 2004: 147). In part, authenticity lay in the use of medical terminology and the accurate portrayal of medical procedures and conditions, leading to the show "being praised by doctors," and gaining sufficient medical authority to have contributed to real world community campaigns, including one about polio (*Daily Mirror* December 1, 1964: 18). Authenticity though was more nuanced than the use of medical dialogue. As a visitor to the television studio noted, the standards and behaviors of cast members had begun to mimic the hierarchical interpersonal relations and cast-iron respect of rank found in actual 1960s hospitals. According to the series producer, "the staff mix only on their own levels; the consultant is regarded as 'God,' which happens in hospitals; the nurses tend to call each other by their surnames" (*Daily Mirror* December 1, 1964: 18). It was still possible to dismiss the program as "pleasant and innocuous" (*Stage and Television Today* December 24, 1963: 8).

Nonetheless, *Emergency Ward 10* was a soap opera, and the human-centered drama meant the private lives of the medical staff could become the narrative focus. In doing so, the program and its portrayal of the nursing profession entered popular discourse in terms of how not only the private lives but also the professional responsibilities of nurses appeared on screen. For example the press caught the story that the nursing head of the

Ambulance Brigade, Major Ralph Raffles, had forbidden his nursing cadets to watch the soap opera. Explaining his reasoning, he said "I think it my duty to make sure my girl cadets, many of whom are likely to become hospital nurses, are not blinded by the glamour of this programme." His comments intersect with different expectations of both actual nursing and the way it appeared on screen. Although the behind the scenes production of *Emergency Ward 10* privileged professional medical insights and sought to ground the plots and dialogue in a plausible medical reality, Major Raffles felt "appalled that nurses should be portrayed as feather-headed fibberti-gibbets who think only of romance. Nurses do not spend all their time having flirtations with handsome doctors and worrying about the private lives of their patients" (*The People* January 15, 1961: 7). His comment though is noteworthy for its emphasis on higher minded expectations of the profession, and was aimed against a program that, despite its patina of medical authenticity, also privileged notions such as the glamour that clung to the young nurses (*Stage and Television Today* February 26, 1959: 9). Beyond the realms of personal opinions, serious and sustained reports into the nursing profession spoke in terms of gender. In 1964 the Royal College of Nursing published a lengthy report criticizing and urging the reform of many aspects of training. One of the animating concerns behind this report was "Nursing is no longer the only profession open to women" (*Press and Journal* June 18, 1964: 6). As a result, both the professional foundations and also the attractiveness of the profession needed reform, but the core point was to relate both problem and remedies to it being a female profession. One solution was even the willingness to re-admit married women to the profession, although that brought concomitant concerns that the married nurse would soon leave again (Dewar, 1978: 401).

Hierarchies

The matron is notable as a constant through these different iterations of nursing in popular culture on both film and television and their cross-overs. One presides over the Nightingale wards of the *Carry On* films, another over the wards of Oxbridge Hospital in *Emergency Ward 10*. To what extent is that leadership model misleadingly invoked in popular culture? Matrons, originally housekeepers or chatelaines but eventually senior nurses, had a long history in British hospitals (Helmstadter, 2002: 328). Although the matron retained currency as a cultural archetype, as an actual member of the nursing profession she fell into obsolescence. The change in leadership, hierarchy, and titles took place alongside other existential changes to nursing practice, such as the gradual replacement of the

Nightingale wards with private or semi-private rooms (Ayliffe and English, 2003: 118) and changing demographics as more men joined the nursing profession, rendering the traditional but sharply gendered terms "matron" and "sister" impractical.

Changes in training, practice and leadership are captured in fine detail in the novel and television adaptation of the novel *Shroud for a Nightingale*. The novel, a 1971 detective story by P.D. James, became a 1984 miniseries made by Anglia Television. The Anglia adaptations of all of James's novels thoroughly and faithfully adapted plots, characters and dialogue, in many instances word for word, in the scripts, and the television version therefore faithfully brought James's story onto the screen. Like most other P.D. James stories, the environment is hermetic. James was herself the product of institutional backgrounds. She had been a hospital administrator and worked in the Home Office, and her novels take place within environments that are close knit in terms of the people but also the physical environment, such as barristers' chambers in the Inns of Court, a clinic, a museum and in *Shroud for a Nightingale*, a hospital and the attached nurses' home and training school.

The 1971 publication of the book made play with the disjunction between homicide and the healing to be associated with nursing, and the book's cover for its first edition was a macabre image of a grinning skull wearing a white nurse's cap. The television adaptation noted and deployed similar imagery; at the climax of the story a nursing sister dies in a fire and viewers see her charred body, surrounded by the burnt remains of her uniform. Both the novel and its faithful television adaptation also create a space for the disjunction between killing and healing, situating murder in the environment of the hospital and even unsettling expectations. The nurse's home (in a converted Victorian mansion) is called "Nightingale House," leading characters new to the scene to reasonably assume it is named after Florence Nightingale. However it is, instead, named after its Victorian builder, a cruel patriarch responsible for a young woman's death a century before. The oddness in naming, the subversion of expectations, the association of the name Nightingale with a cruel male killer rather than the high-minded female founder of nursing, all serve to unsettle the storytelling and the atmosphere.

As the story progresses, the interplay between the nursing hierarchy (the matron, the sisters, and the trainee nurses), the medical doctors, and the patients, gives narrative space to a sustained presentation of nursing training in television. The student nurses at Nightingale House live and eat together in their "pod," attend classes conducted by the sisters at the hospital, and apart from a brief glimpse of a male staff nurse, are exclusively female. The story is a murder mystery, and the murder itself is framed and caused by the abuse of nurse training. A sister, in front of a room full of trainee nurses (all together in their "pod") watches as the clinical sister trains them in naso-gastric feeding of patients who have had a laryngectomy. One nurse plays the patient, other nurses conduct the demonstration, and the entire sequence gives much time and space to portraying the hands on tube feeding training the sister is delivering, including not only the technical aspects of using the Ryles Tube, but the affective also, as the trainee nurse is advised on communicating with and reassuring the conscious patient as the procedure takes place. "Always explain what you are doing and why" instructs the clinical sister. The scenes are grotesque, and the calm inculcation of professional practice and effective communication ends fatally as someone, the as yet unknown murderer, has pushed poison down the Ryles Tube and the extra diegetic music adds chillingly discordant strings over the top of the calm but lethal procedure. The scene, first on the page and then reproduced on screen by the scriptwriters and cast is positively anachronistic for the 1980s. It resembles almost without change a description given of a training session at Dudley Road Hospital in Birmingham in 1966. There, a sister with a room full of student nurses in caps stepped through practical procedures (*Birmingham Post* October 6, 1966: 5). In *A Shroud for a Nightingale* a watching surgeon commentates on the action, explaining the time-honored pedagogical approach as being "the best way. Good for them to learn on each other, better than a seriously ill patient."

The miniseries, more than the written words of the book could do, makes visible the nursing profession as hierarchies and practices change. The nurses, staff nurses, sisters and matron are attired according to rank. Immaculately rendered details such as the style, size and scale of the caps and capes demarcate the ranks and functions. But the series also evokes the nursing profession at a point of change and uncertainty. Both are embodied in the matron, a dominating force in the hospital and in the lives of the student nurses; but as the plot develops, the matron is disgraced when it is revealed that many years ago she had been a Nazi, a past disguised in the present by a new name and an anglicized accent. The matron's suicide is a personal tragedy that foreshadows institutional change. By the end, it is explained by an administrator that she was the last of the line and will be the hospital's last matron. The hospital has at last moved with the times, changing terminology and professional identity.

The changes discussed by characters on screen are repeated from the pages of the novel. The book's 1971 publication meant it was close in time to large scale reports into the ranks of the senior nurses which James, as a civil servant and administrator, would have understood and could deploy as the substance of her fiction. The novel's faithful adaptation into the miniseries meant that the structural, educational and organizational concerns around nursing in the 1970s, the context of the book's publication, came onto the screen in the 1980s. The hospital hierarchy appears on screen at a point of tension and transition. Back in 1968, the real-world Salmon report, issued by a committee chaired by businessman Brian Salmon, reported on a large-scale investigation into the profession, especially its senior ranks. The report, offered in 1967 and piloted from 1967 to 1972 (Allen, 2001: 112), was not the first critical investigation into post-war nursing training. Nor was the training static. A year after the foundation of the NHS, a staff college for Ward Sisters came into existence. A staff college for matrons came into existence in 1953. In post-war nursing, the matron remained a fixed point in a hierarchy, even if the scope of the role varied considerably across institutions. This dual nature—the consistency of title and office, but the inconsistency in the scale of responsibilities—was noted in the Salmon Report. As Dewar noted (1978: 399), a matron could be in charge of 20 beds or 2000 beds, but the title did not differ despite the level of responsibility. The chain of command also differed, for while there would always be a matron, that matron might report to any number of differently titled administrators (Allan and Jolley, 2013: 68). Salmon's report had a controversial impact and afterlife. As Allan and Jolley indicate, the perceived impact of its recommendations was the privileging of bureaucracy and administration, meaning that nurses moved away from clinical work to administrative work, while the recommendations also incurred criticism for stratifying and de-personalizing the nursing profession (Allan and Jolley: 69).

Both the Salmon and Briggs reports had a wider public life. Before, during and after the periods their committees sat and their reports came out, nurses entered public debate on the standards of their profession. Specific instances existed of medical authorities intervening if they found training and standards were deficient. In 1977, the General Nursing Council suspended training in Rugby, on the grounds that the facilities were deficient (*Coventry Evening Telegraph* August 9, 1977: 5).

Conclusion

To conclude, British popular culture, especially the intersecting realms of film and television, presented nurses and nursing to audiences and this essay has considered where this presentation included the training and standards of nursing. Physical and visual exploitation of the actresses portraying nurses is an inevitable component of nursing in popular culture, but alongside glamour and stereotypes this essay also located where scripting, characterization and production realities such as casting changes provided space to show training, and professional expectations were brought

onto the screen. In the real world, nursing was changing and being challenged. Some thought nurses were too clever, others that they were not
clever enough, or else they were too young, or if married would lack commitment. The National Health Service and the Department of Health investigated, questioned and made recommendations about what nurses should
do and what they should learn, and popular culture texts were responsive
to actual shifts in ideas of nursing. Notably the matron still does carry on
and the television series *Getting On* (2009–2012) included a male matron
among the cast, a topical allusion to changes in the NHS and an effort to
restore some reassuringly traditional standards to hospitals but in this
instance presiding a dysfunctional team in a struggling hospital. Having
a man as matron is an intriguing modern adaptation taking the performance of nursing and nursing leadership in popular culture in directions
still responsive to actual NHS developments.

Films and Television Productions Referenced

Angels (1975–1983) BBC.
Carry On Again Doctor (1969) Rank Organisation.
Carry On Doctor (1967) Rank Organisation.
Carry On Matron (1972) Rank Organisation.
Carry On Nurse (1969) Rank Organisation.
Carry On Regardless (1961) Rank Organisation.
Casualty (1986–present) BBC
Emergency Ward 10 (1957–67) ATV.
General Hospital (1972–1979) ATV.
Getting On (2009–2012) BBC.
The Goodies (1970–80) BBC.
Shroud for a Nightingale (1984) Anglia Television.

References

Newspapers and Periodicals

Birmingham Post
Brechin Advertiser
Coventry Evening Telegraph
Daily Mirror
Liverpool Echo
The People
The Press and Journal
Stage and Television Today

Other Sources

Allan, Peta, and Jolley, Moya (2013) *Current Issues in Nursing.* New York: Springer.
Allen, Davina (2001) *The Changing Shape of Nursing Practice: The Role of Nurses in the Hospital Division of Labour.* New York: Psychology Press.

Ayliffe, Graham, and English, Mary (2003) *Hospital Infection: From Miasmas to MRSA*. Cambridge: Cambridge University Press.

Barber, Sian (2013) *The British Film Industry in the 1970s: Capital, Culture and Creativity*. New York: Springer, 2013.

Cooke, Lez (2015) *British Television Drama: A History*. London: Palgrave Macmillan.

Cull, Nicholas J. (2015) Camping on the Borders: History, Identity and Britishness in the Carry On Costume Parodies, 1963–74. In: Monk, Claire, and Sargeant, Amy (eds.) *British Historical Cinema*. London: Routledge, pp. 92–109.

Darbyshire, Philip (2014) Heroines, Hookers and Harridans: Exploring Popular Images and Representations of Nurses and Nursing. In: Daly, John, Speed, Sandra, and Jackson, Debra (eds.) *Contexts of Nursing*. Sydney: Elsevier, pp. 53–70.

Dewar, H.A. (1978) The Hospital Nurse After Salmon and Briggs. *Journal of the Royal Society of Medicine* 71: 399–405.

Feasey, Rebecca (2008) *Masculinity and Popular Television*. Edinburgh: Edinburgh University Press.

Gerrard, Steven (2016) *The* Carry On *Films*. New York: Springer.

Hargreaves, Kevin (2019) *A History of the Male Nurse*. Morrisville, NC: Lulu.

Harper, Sue, and Smith, Justin (2013) *British Film Culture in the 1970s: The Boundaries of Pleasure*. Edinburgh: Edinburgh University Press.

Helmstadter, Carol (2002) Early Nursing Reform in Nineteenth-Century London: A Doctor-Driven Phenomenon. *Medical History* 46, 3: 325–50.

Hunt, Leon (2013) *British Low Culture: From Safari Suits to Sexploitation*. London: Routledge.

Huxley, Dave (2004) Viz: Gender, Class and Taboo. In: Wagg, Stephen (ed.) *Because I Tell a Joke or Two: Comedy, Politics and Social Difference*. London: Routledge, pp. 271–288.

Landy, Marcia (2015) *Cinema and Counter-History*. Bloomington: Indiana University Press.

Merriman, Andy (2011) *Hattie: The Unauthorised Biography of Hattie Jacques*. Aurum.

Petley, J. (1986) The Lost Continent. In: Barr, C. (ed.) *All Our Yesterdays: 90 Years of British Cinema,* London: BFI Books, pp. 98–119.

Purser, Philip (1981) Dennis Potter. In: Brandt, George W. (ed.) *British Television Drama*. Cambridge: Cambridge University Press, pp. 168–193.

Thumim, Janet (2004) *Inventing Television Culture: Men, Women, and the Box*. Oxford: Oxford University Press.

Williams, Kenneth (1993) *The Kenneth Williams Diaries* (ed. Russell Davies). London: HarperCollins.

In Search of Sympathy

Stereotypes and Stiff Upper Lips
in Interwar Nursing

Sarah Chaney

Introduction

In July 1939 the *Nursing Mirror and Midwives Journal* launched a competition to find the "typical" British nurse. Over the summer months, nearly a thousand nurses submitted their portrait photograph in an attempt to "portray the nursing countenance that can be called typical, used in the sense of ideal" ("Typical Nurse Competition: Adjudicators' Report," 1939: 48). The journal was the best-selling nursing publication at the time, and the pictures these nurses submitted indicate something of the variety of British nursing (McGann, Crowther and Dougall, 2009: 44). "This is not a beauty competition in the ordinary sense of the word." The *Nursing Mirror* editors stressed, "It is to find the typical nurse, the nurse whose features suggest not merely beauty of line, but professional capacity and human sympathy" ("Our Typical Nurse Competition," 1939: 616). The journal was careful to publish pictures showing a range of ages, positions and fields, although general hospital nursing predominated. Yet the photographs also show certain common features. All of the nurses pictured were white, while not a single man featured in *Nursing Mirror*'s pages, even though men made up nearly ten per cent of the 1930s nursing workforce in Britain (Abel-Smith, 1960: 257).[1] Nurses in psychiatric and municipal hospitals—more often from working class backgrounds—were also largely absent.[2] Whatever the reality, the middle class white female nurse—with her starched white cap and perfect uniform—firmly represented the nursing ideal on the eve of the Second World War.

The attempt to use a single, striking image to represent nursing in its entirety was nothing new. For over a century after the publication of Charles Dickens' *Martin Chuzzlewit* in 1843–4, the stereotype of the lazy, drunken Sarah Gamp was assumed by nursing reformers and historians alike to represent the realities of private and domiciliary nursing (Summers, 1989). In the second half of the nineteenth century, the romanticized "lady with the lamp," made famous by war reporters and artists in the Crimea, shaped visions of the new Nightingale nurse (Baly, 1997). And, in the First World War, Edith Cavell was neatly transformed into a self-sacrificing saint in the immediate aftermath of her execution (Hallett, 2019: 82–3). All these representations of nursing have been questioned by historians in recent years. However, they have nonetheless shaped both popular perceptions of nursing and nurses' own expectations and self-image in the decades since their inception, as Julia Hallam shows in her analysis of nursing images in the post-war era (Muff, 1989; Hallam, 2000: 8).

In this essay, I place in historical context the three themes identified as important for the image of nursing in the *Nursing Mirror* competition, using nursing textbooks, diaries, memoirs, institutional and committee records and oral histories of nurses who trained in the 1920s and 1930s, largely from the Royal College of Nursing Archive. I begin with "human sympathy," a trait newly emphasized in nursing around the turn of the twentieth century (Chaney, 2020). As I have shown elsewhere, there were definite class overtones to this new framing of nursing care. The emphasis on "finer" feelings such as sympathy was linked to explicit efforts by some reformers—such as Ethel Bedford Fenwick—to turn nursing into a middle-class profession (Rafferty, 1993; Brooks, 2001). The professional status of nursing in Britain was even newer, solidified by the passing of the *Nurses Registration Act* in December 1919. I turn next, then, to "professional capacity." The view of professional identity that followed the introduction of registration was heavily shaped by First World War nursing. As well as the hierarchical structure of military discipline, the Edith Cavell myth popularized the view that *not* to show strong emotion was the hallmark of the modern, professional nurse. Finally, I examine the third theme outlined by the *Nursing Mirror*—beauty of line—in relation to the expectations around femininity and appearance in the interwar period. The good nurse was also a good woman, something visible in both her appearance and her actions.

The interwar period (1918–39) has largely been neglected in the history of British nursing. Existing scholarship has tended to focus on the nursing reforms of the Victorian era, the two world wars and the post-war founding of the National Health Service (NHS). Yet, beginning as it did with the passing of the Nurses Registration Act of 1919, the interwar era is an important moment for the formation of a new nursing identity. While this identity certainly built on prior expectations around class and gender, it was also shaped by changes in education, new freedoms for women, and an increased interest in categorizing so-called "women's work." The nursing image was also affected by changing expectations on women's emotions after the First World War—an avoidance of sentiment, and the desire to show a "stiff upper lip" (Dixon, 2015: 214–6). The image of nursing found in the *Nursing Mirror* can thus be understood as, at one and the same time, an expression of the attitudes of the era, and a means by which nursing leaders actively sought to project a new vision of nursing. The three themes of the competition highlight different elements of this vision.

Human Sympathy: The Emotions of Interwar Nurses

"Sympathy and service is the province of woman" wrote Joseph Johnson, author of several late Victorian advice guides for girls and boys, as the nineteenth century came to an end. "She turns as naturally to sorrow and suffering as the sun-flower to the sun; if she cannot aid by her hand she gives the sympathy of her heart" (Johnson, 1898: 88). Johnson implied that emotion arose from the physical weakness of women, unable to provide aid "by her hand." This form of self-sacrificing sympathy was seen especially in the home, where daughters dutifully attended to sick or aging parents and mothers to their children. The name Joseph most associated with the "serving and loving" of women was Florence Nightingale (Johnson, 1898: 98). No matter that Nightingale had explicitly rejected her family duties, as furiously outlined in her 1852 essay *Cassandra* (Nightingale, 1979). By carefully selecting newspaper quotes, and telling a Nightingale story that ended with her return from the Crimea in 1856, Johnson promoted the popular view of Florence Nightingale as a "ministering angel," smoothing pillows and soothing soldiers with kind words (Johnson, 1898: 100). It was Nightingale's love and service, according to Johnson, and not her efficiency and management skills, which made her the model to induce "many a dear and good girl to become an earnest woman" (Johnson, 1898: 5).

As the twentieth century dawned, this image of the Nightingale nurse remained alive and well. Yet, despite Johnson's choice of words, sympathy was a new addition to descriptions of the ideal nurse, even if a nurse's character and attitude had long been deemed important. "What is a nurse?" asked later editions of Nightingale's *Notes on Nursing*, explaining nursing as a need to move beyond dutiful obedience towards a "calling" which, in some mysterious way, gave one the ability to understand a patient's needs and desires (Nightingale, 1909: 97–9). Eva Lückes, Matron of the London Hospital, broke this skill down into "memory, forethought, cleanliness, calmness, cheerfulness, neatness." These were all traits which could be named but needed little attention or teaching because new recruits knew "without my telling you, how valuable they are, and what a difference all these things make" (Lückes, 1884: 13). Nurses had these skills simply because they were women, and any failing in manner, touch or attitude meant they were "lacking in true womanly pity and tenderness" (Lückes, 1884: 14). A good nurse was simply a good—or earnest—woman.

Although the word sympathy was not often mentioned by nurse leaders in the late nineteenth century, this trait became increasingly associated with nursing in the interwar period (Chaney, 2020). In the 1930s, twice as many nursing textbooks identified sympathy as a valuable trait for nurses as had in the 1920s (although it was still by no means universally mentioned). What, though, did nurses of this era mean by human sympathy? On the one hand, sympathy remained a "natural" female trait, as it had been for Joseph Johnson. On the other, it was a product of a woman's class and education. "The woman who is spoken of as a 'born nurse,'" wrote sister-tutor Alice Jackson in 1934, "will have the same instinctive tendencies as other women, but some of them may exist in her in a particularly strong degree" (Jackson and Armstrong, 1934: 11). "Nature has endowed most women with a natural sympathy for the weak and helpless, great powers of endurance and much tenderness," obstetric physician and bon vivant Comyns Berkeley explained in 1931, "and these qualities, together with the training which is to be obtained at a good girls' school, have given to our country a large body of women who had devoted their lives to social service" (Berkeley, 1931: 9).

While nurse writers of the 1920s and '30s wrote in a more carefully critical vein of the innate womanly sympathy described by Berkeley, most nonetheless tended to agree with him on the importance of training from "a good girls' school." This was a running theme throughout the interwar years, especially by those who viewed nursing as a profession and a career, led by the newly founded College of Nursing. In 1920, a College of Nursing meeting in Leicester described the ideal nursing candidate as having "grace and dexterity through games and exercises—not least by dancing" and "pleasant speech, as well as something to say." The good nurse needed to be able to speak at least one foreign language, keep accounts and write a well-phrased letter while her "good character" meant not only that she was not a liar or thief, "but that she is gifted with social virtues" (*Leicester Mail*, 1920). Most of these skills had little direct relevance for nursing practice. Instead, they were associated with the desire to attract middle- and upper-class girls into the profession.

Voluntary hospitals had begun to recruit matrons and ward sisters from the middle and upper classes in the 1870s. However, well into the twentieth century, large numbers of probationers were still drawn from the working class, especially in provincial hospitals (Maggs, 1983: 73–101;

Hawkins, 2010: 54–5). This led, as Jane Brooks describes it, to a "two-tier system." Throughout much of the interwar period, "gentlewomen" could enter special probationer schemes, undertaking a shorter period of training for which they paid their own maintenance fees (Brooks, 2001). "Working class girls did not go in for nursing." Miss Maden stated in an oral history in the RCN collection, reflecting back on her training in the late 1920s (Maden, 2009). Maden had trained in a fever hospital, where the pay was so low that only those whose parents could afford to subsidize them could manage: most were fellow boarding school pupils.

While other interviewees in this collection found their cohorts more mixed—Sybil Gibbon and Mrs. Pearce, who left school at 16 and 17 respectively, nonetheless found they were better educated than most of their fellow probationers—the nursing elite placed a great deal of emphasis on class (Gibbon, no date; Pearce, 2009). It was by making nursing a middle-class occupation, the College of Nursing believed, that it would be held up as a skilled profession. The College sent representatives to headmistress' conferences to attract privately educated women into nursing, and firmly resisted demands to lower the entrance age from 18, in the hope that working-class girls would be forced to take jobs elsewhere long before they were eligible for admission. As Ellen Musson—chair of the General Nursing Council from 1926 to 1943—put it in 1931, "it is particularly those girls who can remain at school until 18 that we look to for the nursing profession" (RCN7/2/1—folder 3). Nursing organizations made no secret of their elitism, and it hardly seems coincidental that when representatives of these groups began to act in an advisory capacity to filmmakers in the 1930s, depictions of nurses on film were entirely of the middle classes (Hallam, 2000: 39–40)

The new emphasis on sympathy was indicative of this elitism. When society painter George Frederic Watts had depicted "sympathy" in 1892, he painted a stern, well-dressed middle-class woman. Sympathy was not only a female trait but thought to be specific to the so-called "educated" classes (Purvis, 1989: 59–70; Frevert, 2016). After the First World War, nursing textbooks thus shifted their focus away from the domestic skills expected of the working-class woman—cleanliness, orderliness, industry, honesty and thrift—to middle-class ideals of femininity—sympathy, gentleness, patience and tact (Gamarnikow, 1991: 127). Nursing textbooks in the interwar era worried about "manners" and "etiquette" as much as practical skills (Riddell, 1931; Perry and Harvey, 1932; Young, 1932). "This so-called 'hospital etiquette'" explained M. Vivian in 1920, "is little more than the ordinary courtesy to which any well-brought-up girl is accustomed in her own home circle" (Vivian, 1920: 26). The well-mannered middle-class girl made the best nurse—even if, in reality, most nurses were still drawn from the lower middle and upper working class, as the Athlone Committee demonstrated in 1939 (Dingwall, Rafferty and Webster, 1988: 99).

Despite the widespread view that sympathy was a trait natural to middle-class white women, it was not quite the same as the Victorian notion of vocation. Indeed, an over-emphasis on vocation came in for some criticism in this period as having "hampered" the profession (Cochrane, 1930: 11; Pavey, 1930). This led some writers to view sympathy as a skill. According to Violet Young, sympathy came from knowledge and experience—a nurse who had suffered illness herself was better able to understand her patients—as well as observation. "To be thoroughly sympathetic a nurse must study the character and idiosyncrasies of her patient," Young explained, "so that she may be able to bear with the peculiarities which are always accentuated by illness" (Young, 1932: 19) Evelyn Pearce, who wrote the first edition of her popular nursing textbook towards the end of this period, agreed. A patient was in need of "understanding and sympathy" specifically because he could not behave normally while ill. The nurse's sympathy was a psychological skill; her interest in learning to "understand the workings of the human mind" (Pearce, 1937: 2).

These nursing leaders, writing amid a growing interest in psychology in medical circles, placed a new slant on sympathy in their drive to professionalize nursing. While it remained true for them that sympathy was inherent to middle-class white women, it was also a skill that needed to be taught and directed to produce the ideal nurse. The natural sympathy and love of a good nurse "must be directed by intelligence," warned Alice Jackson (Jackson and Armstrong, 1934: 19). If this was not the case, Edgell stressed, "There is a danger that understanding the situation in which another finds himself, we shall read into that situation not his feeling but our own" (Edgell, 1929: 134). While the *Nursing Mirror* was a commercial concern, the competition judges included matrons of London teaching hospitals and a member of the General Nursing Council; all of whom undoubtedly held a similar class and skill based notion of "sympathy" as these nursing textbook authors. The value of human sympathy they aimed to represent, then, was closer to a nurse's professional capacity than we might imagine it to be today. Although it remained a gendered—and class-based—trait, sympathy was also newly presented as an ability that could be taught, rendering nursing a skilled and elite form of women's work.

Efficiency and Order: A Nurse's Professional Capacity

At 7.30 a.m., on 12 October 1915, British nurse Edith Cavell was executed by a German firing squad in Belgium. Cavell had been living in

Brussels since 1907, first as the head of the Ecole Belge des Infirmières Diplomées and, since 1910, as matron of the St. Gilles Hospital as well. Permitted to remain in Belgium after the German invasion which started the First World War, Cavell wrote anonymously in nursing journals of her sympathy for the Belgian people. As a "looker-on," she told readers of the *Nursing Mirror,* "I can only feel the deep and tender pity of the friend within the gates, and observe with sympathy and admiration the high courage and self-control of a people enduring a long and terrible agony" (Our Nurse Correspondent, 1915: 64). Cavell's sympathy was certainly not the passive service described by Joseph Johnson; instead, it drew her into an active role in local resistance networks. She helped more than 200 allied soldiers escape Belgium, and recruited others to the cause (Hallett, 2019: 23). Arrested in August 1915, Cavell was one of just two defendants sentenced to death out of 34 who stood trial on the same day. While she was by no means a leader of the resistance, more recently Cavell's acts have been defined as espionage (Hallett, 2019: 67–8).

In the weeks before her trial and execution, Edith Cavell wrote often from her prison cell to the nurses she had trained. "To be a good nurse one must have lots of patience" she told them drily on 14 September 1915. "Here one learns to have that quality, I assure you!" (Hallett, 2019: 26). Yet Cavell was remembered less for her nursing qualities than for her martyrdom. Her death was quickly adopted for propaganda purposes by British and Allied governments alike, and her genteel, feminine image played an important part in this. "Murdered by the Huns! Enlist in the 99th and help stop such atrocities" read a typical recruitment poster from Essex County, Ontario (Essex County Recruiting Committee, 1915). The Canadian poster featured a photograph of Cavell looking every bit the middle-class English ideal: calm and composed in her neat civilian dress. As Christine Hallett explains in her recent analysis of the Edith Cavell legend, the British government and press quickly produced "a monolithic image" of Cavell as a "patriotic 'martyr'" (Hallett, 2019: 3; 41). In a few years, Cavell had become a national heroine, and remained so throughout the interwar era. In 1932, when Madame Tussaud's asked children which of the famous figures among the waxworks they most wanted to be like when they grew up, Edith Cavell beat male explorers and female pilots alike to take top place (Dixon, 2015: 215).

Edith Cavell offered a new model for nursing in the interwar years, in which human sympathy was part of the nurse's professional capacity. Nursing accounts of her tended to describe Cavell as "calm and composed." Her thin lips, wrote Jacqueline Van Til, who claimed to have been trained by Cavell in Belgium, "denoted strength of will and firmness of character" (Hallett, 2019: 54). This connection between an active, intelligent sympathy and the nurse's professional role helps to explain why sympathy grew in prominence after the passing of the Nurses Registration Act in 1919. Sympathy was, at one and the same time, a skill to be developed and an inborn, womanly trait. As Eva Gamarnikow has argued, the description of nursing as "women's work" was a political strategy employed by nursing reformers in the late-nineteenth and early-twentieth centuries. This tactic enabled them to frame the profession as something separate from and different from medicine, that could only be properly taught and regulated by other women (Gamarnikow, 1991).

The passing of the *Nurses' Registration Act* of 1919 meant greater emphasis was placed by nursing leaders on the development of a nurse's practical skills. The "born" nurse remained a stock character in nursing textbooks, but training was everywhere emphasized as essential. "While some women have a natural aptitude for tending the sick," wrote Charlotte Moles in 1933, "many others have hidden potentialities which can only be developed by training" (Moles, 1933: 1). Other writers stressed that "love, which is a powerful dynamic force, must be directed by intelligence": a nurse who was simply "kind-hearted" might cause "unnecessary pain" by her poor technique (Jackson and Armstrong, 1934: 19). Women still made the best nurses, but only if they were properly educated.

In the post-war period, this emphasis on education also incorporated a newly stressed need to rein in the nurse's natural emotions. Edith Cavell had become a national hero as much for her calm acceptance of her death as for her role in the resistance network. Historian of emotions Thomas Dixon describes her as "one of the first British women to be celebrated for her 'stiff upper lip'" (Dixon, 2015: 216). This new model of calm, stoic womanhood was associated in the press with the very educational background desired by nursing leaders: "boarding-school education and organized games" (Dixon, 2015: 222). Not coincidentally, this had been Edith Cavell's own background, educated first by governesses at home and then at a series of girls' boarding schools between the ages of 16 and 21 (Hallett, 2019: 10). The middle-class female ideal had shifted following the First World War, from the passive sympathy outlined by Joseph Johnson to the calm and practical response demonstrated by Edith Cavell.

Nurse leaders quickly adopted the notion of the no-nonsense modern woman, while admitting that the unemotional nurse—and woman—had her critics. "Accusations have been made from time to time that nurses are hard and callous" noted Mary Cochrane, matron of the Charing Cross Hospital in 1930. She went on to warn, however, about the "vast difference between quiet, knowledgeable, sympathetic help and frothy sentimentality. The calm demeanor of the true nurse does not indicate hardness and insensibility to suffering, only that her training has taught her that emotional outbursts do as much harm during a crisis as anything of a more actively dangerous character" (Cochrane, 1930: 186). Similarly, Manchester matron E. Maude Smith wrote that "Nurses are often said to be 'hard' and callous." Smith drew a distinction between the nurse's inner feelings and outward presentation of them, concluding that "This is never true of a good nurse, but outsiders do not always realize that if a nurse did not control her feelings, she would be of little use to her patient in helping him to bear his sufferings, dread of an operation, etc., bravely and cheerfully" (Smith, 1929: 16).

Emotional restraint became an important—and visible—sign of professional capacity in nursing in this period. "I cried in the kitchen towel more than once" Mrs. Pearce recalled of her training at a Poor Law hospital. Even though it was "heartbreaking" to lose patients, "You don't let anybody see you. You might let the other nurses see, but you don't let the patients see" (Pearce, 2009). The interwar nurse was sympathetic but efficient. She had a good store of womanly sympathy but her training had equipped her with professional control and the ability to appear outwardly calm: that famous stiff upper lip.

The stereotype of the stiff upper lip had itself emerged from the upheaval of war. It came to prominence in Britain during the Boer War (1899–1902) and, by the First World War, was widely presumed to be part of the English national character (Dixon, 2015: 201–3). Some interwar nurse leaders—including founding members of the College of Nursing—had served in the Boer War, while others came to prominence during the First World War, when 17,000 trained nurses served in the armed forces. From 1914 to 1918, these nurses worked close to the front lines for the first time, in Casualty Clearing Stations, on ships and trains as well as in base hospitals, part of a military system that valued strict hierarchy and controlled efficiency (Hallett, 2014). These matrons and nursing leaders carefully avoided "frothy sentimentality"—the most commonly mentioned of all undesirable traits in interwar nursing textbooks—and emphasized the practical side of nursing. Emotional restraint was the hallmark of the modern woman. So too, however, was her appearance.

Beauty of Line: Womanly Love and the Attractive Nurse

"Wipe that rouge off your face!," Dr. Wylie, Head Resident Surgeon, roars at new student nurse Cherry Ames on her first day at Spencer School in the early 1940s (Wells, 2006: 32). But nurse Cherry isn't actually wearing make-up. Her cheeks naturally glow red with health, her dark brown curls glisten, and she is groomed to "crisp perfection." Cherry is slender, healthy and well-built. She moves with grace and looks "vivid as a poster" in her red wool sports outfit, the best-looking suit in her hometown of Hilton (Wells, 2006: 2). While "beauty of line" was certainly not the only quality expected of a nurse in the 1930s—as the *Nursing Mirror* editors had stressed—these descriptions of the fictional Cherry Ames emphasize the importance of appearance for both nursing and young women as the Second World War began. After the war, nursing recruitment literature similarly showed nurses as "young, attractive and fashionable" (Hallam, 2000: 96).

While Cherry Ames—first published in 1943—and her fictional nursing sister Sue Barton—first published in 1937—were both American heroines, their adventures quickly became available on both sides of the Atlantic (Hallam, 2000, p. 33). Their experiences seemed universal to many readers; Julia Hallam recalled being surprised to later discover that the fictional nurses she had grown up with were American, and not British (Hallam, 2000: 48–9). Sue Barton was invented by nurse Helen Dore Boylston, who nursed with the British Expeditionary Forces during the First World War (Hallam, 2000: 48). The author of the early Cherry Ames books, Helen Wells, was a social worker by background. Both applied themselves to the task of writing career novels for young women. The books were extremely popular, especially among their target audience of teenage girls. Over 5 million Cherry Ames books were sold, and Sue Barton sold even better (Finlay, 2010: 1189). It does not, however, seem as if they necessarily led these young women into nursing. Only one of the nurses Julia Hallam interviewed who had trained in the post war period, only one remembered being an "avid reader" of Sue Barton, but even she didn't think it had influenced her choice of career (Hallam, 2000: 152).

In these books, appearance was presented as something that interests young women—Cherry dresses well inside the hospital and out—as well as central to being a nurse. The first thing Sue Barton and her friends learn is how to put on their uniforms correctly, and their first class begins with a stern inspection. "If that's the way you put on your clothes at home," Miss Cameron, their tutor rebukes her charges, "I'm surprised that your family allowed you to go out of the house" (Boylston, 1981: 32). Appearance, like sympathy, was about class as much as gender. Tidy hair, a perfectly pinned collar and a straight apron were the mark of a well-brought up girl. Vivian Warren, one of the few working-class students in Cherry's school, has "cold eyes and [an] overrouged mouth" which "did not seem to belong here" (Wells, 2006: 26). Vivian struggles to fit in, until she finally confides in Cherry and relaxes her guard. In oral histories of nurses who trained in the 1920s and early 1930s, collected by the Royal College of Nursing, appearance was a running theme—more so than emotion, if a little less frequently discussed than practical nursing skills. Miss Maden remembered being told by the matron not to use the front entrance of the hospital because the matron disapproved of her bright blue pill box hat, thinking she looked like an actress. The same matron demanded her nurses wear bright white shoes and stockings—"difficult to buy and so expensive!" (Maden, 2009).

The bright white of nursing uniforms symbolized the sexual purity of the nurse—quite the opposite of the stereotypes associated with actresses. Sybil Gibbon remembers feeling safe when going out as a district nurse late at night because of it: "your uniform was your protection" (Gibbon, no date). It was in part because of these connotations that a nurse must be "careful to wear her uniform with spotless cleanliness, neatness, and simplicity" warned Millicent Ashdown in 1922. Her hair should be tidy, and "her general bearing that of military smartness" (Ashdown, 1927: 1). Even into the 1970s, Julia Hallam notes, "respectability" in nursing was signified by tidy hair, pinned up above the collar, sensible shoes and an absence of jewelry and make-up (Hallam, 2000: 171).

Make-up and jewelry implied loose morals—like that bright blue hat owned by Miss Maden—a significant concern for interwar nursing leaders in Britain, who made no secret of their desire to "keep the register pure" (General Nursing Council, 1922, sec. 02/02/1928). Most of the cases brought before the General Nursing Council Disciplinary Committee in the interwar period dealt with sexual indiscretions—from illegitimate children to affairs with married men—rather than professional misconduct (Chaney, 2019). This was one of the reasons for the imposition of strict discipline in nursing training, which was increasingly described as outdated in the 1930s. When Sybil Gibbon asked for a sleeping out pass to attend a dance, it was nearly refused. "You would have thought I was going out on the streets or something!" She reflected (Gibbon, no date). Sexuality was also a concern for nurse leaders. Matron Lucy Duff Grant recalled in an oral history that disciplinary cases dealing with homosexuality in male nurses—illegal in Britain until 1967—might be judged on the appearance and mannerisms of the accused (Duff Grant, 1983).

It was also assumed that nurses were almost invariably white women. Sue Barton and Cherry Ames both have white friends with Anglo-Saxon names almost all of whom are from comfortable backgrounds (Philips, 1999: 68)—although Cherry does make friends with one Chinese student, Mai Lee. This was also the case in British nursing in the 1930s. While matron of the Manchester Royal Infirmary in 1937, Duff Grant openly refused to take "coloured nurses" for training (Eddo-Lodge, 2017). Black nurses did not appear in British film, even in minor roles, until the 1950s (*Doctor in the House*, 1954, and *Sapphire*, 1959), while the first black nurse in romance literature appeared in 1960. Julia Hallam, in her analysis of images of nursing, notes that these nurses tended to be given a white, middle class identity and a well-spoken English accent (Hallam, 2000: 158). Even in the 1980s, Pam

Smith found that hospital recruitment brochures showed only pictures of young, white, female nurses—at odds with the actual make-up of hospital staff—and physical appearance remained important (Smith, 2012: 44–5). Race and class also intersected. When a Miss Windsor asked if she might entertain her "coloured friends" at the Nation's Nurses and Professional Women's Club (later the Cowdray Club) in 1924, she was quick to inform the committee that these were "men and women drawn from the cultured and educated class." Miss Windsor's request was approved and she thanked the committee for being "so broad-minded" ("Cowdray Club House Committee Minutes, April 1922–December 1927," 1922: 139).

The ideal interwar nurse—for the nursing elite, at least—was white, youthful and middle class. Her perfectly pinned hair and clean, starched uniform made the standards of human sympathy and professional capacity visible, even if ideal appearance was harder to achieve than prescriptive texts might assume. Several oral histories in the RCN archive complain of the cost of uniforms: "I think most of our money went on shoes," Mrs. Pearce recalled (Gibbon, no date; Pearce, 2009). Muriel Hibbert, who began her training at King's College Hospital in 1941, struggled to maintain her uniform during the busy working day a decade later. "Much against my will I had to make up a clean cap," she wrote in her daily diary for 9 January 1952, "the one I have been wearing is so dirty that I dare not even wear it for the last two days of my practical work. I feel that I have abused the King's uniform enough already this fortnight without making matters worse by wearing it looking pale grey when it should be white" (Hibbert, 1952).

It becomes hard to disentangle the physical appearance of the ideal interwar nurse—her "beauty of line" as it were—from her professional and emotional capacities. As Adrienne Finlay describes it, the fictional Cherry Ames' "appealing looks, youth, and wholesomeness allow her to fulfil a dual role as chaste pin-up girl and nurturing caregiver" (Finlay, 2010: 1196). Finlay concludes that, by "renouncing men, sex, and actual motherhood," Cherry becomes the "ultimate mother" (Finlay, 2010: 1204). The efficient, educated but emotionally reserved middle-class nurse was similarly expected to treat her patients as her children: giving them her love and sympathy, but within carefully controlled limits to ensure order was maintained on the ward. "The relationship of the nurse and patient should be characterized by firmness and sympathy without familiarity" cautioned Margaret Riddell in 1931 (Riddell, 1931: 11).

The image of the nurse as mother was particularly important because most nurses were *not* mothers. Before the war, nursing training had frequently been associated with a woman's role in society, especially by medical men and hospital managers; it was work performed before marriage or after widowhood (Hawkins, 2010: 22). "A little training in nursing in the school," psychiatrist James Crichton-Browne suggested in 1904, made "the girl a better wife and mother" (Committees, 1904: 54). Interwar nursing writers continued to see nursing skills as innate, but newly claimed that nursing itself could satisfy the biological maternal instinct, while simultaneously giving a nurse the "knowledge of a job well done" (Edgell, 1929: 125). This retained the idea of nursing as women's work but made it an alternative to a life of domesticity.

Sister-tutor Alice Jackson drew on the psychological theory of sublimation to explain that nurses were able to use their "natural" instincts for purposes other than that of husband and home. "The maternal instinct, often particularly strong in those who choose the profession of nursing," she suggested, "may be redirected or sublimated, so that the nurse gives to her patients a love akin to that which she might have given to her own children if she had been a mother" (Jackson and Armstrong, 1934: 13). "Sublimation" as a psychological term was used in the 1920s by psychologists like William McDougall and W.H.R Rivers to argue that "instinctive tendencies out of harmony with the needs of social life" did not necessarily cause pathology but could lead to "success in all the higher accomplishments of life, especially in art, science, and religion" when diverted (Rivers, 1920: 156). Jackson used this notion to argue that nursing was a very definite career for women, which had as much value as motherhood itself.

It was important to these nursing leaders that the ideal nurse appeared as a womanly, mothering figure. They were fighting against the pre-war panic that a declining birth rate and increasing infant mortality would damage the prosperity of the nation (Davin, 1978; Hunt, 1991, p. 25). This had led to unmarried women being viewed more negatively than they had in the Victorian era (Jeffreys, 1985: 134–5). In one particularly virulent pre-war example, the biologist Walter Heape referred to spinsters as "the waste products of our Female population" (Heape, 1913: 308). Many nurses, especially those who rose to the level of matron, did not marry; the marriage bar in hospitals meant that those who wished to work after marriage were usually pushed into private nursing. The appearance of these women became all the more important—in the absence of a husband and children—in proving them to be "ideal" women.

Conclusion

The judging of the *Nursing Mirror*'s "typical nurse" competition was interrupted by the outbreak of the Second World War. The winners were not announced until 14 October, in a double page spread ("The Typical Nurse," 1939: 38–9). All winners were in uniform—though not all entries had been—and all were white women. Most—like the second and third prize winners—were also young. Yet the photograph of the winner—Miss Violet Dargan, Deputy Sister at the Southern Grove Hospital—suggests a few of the changes that had taken place in the image of nursing since the meek and youthful Nightingale nurse was pictured in the *British Journal of Nursing* some fifty years before. More mature than her fellow prize winners, Miss Dargan looks tall and imposing in her stiff white veil. Her arms are folded over the spotless uniform that symbolizes her professional capacity, and she stares directly into the camera in quiet determination. Her human sympathy is not shown in a smile but in her almost stern restraint; it is difficult to know what she is really thinking or feeling.

The posed photographs of these interwar nurses, with starched uniforms, and calm, reposed faces—offer a telling glimpse into the place of nursing in the early twentieth century. *Nursing Mirror* editors sought human sympathy in the nurses they pictured which, as we have seen, was a newly emphasized trait in twentieth-century nursing. This sympathy was associated with the gender of the nurse and, perhaps even more strongly, with her class. Middle-class women had sympathy, while their working-class counterparts were not expected to possess the same fine feelings as their educated sisters. Yet sympathy was nonetheless presented as more of a skill to be learned than a vocation. It was also, in the interwar era, a trait more associated with Edith Cavell than Florence Nightingale. In this new nursing ideal, human sympathy became part of a nurse's professional capacity. Her practical skills were important, but so too was her ability to restrain her emotions.

Although the image of the nurse—and woman—with the stiff upper lip was new to the interwar period, it was nonetheless used within the nursing elite to justify a continued focus on feminine qualities that appeared increasingly old-fashioned to those outside the profession—and new nursing in training. Some things in nursing, then, did not change even as the place of women—and the work they were able to take up—altered following the First World War. While the image of the interwar nurse was, in some ways, that of the modern working woman, it also continued to draw on long-held beliefs about the need for a vocation and calling within the profession. This placed nursing a little at odds with a new society, in which "the modern woman," as Dr. Hadley put it to the College of Nursing in 1929, "is able to think and act and vote for herself!" (Hadley, 1929: 6).

Both sympathy and professional capacity were, it was assumed, visible in the appearance of the interwar nurse. Her "beauty of line" was not simply an afterthought of the *Nursing Mirror* judges, but a means of quickly evaluating a nurse's worth. A well-presented appearance reflected the expectation that white, female, middle- and upper-class women made the best nurses. Yet this was also associated with changing expectations of women. As nurse leaders began to argue that a career in healthcare might prove a valuable alternative—and not a preliminary—to marriage and motherhood, they had to counter pre-existing negative stereotypes of the spinster as an "unwomanly" being. The nurse was thus presented as the ultimate mother, her womanliness developed, rather than stunted by, her nursing training. "Sister-tutors are always helping to produce, not merely nurses, but women." Alice Jackson told her fellow tutors in 1934 (Jackson and Armstrong, 1934: 5). Yet the kind of women these sister-tutors were hoping to produce was subtly changing. Restrained, efficient but quietly emotional, the ideal interwar nurse was not quite the same as her Victorian and Edwardian predecessors.

Notes

1. There were also black nurses working in the UK at this time. In 1937, Harold Moody's "League of Coloured Peoples" (founded in 1931) protested against the discrimination these nurses faced in hospital employment (Eddo-Lodge, 2017, pp. 15–17).

2. Only two mental health nurses appeared—the editors were so unfamiliar with psychiatric hospitals that they spelt the name of one of them wrong, with Croydon's Warlingham Park Hospital becoming Warlington Park.

References

Abel-Smith, B. (1960) *A History of the Nursing Profession*. London; Melbourne; Toronto: Heinemann.

Ashdown, A.M. (1927) *A Complete System of Nursing*. London: Waverley Book Company.

Baly, M. (1997) *Florence Nightingale and the Nursing Legacy*. 2nd edition. London: Whurr.

Berkeley, C. (1931) *A Guide to the Profession of Nursing: Before and After State Registration*. London: George Newnes.

Boylston, H.D. (1981) *Sue Barton: Student Nurse*. Sevenoaks, Kent: Hodder & Stoughton.

Brooks, J. (2001) Structured by Class, Bound by Gender: Nursing and Special Probationer Schemes, 1860–1939. *International History of Nursing Journal* 6, 2: 13–21.

Chaney, S. (2019) "Purifying the profession": Good Character and the General Nursing Council Disciplinary Committee in the Inter-War Period. *Women's History: The Journal of the Women's History Network* 2, 13: 9–13.

Chaney, S. (2020) Before Compassion: Sympathy, Tact and the History of the Ideal Nurse. *Medical Humanities*. doi: 10.1136/medhum-2019–011842.

Cochrane, M.S. (1930) *Nursing*. London: Geoffrey Bles.

Committees, Great Britain Parliament. House of Commons (1904) *Report from the Select Committee on Registration of Nurses*. London: HMSO.

Cowdray Club House Committee Minutes, April 1922–December 1927 (1922) London Metropolitan Archives, London, A/COW33.

Davin, A. (1978) Imperialism and Motherhood. *History Workshop Journal* 5: 9–65.

Dingwall, R., Rafferty, A.M., and Webster, C. (eds.) (1988) *An Introduction to the Social History of Nursing*. London: Routledge.

Dixon, T. (2015) *Weeping Britannia: Portrait of a Nation in Tears*. Oxford: Oxford University Press.

Duff Grant, L. (1983) Interview with Lucy Duff Grant by Bill Kirkpatrick, Royal College of Nursing Archive, Edinburgh, T/31.

Eddo-Lodge, R. (2017) *Why I'm No Longer Talking to White People About Race*. London: Bloomsbury Publishing.

Edgell, B. (1929) *Ethical Problems: An Introduction to Ethics for Hospital Nurses and Social Workers*. London: Methuen.

Essex County Recruiting Committee (1915) Murdered by the Huns. Ontario, Canada, Imperial War Museum Collection.

Finlay, A. (2010) Cherry Ames, Disembodied Nurse: War, Sexuality, and Sacrifice in the Novels of Helen Wells. *The Journal of Popular Culture* 43, 6, 1189–1206.

Frevert, U. (2016) Empathy in the Theater of Horror, or Civilizing the Human Heart, in Assman, A., and Detmers, I. (eds.) *Empathy and Its Limits*. London: Palgrave Macmillan, pp. 79–99.

Gamarnikow, E. (1991) Nurse or Woman: Gender and Professionalism in Reformed Nursing 1860–1923. In: Holden, P., and Littlewood, J. (eds.) *Anthropology and Nursing*. New York: Routledge.

General Nursing Council (1922) Disciplinary Committee Shorthand Notes. London.

Gibbon, S. (no date) Interview with Sybil Gibbon (née Johnson), Royal College of Nursing Archive, Edinburgh, T/14B.

Hadley, D. (1929) Reform in the Training of Nurses. Royal College of Nursing Archive, Edinburgh, RCN7/2/1.

Hallam, J. (2000) *Nursing the Image: Media, Culture and Professional Identity*. Abingdon, Oxon: Taylor and Francis. Available at: https://ebookcentral.proquest.com/lib/gmul-ebooks/detail.action?docID=165601 (Accessed: 16 November 2020).

Hallett, C. (2014) *Veiled Warriors: Allied Nurses of the First World War*. Oxford: Oxford University Press.

Hallett, C.E. (2019) *Edith Cavell and Her Legend*. London: Palgrave Macmillan. Available at: https://www.palgrave.com/gp/book/9781137543707 (Accessed: 16 November 2020).

Hawkins, S. (2010) *Nursing and Women's Labour in the Nineteenth Century*. Abingdon, Oxon: Routledge.

Heape, W. (1913) *Sex Antagonism*. London: Constable and Company Ltd.

Hibbert, M. (1952) Diary for 1952. Royal College of Nursing Archive, Edinburgh, C780/1/19.

Hunt, F. (1991) *Gender and Policy in English Education*. Hemel Hempstead: Harvester Wheatsheaf.

Jackson, A.M., and Armstrong, K.F. (1934) *Teaching in Schools of Nursing*. London: Faber & Faber.

Jeffreys, S. (1985) *The Spinster and her Enemies: Feminism and Sexuality 1880–1930*. London: Pandora Press.

Johnson, J. (1898) *Earnest Women: Their Efforts, Struggles and Triumphs*. London: T. Nelson.

Leicester Mail (1920) The Perfect Girl, Royal College of Nursing Archive, Edinburgh, RCN17/4/29, 12 July.

Lückes, E.C.E. (1884) *Lectures on General Nursing: Delivered to the Probationers of the London Hospital Training School for Nurses*. London: Kegan Paul, Trench, Trubner & Co.

Maden, M. (2009) Interview with Miss Maden, Royal College of Nursing Archive, T/14A.

Maggs, C. (1983) *The Origins of General Nursing*. London: Croom Helm.

McGann, S., Crowther, A., and Dougall, R. (2009) *A Voice for Nurses: A History of the Royal College of Nursing 1916–90*. Manchester: Manchester University Press.

Moles, C.L. (1933) *Nursing as a Career*. London: Pitman.

Muff, J. (1989) Of Images and Ideals: A Look at Socialization and Sexism in Nursing. In: Jones, A.H. (ed.) *Images of Nurses: Perspectives from History, Art, and Literature*. Philadelphia: University of Pennsylvania Press.

Nightingale, F. (1909) *Notes on Nursing*. London: Harrison.
Nightingale, F. (1979) *Florence Nightingale's Cassandra*. Edited by M. Stark. New York: The Feminist Press.
Our Nurse Correspondent (1915) Brussels Under the German Rule. *Nursing Mirror and Midwives Journal*: 63–4.
Our Typical Nurse Competition (1939) *Nursing Mirror and Midwives Journal*: 616.
Pavey, A. (1930) Nursing as a Profession. *The Zodiac*.
Pearce, E.C. (1937) *A General Textbook of Nursing*. 1st edition. London: Faber.
Pearce, M. (2009) Interview with Mrs Pearce (nee Robertson), Royal College of Nursing Archive, Edinburgh, T/20.
Perry, A., and Harvey, D. (1932) *General Nursing: A Textbook for the State Examination*. London: Edward Arnold.
Philips, D. (1999) Healthy Heroines: Sue Barton, Lillian Wald, Lavinia Lloyd Dock and the Henry Street Settlement. *Journal of American Studies* 33, 1: 65–82.
Purvis, J. (1989) *Hard Lessons: The Lives and Education of Working-Class Women in Nineteenth-century England*. Cambridge: Polity Press.
Rafferty, A.M. (1993) Decorous Didactics: Early Explorations in the Art and Science of Caring, circa 1860–90. In Kitson A. (ed.) *Nursing: Art and Science*. London: Chapman & Hall, pp. 48–60.
Riddell, M.S. (1931) *A First Year Nursing Manual*. London: Faber & Faber.
Rivers, W.H.R. (1920) *Instinct and the Unconscious*. Cambridge: Cambridge University Press.
Smith, E.M. (1929) *Notes on Practical Nursing*. London: Faber and Gwyer (The Scientific Press).
Smith, P. (2012) *The Emotional Labour of Nursing Revisited*. Basingstoke: Palgrave Macmillan.
Summers, A. (1989) The Mysterious Demise of Sarah Gamp: The Domiciliary Nurse and Her Detractors. *Victorian Studies* 32, 3: 365–86.
The Typical Nurse (1939) *Nursing Mirror and Midwives Journal*: 38–9.
Typical Nurse Competition: Adjudicators' Report (1939) *Nursing Mirror and Midwives Journal*: 48.
Vivian, M. (1920) *Lectures to Nurses in Training*. London: The Scientific Press.
Wells, H. (2006) *Cherry Ames: Student Nurse*. Edited by H.S. Forman. New York: Springer.
Young, V. (1932) *Talks to Probationers*. London: Arthur H. Stockwell Ltd.

Nostalgia for Spiritual Community Care

Midwifery as Religious Calling
in Call the Midwife

MORAG MARTIN

> God isn't in the event … he is in the response to the event.
> In the love that is shown, in the care that is given
> —Sister Julienne in *Call the*
> *Midwife* Season 3, episode 4

Introduction

The television show *Call the Midwife* (CTM) (BBC 2012–present) has been popular in both Britain and abroad for its nostalgic depiction of 1950s working-class London Docklands, focusing in on the reproductive lives of women in ways that are not usually highlighted in film and television. CTM begins in 1957, nine years after the advent of the National Health Service (NHS) which gave British citizens access to healthcare, including pre- and post-natal care. At the moral center of the show are the religious sisters who run a midwifery training home. Their work as midwives is anchored in the community by an ethos of Christian unconditional love. As in Jenifer Worth's memoirs, on which it is based, the show's characters are caught between tradition and modernity. They adapt to new medical technology as well as cultural norms, while holding on to their rituals and beliefs. The show contrasts a family centered 1950s with examples of how difficult life was for working class mothers before the advent of reliable contraception, abortion rights, maternity leave, and professional opportunities.

This essay covers the first six seasons of the show when it most closely follows the period of Jennifer Worth's memoirs (2002, 2005, 2009). The show uses historical advisors, including sisters from the Anglican order of St. John the Divine (in the show called Sisters of St. Raymond Nonnatus) and healthcare advisors, to fully evoke the period setting. The 1950s is described by historians as a golden age for domiciliary midwives, who gained status and independence under the NHS (McIntosh, 2012). Yet, this period is also one when the public perception of the primarily white nurse-midwife was of a "ministering angel," a respectable woman sacrificing herself (and her traditional roles as mother and wife) for the good of the community (Hallam, 2000: 133–135). Even today, many still see nursing, and with it midwifery, not just as a profession, but as a calling which combines skills with emotional or spiritual succor.

The vision of nursing, particularly midwifery, as a calling, mimics that of the active sister, whose vow of obedience positions her as willing to take on the most difficult community care. The Sisters of Nonnatus House by default embody obedience and self-sacrifice, subservient to their dual callings. Yet the show complicates their obedience by showing the Sisters standing up to secular authorities and the leadership of their own religious order in the name of medical practice and selfless love or "agape." The Sisters work for the newly created NHS, yet are outside its technocratic tendencies, allying themselves with their patients before the state. They are also often in tension with their own Motherhouse, aligning themselves with nursing/midwifery when their religious rites clash with their professional responsibilities. As the kind and wise head of the house Sister Julienne says in the first episode, "we are all nurses first, and midwives foremost." They take a vow of obedience, but they interpret and enact that vow in ways that sets them apart from the Church, the larger system of healthcare of the period, and ultimately our own current view of birthing as well. This essay argues that the show creates a utopian community of caregivers who are anchored in the governing systems of the NHS and the Church of England, but also rebel against both systems. Lovingly recreating 1950s London Docklands, the show presents the Sisters as both within and outside history—ideal attendants in a rapidly changing landscape both for their patients and the viewer.

A Short History of the Sisters of St. John the Divine

The late 1950s setting of the show yokes its working-class female characters to marriage and motherhood, often with no ability to keep jobs or control pregnancies. The mostly middle-class midwives and Sisters, however, have a professional life outside of marriage and motherhood. When the Anglo-Catholic movement of the mid-nineteenth century established the first Anglican sisterhoods, these women too were pushing back against traditional expectations of womanhood and Protestantism (Reed, 1988). For Victorian women, joining a religious community provided an option for participating in a socially useful profession, such as nursing or teaching (Mumm, 2001).

Though the Protestant wing of the Anglican Church frowned on the creation of religious orders, the emergent Oxford Movement promoted them as a means of helping working-class families during the Industrial Revolution. The movement founded a small group of female religious orders starting in the 1840s, which provided charity for women and children (King, 1999). One of these newly formed institutions was St. John's House, established in 1848 by physician Robert Bentley Todd in order to improve nursing in London's hospitals (Helmstadter, 1993). In this period, both hospitals and nurses had poor reputations, with little training or pay given to staff. The Sisters of St. John, as they were first called, would remedy this lack. As respectable women they oversaw the training of lay working-class nurses for King's College Hospital London or for work as district nurses in private homes (Mumm, 2001).

From the start, the Sisters of St. John wished to take yearly vows of obedience, chastity, and poverty. The male leadership, however, resisted allowing any of the newly formed orders to take vows, as this mimicked too closely the Catholic tradition (King, 1999). In 1862 the Bishop of London allowed the Sisters of St. John a special prayer and a promise of obedience, but nothing more. The Sisters also wished for more independence from the council of St. John's House which oversaw their nursing work. In 1883, Mother Caroline broke off from King's Hospital and St. John's House Council, taking with her all the sisters and nurses to form a new independent order, the Community of the Nursing Sisters of St. John the Divine (Moore, 1988). They expanded their purview, founding St. John's Hospital, as well as a number of other smaller institutions, and continued district nursing. By the turn of the century they opened a small district home in the London neighborhood of Poplar, where they trained nurses for home healthcare. Their goal was to give "ladies and respectable women sound training under a superior and Sisters, with a comfortable and well-ordered home when unemployed" (Southall-Tooley, 1906: 73–74).

The changing state of nursing in Britain led to the Sisters shifting their professional calling to midwifery. When the government created the status of State Registered Nurse in 1920, the Sisters could not compete with the increasing number of secular nursing agencies. By 1923, with only five

Sisters remaining, they gave up running St. John's Hospital and wholly focused on their district nursing work in Poplar and Deptford. In 1930, when Sister Frances, who had been superintendent at a school for midwives, joined the order, they shifted focus to births: they opened three new locations in Poplar specializing in midwifery with a focus on pre and post-natal care (Cartwright, 1968). Sister Frances, who became mother superior in 1933, wished also to embrace "more fully the religious life." She led the order to take life (rather than yearly) vows of poverty, chastity, and obedience for the first time (Csjdivine). Thus the increase in religious obedience occurred simultaneously with the adoption of midwifery, a highly time-consuming profession.

The Sisters' new vocation came under the auspices of the government, as the state in the 1930s moved to regularize midwifery and eliminate the use of untrained matrons. The 1936 Midwives Act set up paid positions run by local councils. This led to greater demand for midwifery education that the Sisters could fulfill. The Central Midwives board recognized the Sisters' training school in 1932 and their post-graduate program in 1938, which included housing for students (Cartwright, 1968). The founding of the National Health Service in 1948 fully transformed midwives into state employees who increasingly worked under the direction of GPs and hospitals rather than as independent practitioners (Hunter 2012). The Sisters worked on an agency basis for the NHS, paying only 10 percent of their costs, with the rest covered by the councils of Poplar and Deptford (Cartwright, 1968). Though this meant they no longer had to depend on charitable donations and private patients, they had to abide by new regulations both in care and in the training of students.

Over time, government agencies looked to increase their oversight. The 1962 Local Government Act gave borough councils control over health services, leading to the closure of the Deptford home in 1966. Poplar was also rapidly changing: the closing of the docks and the advent of the birth control pill shifted the demographics of the area. The midwives went from attending 100 births a month to only four or five (Worth, 2009). Nevertheless, the Sisters continued to run their midwifery training school, as well as teaching at Mile End Hospital (Cartwright, 1968). Declining numbers, both of infants and recruits to the order, eventually forced the Sisters to close their Poplar home in 1978. Today, the Sisters are located in Birmingham with each individual sister choosing her own professional calling (Csjdivine). Thus, the order is no longer associated with midwifery as a secular calling linked to religious life. Across both Anglican and Catholic religious orders, the combination of bureaucratization of healthcare and declining numbers of postulants has led to most orders focusing on individual career choices rather than a unified calling.

Traditional Midwifery and the NHS

While CTM overall presents the NHS as a hugely positive force that gave working class families access to healthcare for the first time, it is also presented as an impersonal force, separating the residents of Poplar from their homes and traditions. Hannah Hamad (2016) argues that the show first aired at a time when the Tory government harshly criticized the quality of NHS services, undermining its credibility with the public. In contrast, CTM presents nurses who provide a standard of care no longer available in the contemporary world, emphasizing their "affective labor." That nostalgic care, however, is presented as outside the purview of the NHS, making the argument that the bureaucracy itself was already tarnished even in its early years. CTM presents an alternative system of complete healthcare that transcends what the NHS can offer. The Sisters provide not just midwifery for Poplar, but nursing visits and a close collaboration with the local GP. Together with the neighborhood police and curate (both of whom are romantically involved with secular midwives), they create an idealized vision of comprehensive social, emotional, and medical care focused on community yet paid for by the state.

Both Worth's memoirs and the show make clear that the experienced duo of elderly sister-midwives, Julienne and Evangelina, are highly effective teachers, who support young trainees with personal care and encouragement that goes beyond what the NHS hospital system offers. The Sisters provide a hot cup of tea and abundant amounts of cake at any hour for midwives returning from night deliveries. In contrast, Worth describes the hospital wake up calls as "a bang on the door and that would be that," summarizing her nurses training as "four years of tyranny from hospital nursing hierarchies…" (Worth 2002: 29, 27). Indicative of the appeal of communal living and training, in Season 3, Jenny (the main character based on Worth's lived experiences), lures nurse Patsy from the London Hospital to train in midwifery, despite Patsy's antipathy towards Catholic orders (episode 5). Yet, during the 1950s, midwifery became increasingly a sub-specialty of nursing, losing some of its independence. Few nurses who trained as midwives ever finished the course, leading to shortages of midwives (McIntosh, 2012). On CTM, in contrast, the secular nurses may laugh at the Sisters' habits and rituals, but they value the support they receive from them and remain deeply loyal to their system of care.

Importantly for their students, the Sisters still teach and use hands-on midwifery for such complications as breech births, skills increasingly left out of hospital training programs. In Episode 1, Season 2, secular midwife Trixie is faced with fixing a prolapsed cord of an obese mother stuck on a cargo vessel. Her previous training failed to address such an emergency, under the assumption that the patient would undergo a C-section in a hospital setting. Due to an injury, Sister Evangelina cannot assist, but her years of experience means that she is able to both pray for the child and coach Trixie to a happy ending. Not only do the trainees learn new skills from the Sisters, so does local G.P., Dr. Turner, who often defers to their greater experience. Rightly so, as during the 1950s–'60s, most G.P.s learned obstetrics by shadowing a midwife.

Despite depending on traditional birthing techniques increasingly abandoned by the NHS, the Sisters adopt and teach new medical procedures. For instance, they administer enemas and pubic shaving, as well as injecting pethidine for pain. Yet, the Sisters do push back against innovations that they feel are either unrealistic for their patients or potentially harmful. In an episode set in 1958, CTM first introduces the use of gas and air, even though by 1952, 62 percent of births already used it whether attended by doctors or midwives (McIntosh, 2012). Since the midwives do not have a car to transport the machine to homes, Dr. Turner must cope with the increasing demand for pain relief (Season 2, Episode 1). Sister Evangelina is reluctant to promote this new-fangled device as it places a burden on the already overworked Dr. Turner and sidelines the midwives. Despite introducing us to a new form of pain relief that mothers enthusiastically adopt, by the next episode the focus returns to the Sisters' hand skills and emotional succor, coaching all types of mothers through an unmedicated and successful birth.

The show often plays Sister Evangelina's reluctance to adopt new ways for laughs. But her stubbornness becomes lethal when she pushes back against bottle feeding. In her memoirs Worth explains that the Sisters ignored NHS promotion of bottle feeding because keeping the bottles clean was unworkable for women living without running water (Worth, 2002). On the show, there is no such explanation. Instead Evangelina states categorically "breast is best" (season 4, episode 1). Twenty-first-century viewers may sympathize with Sister Evangelina's fight against aggressive powdered-milk companies and the enthusiasm of younger midwives and mothers for fads. Unfortunately, Evangelina's unwavering focus on breastfeeding is interpreted as dogma by an insecure mother, which endangers the life of a newborn. Evangelina retreats to the Motherhouse in shame for having forgotten her vow to protect her patient and act as a "vessel for God" (in season 5, episode 2). Despite this reckoning with her own flaws, Evangelina's heart and purpose remain pure. The traditional means of hands-on midwifery and focus on mother-infant bond represented by the Sisters stand out as the gold standard lost today alongside enemas and pubic shaving.

The engaged and cathartic births supervised by the Sisters reinforce the image that homebirths provide the ideal place for bringing a new life into the world. Nonnatus House has a very low rate of mortality and no newborns perish in the Sisters' hands. TV shows prior to CTM often depicted midwives as the choice of hippies, inevitably associating home births either with humor or disaster (Kline, 2007; Luce, et al, 2016). Along with a number of more recent reality television shows documenting the work of actual midwives, CTM provides a counter to that vision, showing home births to be safe and preferable to hospital births (Takeshita, 2017).

The show's positive depiction of home births contrasts with the bureaucratic care shown in NHS funded hospitals. The women of Poplar fear the hospital due to its historical resonances with the poor house, preferring the capable hands of the Sisters of Nonnatus. CTM juxtaposes the warmth and joy of home births, to the cold, impersonal experience of hospital births. Jenny experiences this first hand when she returns to the London Hospital for a stint in the maternity ward. The 1960s was a period in which hospital care became fragmented—with delivery suites and recovery rooms (Hunter, 2012). Jenny is dismayed by the strict time table, separation of units, and brisk treatment of patients. Unable to follow an anxious patient into the delivery room, she returns to Nonnatus in order to emotionally and physically support her patients throughout the birth process (in season 3, episode 7).

Hospital births, however, were on the rise by the 1930s, and many women who lived in poverty preferred them to giving birth in their less than ideal living conditions. As early as 1935, 58 percent of the women in Poplar had hospital births. Increasingly, working-class women wanted to be taken care of in free teaching hospitals, unlike the women on the show who prefer to give birth at home no matter their circumstances (Marks, 1996). The Royal College of Obstetricians and Gynecologists set a goal of 70 percent hospital births in 1944. The main reason they did not get to 100 percent by the 1960s was lack of beds, rather than lack of will from the medical community or lack of demand from mothers (Rivett, 2019). The show does underline that, for some women, hospital births are preferable: women who need rest from their large families as well as women with complications (in episode 8, season 2). Despite these exceptions, throughout the first six seasons the show depicts hospitals as unnecessary for most and certainly not as comfortable as home.

The solution to impersonal hospital care and the often unhygienic and cramped conditions of homes in Poplar is the creation of a maternity home. Maternity homes were common in the 1950s and many trained midwives. In season 3, Dr. Turner sets one up, ostensibly for patients who need more monitoring. Rather than being in competition with Nonnatus House, as it would have been historically, the maternity home works in tandem with the midwives. The show creates a model system of healthcare, where GPs, nurses, and midwives cooperate and work together as a loving family. No mention is made of how these different systems are funded and administered. Unlike Worth's portrayal of multiple and anonymous GPs, Dr. Turner is the only one available for countless patients. The community of care the midwives and Dr. Turner represent provide personal, supportive, and holistic care for not just pregnant women, but the entire population of Poplar. Historically, however, due to shortages of midwives in the 1950s, GPs took on more births, while midwives focused instead on antenatal and postnatal care. This division of work often created gaps between providers, rather than create a coordination of care (Hunter, 2012).

The Sisters provide total care: pre-natal, births, and post-natal. That continuity of care, however, also imposed extreme work hours and hardships on midwives who took it on. District midwives of the 1950s were perpetually over-worked and over-booked due to high numbers of births as well as the growing burden of doing pre- and post-natal visits provided by the NHS. On CTM, this extreme work-ethic is used to mend broken hearts (Jenny) or delay reckoning with addiction (Trixie). In the show, many young, unmarried women who became domiciliary midwives lived together in small communities. Most midwives were single since traditional marriage clashed with the long hours that the profession required (McIntosh, 2012). The camaraderie and somewhat enforced celibacy represented in the show reflects the larger world of midwifery.

The community of care depicted in the show stands in contrast to the bureaucratization of the NHS and in solidarity with the working class community of Poplar. Tania McIntosh (2012) argues, however, that by the 1950s the professionalization of midwives distanced them from families in poorer districts. The matron who had been one with the community disappeared to be replaced by a middle-class, hospital trained midwife who often bullied and looked down on her patients. The main secular midwives on CTM, including Jenny, Trixie, Cynthia, Chummy, and Barbara, are very much fish out of water in the East End, failing at times to empathize with their patients' extreme hardships. The Sisters have little patience for the secular midwives' revulsion towards their patients' living conditions (in season 1, episode 1). The Sisters provide an entry to this foreign culture by being both medical and spiritual anchors to the community. Their habit keeps them separated from the drink, sex, and sometimes violence which envelops the lives of their patients, but they are not unwanted do-gooders. Sister Evangelina, from a working-class background, bonds directly with her patients through humor and bluster, but even the more aristocratic Sisters are trusted by the population. In a telling scene, an older woman, whose husband is being cared for by Sister Winifred, feels threatened by the arrival of Nurse Barbara Gilbert (in season 4, episode 7). She mistakes Barbara for a government worker come to interfere with her home. Only when Sister Winifred visits alongside Nurse Gilbert does the older woman relax. Residents of Poplar fear government intervention in housing, hygiene, and traditions even as they welcome medical care. The Nuns, in their wimple and whites, represent the traditional means of care, given by charity and the Church, not government agencies. In this way they are both working for the NHS, but remain perceived as outside it by their patients.

The coverage of disability illustrates one of the ways the Sisters supplement and supersede the sometimes callous services provided by the NHS. The Sisters embody the belief that patients are more than their diagnoses, respecting the life of any child. When juxtaposed with medical procedures, the Sisters' prayers underline the show's message that life is never without hope, even if raising a disabled child in 1950s Docklands remains a daunting task (Wilder, 2017). When Sister Julienne discovers a thalidomide infant (born with phocomelia and only as a trunk) left by hospital staff alone to die, she is shocked by the cruelty of this act. She prays for the dying baby (from Isaiah 43:1) and lies to the mother about its death as there is "no virtue in truth that is cruel" (in season 5, episode 4). Since God did not cause this baby's suffering and the doctors cannot heal it, they are left with the words of the medieval mystic Hildegard of Bingen: "God hugs you, you are encircled by the arms of the mystery of God." By inserting spirituality into the limited medical options for children with disabilities, including those caused by unnatural means such as the administration of thalidomide for morning sickness, CTM gives hope to both the characters and the audience that goes beyond the offerings of the NHS system of medicine (Nussbaum, 2015).

Midwifery and the Religious Life

That hope based in spirituality is what makes the Sisters' community exceptional both in the 1950s and today. Yet, in order not to alienate more secular audience members, the Sisters only vocalize their religious beliefs with permission from their patients. Though they work closely with Tom Hereward, the local curate, they are not integrally placed within the larger Anglican Church and the show hardly ever shows church services led by clergy, other than for major life events like weddings and baptisms. Just as the show creates a fully supportive community of healthcare professionals, aided by the larger community, it provides an alternative model of religious life outside the rigors and judgment often associated with church institutions. The Sisters provide care with love and compassion without question, accepting their patients for who they are. Though midwifery historically clashed with religious vocations, CTM makes the connection seem natural and long-lasting. Ultimately their vow of obedience focuses outwards to the health of their community, rather than inward to their religious vocation.

Instead of prayers over infants or admonitions to attend church, the show uses shots of the Sisters singing at Compline to illustrate how their faith ties to their patients' struggles, be they moral or physical. The psalms they sing match what we watch unfolding: forgiveness and love for those who have entered prostitution, had an abortion, or fallen on hard times, but judgment (albeit kind) for the men who trapped women into these situations. As the show progresses, more and more of the secular midwives sit outside the chapel listening to the chanting in order to investigate their own hearts and souls: Chummy when she is considering going to Africa as a missionary, Jenny when she is tempted to return to her married lover. The shots of the chapel remind us that the medical work done by these women is girded by faith.

The prayers are aimed at providing hope rather than admonitions for patients in difficult and often morally complex situations. The Sisters look past their patients' circumstances because their central motto is "mothers and babies first," focusing their gaze foremost on healthcare. The Sisters have lived long enough in Poplar to have seen all aspects of human misery and suffering. The older Sisters do not bat an eye at a whole host of sinful behaviors: incest, bigamy, abortion, prostitution, gambling, homosexuality, and more. Instead they focus on the medical issue at hand. Only young novice Sister Winifred is shown struggling with her religiously taught aversion to homosexuality and pre-marital sex (in season 4, episodes 3 and 4). The Anglican Church in some quarters will adapt its beliefs to historical circumstances, giving it more flexibility towards issues of reproduction, contraception, and sexuality than the Catholic Church (Creighton, 2009). The Sisters may frown on unmarried women accessing the newly developed birth control pill, but they accept that many married mothers will benefit from contraception. Though the Sisters do struggle to adapt to some of the rapid social changes occurring in the 1960s, they do so in the context of their community. Ultimately they view the world through the eyes of that community, rather than through a lens of moral censorship.

As well as being open-minded, the Sisters know they have limited means to reform their patients so they must accept them as they are. Sister Julienne tells Jenny that she could not have stopped a desperate woman's abortion attempt. She argues, furthermore, that focusing on the illegal nature of the act once it is done would destroy a family rather than make things right (Season 2, Episode 5). The show stresses that the Sisters' general approach of giving attention, love, and prayer is what helps families take responsibility and heal their souls. Sister Julienne stresses to her more romantic charges that they cannot save every patient. On only one occasion does she break her own rule, interfering in the life of a pregnant prisoner. In this case, Julienne makes clear that her meddling is based neither in sentimentality nor ignorance of the world's harsh realities, but on a strong feeling that this one patient can be saved (in season 3, episode 3). Ultimately, this one individualized act reinforces the Sisters' focus on the patient's well-being, rather than taking on larger systemic problems in the community. They always provide hope and love, as well as medical care, but do not assume that their faith will bring healing for all.

The Sisters never question that their medical work is girded by faith, demonstrating that religious and professional callings can function in harmony. Yet, the media image of the sister-nurse stresses a woman whose dual sacrifices lead to explosive tensions. In films, that notion of sacrifice of self is often threatened by the presence of a handsome leading man— such as *White Sister* (1923, 1933), *The Sin* (1972), and *Change of Habit* (1969). The important exception to this theme of romantic love overcoming faith is the *Nun's Story* (Zimmerman, 1959). Though the film attempts to show religious life sympathetically, its heroine Sister Luke leaves the order when her vow of unquestioning obedience clashes with her medical calling during World War II and she is accused of "singularizing" herself. By the time of the film's release, some nuns criticized it for representing an old-fashioned, austere version of religious life, no longer relevant to their experiences (Sullivan, 2005: ch. 3).

Historically, the practice of midwifery has been even harder to ally with religious calling than nursing. Before the nineteenth century, midwives were mostly married post-menopausal women, who had experience with their own childbirth. A virginal sister midwife did not fit social expectations. The Catholic Church specifically refused to recognize orders which mixed midwifery with religious vows, because it saw birth as too carnal. Many religious congregations of nurses refused to even care for pregnant patients, as to interact with a sexualized body might threaten their own well-guarded purity. Only in 1936 did Pope Pius XI authorize religious sisters to take on midwifery training in the context of missionary work (Martin, 2018). By contrast, the Anglican Church never had a specific ban against midwifery or work with pregnant patients. The Sisters of St. John had a long history of caring for pregnant patients and overseeing midwifery by secular nurses, but they did not train or practice it themselves until the 1920s (Cartwright 1968). CTM avoids allusion to the tension between birthing and the vow of chastity, implying that midwifery had been an integral part of the community since its founding in the 1890s.

The professions of both nursing and midwifery clash with religious life in their competition for time. Religious orders require regular time for prayer, contemplation, and fasting. In the *Nun's Story*, Sister Luke's religious commitments compromise her nursing work (Babini, 2012). Even more than nursing, midwifery demands flexibility of time and commitment. Recognizing this, the male spiritual head to the Sisters of St. John the Divine gave them a shorter Daily Office book in 1942, since as an active order they did not have the time to do the complete Breviary (Cartwright, 1968). In CTM, time conflicts between the two callings are quickly solved. The Sisters interrupt their time of silence or moments of prayer to take on a crisis or even a new health focus. For instance, Sister Winifred receives permission to skip Compline so she can educate prostitutes on the use of condoms (in season 4, episode 3). As seen in their unwavering support for the entire community, theirs is a professional calling that often takes precedence to their religious rituals.

The duo of experienced midwives, Sister Julienne and Sister Evangelina, never question the relationship between their faith and their medical calling. It is the young recruit, Sister Winifred, who makes visible the tension between her religious vocation and the practice of midwifery. Originally trained as a teacher, Sister Winifred finds adapting to midwifery hard since it was not her original calling and is not directly linked to her faith. Yet, she perseveres and finds the joy that other characters feel at births (Season 3, Episode 4). From their inception, Anglican orders put a strong emphasis on members having the ability to do the work asked of them, not simply having a religious vocation. Sisterhoods, however, stressed that religious vows should come first: "her life in God always comes before the thought of her work for God" (Mumm, 2001: 19). Yet, in CTM, not having a calling as a midwife would mean rejection from the order. Fortunately, Sister Winifred becomes a competent midwife, as all the characters do in the show. The show leaves out not just the high number of nurses who trained in midwifery yet never practiced, but also the postulants who never took their final vows (Mumm, 2001).

If the Sisters' ability to be true to both their patients and their God is at the center of the utopian spiritual community, this is because the show makes clear that their obedience should not be focused on institutional structures and rigid rules. The vow of obedience taken by the Sisters, as with more modern orders, stresses the root meaning of obedience "to listen," rather than to obey without thought. The nuns of CTM integrate their vow of obedience, as well as poverty and chastity, into their professional calling as midwives, underlining the importance of their medical independence. Obedience plays out at Nonnatus as a focus on the health of the community, embodied by Sister Julienne's authority over which patients are prioritized and which midwife/nurse is assigned to a given job. Unlike the bureaucratic division of labor at the hospital, Julienne's assignments are undergirded by her faith and her focus on love, emphasizing for the secular midwives that they too are committed to a calling. Though the secular midwives sometimes push back against Julienne's rule over their day-to-day lives, her touch is always benevolent.

In contrast, the larger Church hierarchy (be it Catholic or Anglican) as well as the Motherhouse function as distant and sometimes unthinking forces in the lives of the Sisters and midwives. In a key series of episodes (Season 6, Episodes 1–3), the Motherhouse sends Sister Ursula to replace Sister Julienne. Ursula has none of Sister Julienne's patience, warmth, or flexibility. Sister Ursula hopes to save Nonnatus House from government interference by imposing efficiencies which end up endangering the life of a newborn. Sister Julienne refuses to obey Sister Ursula's rules, modeling rebellion for the younger Sisters and midwives. In this way she pushes back for today's audience against the aspects of religious life that seem most onerous; not the prayers and rituals but the need to obey a distant and often cold hierarchy represented by the Motherhouse. Ultimately, Ursula retreats to the Motherhouse, leaving Nonnatus once more under the benign rule of Sister Julienne, but not before predicting that the time-consuming care given to patients will soon clash with the bureaucracy of the NHS.

The tensions between the Motherhouse and Nonnatus is also stressed in the episode arc surrounding Sister Mary Cynthia's depression (in season 6, episodes 3–6). Sent to the Motherhouse to heal, she apparently disappears. She is found by elderly and eccentric Sister Monica Joan in a grim, impersonal insane asylum, forced to undergo Electroconvulsive Therapy without her consent. Monica Joan cries out in horror, exhorting that they must "muster our cohort, we must instruct our troops—an innocent is in danger." This cry to battle could be the motto for the entire show, since it embodies the ethos of unity and solidarity that Nonnatus represents for both inhabitants and patients. In contrast, the show depicts the Motherhouse as an impersonal force, making poor medical decisions about a fellow Sister that do not take into consideration the tropes of love and compassion. Only when Julienne frees her from the asylum, does Cynthia receive care that is of a standard we would find acceptable today. Here, as in many other episodes, it is the community of health professionals, including Dr. Turner, who make this transfer possible—reinforcing the way this pseudo-family of practitioners creates the best possible model of spiritual healthcare not only for their patients, but for themselves as well.

Conclusion

Despite the many ways midwifery and religious vocations have clashed historically, CTM presents an image of active sisters whose work is essential to both the physical and spiritual health of mothers and infants. It presents the twin vocations as an essential part of community oriented healthcare based in love, forgiveness, and hope. The sisters work for the newly created NHS, but are firmly outside its technocratic tendencies, embracing tried and true traditions while nevertheless providing the best care possible. They push back not only against the state, but against the larger church system as well, underscoring that their healthcare is part and parcel of their spiritual calling and vows, rather than separate from it. The show depicts a utopian community of caregivers rebelling against systems of control, while at the same time foreshadowing the dismantling of this community.

Midwifery became increasingly secularized and bureaucratized since the SJSD left Poplar in the 1970s, with the majority of midwives today working within the hospital system. Recently both scholars and activists have questioned if birth attendants need to be distinct and divided from spirituality. Indigenous communities have called for a return to spiritual practices in births, either through the use of local midwives or the incorporation of rituals in hospital settings. Western secular systems of care have also started promoting the nurse-midwife as integral to the spiritual care of patients (Delaporte and Martin, 2018). CTM, though set in a nostalgic past, reimagines how midwives can support mothers and their families through personal bonds, spiritual understanding, and unending amounts of tolerance and love. Though it is not entirely a realistic vision of how births occurred in the past or can occur in the future, it provides an ideal that may allow mothers to rethink and resist the current systems of hospital obstetrics as effectively as other forms of activism.

FILMS AND TELEVISION PRODUCTIONS REFERENCED

Call the Midwife (2012–present) BBC.

REFERENCES

Babini, Elisabetta (2012) The Representation of Nurses in 1950s Melodrama: A Cross-Cultural Approach. *Nursing Outlook*, Supplement Issue: Nursing and the Media, 60, 5: S27–35.

Cartwright, F. (1968) *The Story of the Community of the Nursing Sisters of Saint John the Divine*. Leighton Buzzard: Faith Press.

Community of Saint John the Divine Website. https://www.csjdivine.wordpress.com/history/.

Creighton, Phyllis (2009) Anglican Faith and Reasoning: Wrestling with Fertility Issues. In Blyth, Eric, and Landau, Ruth (eds.) *Faith and Fertility: Attitudes Towards Reproductive Practices in Different Religions from Ancient to Modern Times*. London: Jessica Kingsley Publishers, pp. 57–85.

Delaporte, Marianne, and Martin, Morag (eds.) (2018) *Sacred Inception: Reclaiming the Spirituality of Birth in the Modern World*. Lanham, MD: Lexington Books.

Hallam, Julia (2000) *Nursing the Image: Media, Culture and Professional Identity*. London: Taylor & Francis Group.

Hamad, Hannah (2016) Contemporary Medical Television and Crisis in the NHS. *Critical Studies in Television* 11, 2: 136–50.

Helmstadter, Carol (1993) Robert Bentley Todd, Saint John's House, and the Origins of the Modern Trained Nurse. *Bulletin of the History of Medicine* 67, 2: 282–319.

Hunter, Billie (2012) Midwifery, 1920–2000: The Reshaping of a Profession. In Borsay, Anne, and Hunter, Billie (eds.) *Nursing and Midwifery in Britain Since 1700*. London: Palgrave Macmillan, pp. 151–176.

King, Peter (1999) *Western Monasticism: A History of the Monastic Movement in the Latin Church*. Kalamazoo, MI: Cistercian Publications.

Kline, Kimberly N. (2007) Midwife Attended Births in Prime-Time Television: Craziness, Controlling Bitches, and Ultimate Capitulation. *Women and Language* 30, 1: 20–29.

Luce, A., Cash, M., Hundley, V., Cheyne, H., van Teijlingen, E., and Angell, C. (2016) "Is it realistic?": The Portrayal of Pregnancy and Childbirth in the Media. *BMC Pregnancy and Childbirth* 16, 1: 40.

Marks, Lara (1996) *Metropolitan Maternity: Maternal and Infant Welfare Services in Early Twentieth Century London*. London: Rodopi.

Martin, Morag (2018) Midwifery as Religious Calling: The Struggle for Church Recognition by the Sœurs de la Charité Maternelle of Metz in the Nineteenth Century. In Marianne Delaporte and Morag Martin (eds.), *Sacred Inception Reclaiming the Spirituality of Birth in the Modern World*. Lanham, MD: Lexington Press, pp. 3–22.

McIntosh, Tania (2012) *A Social History of Maternity and Childbirth: Key Themes in Maternity Care*. London: Routledge.

Moore, Judith (1988) *Zeal for Responsibility: The Struggle for Professional Nursing in Victorian England, 1868–1883*. Athens: University of Georgia Press.

Mumm, Susan (2001) *Stolen Daughters, Virgin Mothers: Anglican Sisterhoods in Victorian Britain*. London: Bloomsbury Publishing.

Nussbaum, Emily (2015) *Call the Midwife*, a Primal Procedural. *The New Yorker* June 20. https://www.newyorker.com/magazine/2016/06/20/call-the-midwife-a-primal-procedural.

Reed, John Shelton (1988) "A female movement": The Feminization of Nineteenth-Century Anglo-Catholicism. *Anglican and Episcopal History* 57, 2: 199–238.

Rivett, Geoffrey (2019) 1948–1957: Establishing the National Health Service. Nuffield Trust. 2019. https://www.nuffieldtrust.org.uk/chapter/1948-1957-establishing-the-national-health-service.

Southall-Tooley, Sarah (1906) *The History of Nursing in the British Empire*. London: S.H. Bousfield.

Sullivan, Rebecca (2005) *Visual Habits: Nuns, Feminism, and American Postwar Popular Culture*. Toronto: University of Toronto Press.

Takeshita, Chikako (2017) Countering Technocracy: "Natural" Birth in *The Business of Being Born* and *Call the Midwife*. *Feminist Media Studies* 17, 3: 332–46.

Wilder, Courtney (2017) Television Dramas, Disability, and Religious Knowledge: Considering *Call the Midwife* and *Grey's Anatomy* as Religiously Significant Texts. *Religions* 8, 1: 209.

Worth, Jennifer (2009, originally 2002) *The Midwife: A Memoir of Birth, Joy, and Hard Times*. London: Penguin.

Worth, Jennifer (2009) *Farewell to the East End*. London: Penguin.

Media Representation of the Nursing Queen Archetype in Its Socio-Cultural Context

MERLE TALVIK, TAIMI TULVA,
ÜLLE ERNITS *and* KRISTI PUUSEPP

Introduction

This essay analyzes the emergence and development of the Nursing Queen Archetype and its media representation, specifically in Estonia, a subject matter and place generally unfamiliar to English-language scholarship. The media creates heroes and idols and represents them over time and change. The Nursing Queen archetype can be used to understand different nursing cultures in different periods of historical and social development (Talvik, Tulva & Ernits, 2021). The archetype of the Nursing Queen is first traceable and applicable to Florence Nightingale (1820–1910) (see also Richard Bates's essay in this volume). Living and working in Victorian England, she influenced the whole of Europe. In Estonia, the Queens of Nursing as a distinctive type of nursing leader emerged at times of rapid and profound changes. During the first Estonian Republic (1918–1940), society modernized and various professions developed rapidly. Two Nursing Queens were recognized at that time. Nurse Anna Erma began to disseminate the ideas of Florence Nightingale. Anette Massov was a leader of practical nursing in the first Republic of Estonia. During the Soviet period (1940–1991), nursing came under ideological pressure. Nevertheless, a new Queen, Ilve-Teisi Remmel, appeared and continues working in re-independent Estonia (since 1991). For the record, The Soviet occupations of Estonia were in 1940–1941 and 1944–1991, when the territory of the Republic of Estonia was occupied by Soviet Russia and later by the Soviet Union. During the occupation that lasted from 1940 to 1941, the Estonian SSR was annexed to the

Soviet Union. In 1941, the Soviet occupation of Estonia was replaced by the German occupation. In 1944, Soviet troops conquered Estonian territory and the second Soviet occupation began.

Socio-Cultural Background to the Queens of Nursing

Ideas spread through personalities. Together with the mental models of individuals, social representations are part of the cognitive interface of social structure, group membership and discourse (Dijk, 2005). When an individual speaks or writes as a member of a group, his or her membership begins to influence the context through the social representation that the group shares, that is, in the form of group knowledge, attitudes, and ideologies (Dijk, 2005). Social representations are created through communication and collaboration. They are social constructs that emerge and are preserved in a specific cultural and historical context (Wagner, et al., 1999).

Representations are manifested in people's speech, thinking and behavior (Bauer & Gaskell, 1999), but also in cultural products (such as images, texts, and discourses). These cultural products are physical objects that reach us, which we can also observe and analyze from a distance. These objects have acquired meaning based on the context and manner of use. The concept of historical discourse is important in Foucault's approach and is relevant here. Stuart Hall (1997: 46) notes: "Foucault argues that things mean something and are true only in a specific historical context." Teun A. van Dijk (1998, 2005) further develops the meaning of context and its role in representation, introducing a new understanding and concept to discourse analysis. The rules and norms of discourse are socially common (Dijk, 2005). Thus, an understanding of interpretation and representation is not possible without a context that in turn arises and is influenced by the culture in which the communication takes place.

The media is linked to ideology and is considered an essential condition for successful propaganda (McQuail, 2000; Hiebert & Gibbons, 2000). Texts, concepts and images that have an ideological content or aspect cannot be understood, regardless of who uses them and why. In representation, van Dijk considers ideologies to be decisive. He creates a theoretical conceptual zone in which ideology is the basis of social representations (Dijk, 2005). In his opinion, no group can exist or function socially without the identity of the group and the ideological beliefs shared by the members of the group (Dijk, 2005).

The points regarding nursing made in this essay are taken from research into and interpretation of images, media coverage and biographies. Data collection and analysis were conducted from 2018 to 2020. The media coverage included newspapers and journals, and biographical material comes from the collections of the Estonian Health Museum and Estonian History Museum, as well as from church books. Historical images offer opportunities to discuss the cultural specifics of nursing development and characterize the subjective journey of personalities. The photograph carries signs and meanings from which the peculiarities of the era and the encounters of cultures can be read (Frank & Lange, 2015). The socio-cultural and historical context provides a framework for the analysis of the media representation of the story of nursing. This story's interpretation takes into account Pierre Bourdieu's theory that "Understanding begins primarily with understanding the field what we have developed into and in opposition to" (Bourdieu, 1993: 38). Bourdieu analyzes not only the "fields" but also the people in these fields, particularly the reasons why they act the way they do. Bourdieu discusses artists, writers and other people working in the field of culture, but is theory can also be taken more generally, that is, to think of a person in any field working in a social space as an "agent." Social "agents" do not exist in a vacuum, but in a complex institutional network that empowers, enables and legitimizes their activities. The agents are free in their decisions and choices only insofar as the field allows. The field offers space for possibilities for everyone involved. Due to this space of possibilities, the agents of a certain era are established in space and time and are relatively dependent on the direct conditions of the economic and social environment. The possibilities offered by history determine what is possible or impossible to do or think in one given field at a given moment in time (Bourdieu, 2003).

The biography, the trajectory of human life (Bourdieu, 2003), is a chain of positions occupied one after the other in successive stages of the social field, formed as a result of the interaction of both social conditions and subjective personal experiences and situations. Thus, it is very difficult to answer the question of why one or another person chose a particular path, but given the person's life trajectory, relationships, affiliation and position in the social field and the choices that life could offer at any given time, it is possible to construct an analysis of representation of the Nursing Queen archetype in Europe, including Estonia.

This essay is framed by a biographical approach. "Biographical turn" means the rapid spreading of biographical research as a recognized critical scientific research method. "The individual's point of view and human experience are used as a methodological tool" (Renders, Haan & Harmsma, 2017: 3). Thus, in this present essay, the era, events, and participants in them are constructed on a mental level using primary sources, and the story is interpreted accordingly. The focus is on media presentations and the development of the Nursing Queen archetype in this process.

The Archetype of the Nursing Queen and Its Representation

An archetype is a permanent structure that has developed in the collective subconscious and that manifests in the consciousness as a universal motif or image. The archetype has been formed because of the common imagination of many people and has thus acquired a concrete form. It is one way of dealing with personality and its conduct. Behavioral role models are also important (Jung, et al., 1968). In the following, the archetype of the Nursing Queen will be opened on the personal background of the charismatic pioneers of nursing.

Florence Nightingale as the World's First Nursing Queen

Florence Nightingale, widely acclaimed as the founder of modern nursing, is called in some quarters and according to some representational models, the Queen of Nurses (Shetty, 2016). The prerequisites for her becoming this figurative queen were her good education and the ability to speak many languages; her participation as a nurse in the Crimean War (1853–1856); being the first nursing theorist; her pioneering role in conceptualizing nurse education; initiating health and sanitation reform; being a methodological researcher and futurist; and finally writing about 200 books. Following her enthusiastic activities in the Crimean War, Florence Nightingale has become a symbol of patience and caring for the sick and wounded in difficult conditions (Talvik, et al., 2021), although, for women of Florence Nightingale's social status, becoming a nurse was not considered appropriate. In Britain in the mid–1800s, nursing was not a highly respected profession. Hospitals were dirty, unpleasant places, and to the wealthy parents of a young woman of higher social status, such an endeavor seemed like a nightmare (Selanders, 2020).

Nightingale is one of the most obvious and most represented nurses in the world, and her actions have fed an enduring iconography. In Crimea, she walked the wards at night, offering support to patients; with this, she earned the nickname "Lady with a Lamp" because that is how, with a lantern in her hand, she went to check the health of wounded soldiers. "She is a guardian angel in these hospitals without any exaggeration, and so soon as her slender body glides down the corridor, the relief and gratitude are seen in the face of every soldier," was an account written in *The Times* during the Crimean War (cited in Sarapuu, 2020: 2).

The "Lady with the Lamp" is the most stereotypical image of Nightingale, in the closest connection with which the archetype of the Queen of Nursing has developed. Such an image of Nightingale is represented in many works of art. The artist who created the most influential painting is Henrietta Emma Ratcliffe Rae (1859–1928). She was a prominent English painter of the late–Victorian era, who specialized in classical, allegorical, and literary subjects. "The Lady with the Lamp" (1891), depicted Florence Nightingale at Scutari in Crimea (Seibert, ca. 2012). The Mary Evans Picture Library (Evans, n.d.), a collection of historical images, contains a total of 63 different images of Florence Nightingale, of which 15, or nearly 24 percent, depict her walking between the rows of beds or nursing the sick in the barrack hospital at Scutari.

Nightingale's activities were noticed and acknowledged during her lifetime. In 1855, Queen Victoria donated a gold enameled brooch to Florence Nightingale. This brooch, the design of which was supervised by Prince Albert, is engraved verso with a dedication from Queen Victoria "To Miss Florence Nightingale, as a mark of esteem and gratitude for her devotion towards the Queen's brave soldiers, from Victoria R. 1855" (Evans, n.d., 1119386). The brooch plays an important role in noting the iconography of Nightingale as the Nursing Queen, showing that her work was recognized by the state.

Nightingale is also reflected as a pioneer in visualizing data. Using infographics, she effectively distinguished statistical data. In addition to her Nursing Queen status, Nightingale has also been considered a "Design Hero" (Andrews, 2019) because she presented her arguments in the form of easy-to-understand graphical images.

Apart from being a dedicated nurse, Florence Nightingale was noted for her writing and also for the nursing school she established. Florence Nightingale was one of the most prolific nursing writers of the nineteenth century (Hallett, 2020). In 1859 Nightingale wrote *Notes on Nursing: What It Is and What It Is Not*, the first textbook of modern nursing (Nightingale, 1859). This book has been published repeatedly around the world. Nightingale set up a nursing school at St Thomas' Hospital in 1860 (Andrews, 2019). The school, which was the first professional nursing school in Europe, operated for 31 years (Lewis, 2019). The Nightingale School was very popular—students came from all over the world to attend the school. After graduating, they returned to their homeland, mainly as managers and trainers (Talvik, Tulva & Ernits, 2020b).

Nightingale was an independent, economically secure civilian, who did not submit to official military and medical hierarchies but carried out a revolution in health care. Men in high positions did not believe in her ideas, fearing admission of their own carelessness, mistakes, and incompetence

(Talvik, et al., 2021). She became a popular hero, a queen, whose writings, photographs and other images were constantly published in newspapers and magazines.

Nightingale's thoughts were characterized by rational optimism and an attempt to move towards a more decent world. According to Nightingale, humanity provides a constant opportunity for development and improvement. Swedish researcher Hans Rosling called such people "possibilists," meaning people who have a clear idea of things, a conviction and hope that further development is possible. Mankind can constantly improve itself (Andrews, 2019). There are 10 monuments and memorials dedicated to Nightingale in various European cities (*Monuments and memorials*, 2020). It is no coincidence that two Latin words have been carved in stone above one of her monuments in London relating back to her dominant iconography of the lamp, but also evoking scriptural associations: FIAT LUX: "Let there be light."

The Queens of Estonian Nursing

Florence Nightingale's principles and ideas have been applied in Estonia. The implementation of these ideas has been mainly led by three pioneers of Estonian nursing—Anna Erma, Anette Massov and Ilve-Teisi Remmel (Talvik, et al., 2020b). In Estonia, nursing began in churches and monasteries in the 1700s. In the mid-eighteenth century, the first nurses trained in Russia came to work in the newly opened hospitals in Estonia (Sooväli, 1998). Later, several nursing homes and nursing schools were opened. During the period of the first Republic of Estonia (1918–1940) nursing grew into a profession and enjoyed high prestige. Continuous training of nurses began, facilitated by the formation of the Estonian Nurses Association. At periods of change people recognizably need heroes and two Nursing Queens were recognized in Estonia. They precisely understood the nature of the era, were receptive to Nightingale's ideas and carried out developmental leaps in Estonian nursing. This process has been mediated to us by the media in its various manifestations.

Anna Erma (1884–1974), referred to as "the mother of Estonian nurses" (Reinart, 2019: 12), was educated at the Bethesda Strelna Deaconess House in St. Petersburg. From 1907, she worked as a deaconess in Germany, Russia and Finland. She was a surgical nurse in German military hospitals during the First World War (active 1914–1917) and the head nurse at Tallinn Military Hospital during the Estonian War of Independence (from 1918 to 1920). Erma also stayed in France and Switzerland for a while to become acquainted with the work and care of the hospitals there (Reinart, 2019).

Like Nightingale, Erma devoted her entire life to her profession; she was one of the founders of the Estonian Nurses Association in 1923 (A.H.L., 1974). One of the first and most important tasks of the association was to establish a nursing school, as various nursing courses could not replace the traditional school. Thus, the school for nurses at the University of Tartu was opened in 1925 (Talvik, et al., 2021). Anna Erma was invited to be the head of the boarding school, which operated there until the school was closed in 1941 (*Anna Erma*, n.d.).

Anna Erma has been of interest to the Estonian media mainly in connection with this nursing school (Otsasoo, 1940; Reinart, 2019). The articles written about her are indicative of attitudes espoused at the school, the ideology of training of nurses, the practices in the school down to the descriptions of the school uniform. Photos from the Estonian Health Museum show Anna Erma with colleagues and alumni of the school. The education at the nursing school was based on religious principles, as Anna Erma herself had experienced. The meals began and ended with a prayer, and spiritual songs were sung in the hall. The school and boarding school had certain rules that were followed by both the students and teachers (Talvik, et al., 2021).

Like Nightingale, Erma considered it important that theory should be closely linked to practice and said that "there is no time to study at the sick-bed" (cited in Reinart, 2019: 14). Erma's School of Nurses laid the foundation for the further development of nursing principles for future generations. Therefore, Anna Erma can be considered the first Queen of Estonian Nursing. She was also recognized by the state. The Estonian state awarded her with the medal of the Red Cross for participating in the Estonian War of Independence (*Anna Erma*, n.d.).

During the same period, another Nursing Queen arose out of and was highlighted by the Estonian media. She was Anette Massov (1883–?), who also received her first education in St. Petersburg. Later Massov studied at the Red Cross School of Nurses in Tallinn. Immediately after graduating (1904), she went to the Russian-Japanese war, taking part in it as a front-line nurse (*Rahvusvaheline teenetemärk*, 1939). She operated in the ambulance train of the Grand Duchess Maria Pavlovna of Russia. Massov received several awards for her activity during the war: Maria Pavlovna and the Russian Tsar Nikolai II awarded a silver and a gold medal to Massov (Kikas, 2018; Talvik, et al., 2021). Thus, she was respected and figuratively crowned queen even before the foundation of the first Estonian Republic (1918).

After 1914, nurse Massov took part in the First World War, staying on the front-line part of the time (*Rahvusvaheline teenetemärk*, 1939) and she was awarded the George Cross fourth degree (Kikas, 2018). In 1919 Massov was appointed a head nurse at the Central Hospital of Tallinn. She worked continuously in Tallinn hospitals, being one of the few nurses who had taken part in the two wars and also treated soldiers wounded in the War of Independence (*Rahvusvaheline teenetemärk*, 1939). Together with her studies, Massov worked as a head nurse for 37 years. Like Nightingale, she had to go through very difficult trials, especially in the Far East and in the First World War, where her work sometimes resulted in her coming under fire. On May 12, 1939, Anette Massov was awarded the Florence Nightingale Medal and given a photo of Florence Nightingale. The medal was awarded for services performed on the battlefield and during peacetime by the Florence Nightingale Society, based in Geneva (Kiviranna, 1939; Talvik, et al., 2021).

The articles about Massov published in the Estonian newspapers and in the Estonian nursing magazine "Eesti Õde" are mainly related to the Nightingale Medal awarded to her (*Rahvusvaheline teenetemärk*, 1939; Põder, 1997), connecting one queen to another. Anette Massov was and is the only Estonian to receive the Nightingale Medal. The tradition could not continue, because the Soviet occupation interrupted the continuity in Estonian nursing. The career of both Nursing Queens of the first Estonian Republic ended with the arrival of Soviet occupation: Erma emigrated together with many Estonian intellectuals and Massov disappeared without trace during Second World War.

Together with the arrival of Soviet power, the image of nursing and the stereotype of a nurse also changed. For the Soviet regime, health care was not only an individual right but also a "political act" (Starks, 2017: 1718). Health care was politicized according to the communist ideology of the Soviet state. Next to the figures of a female tractor driver and an astronaut, a nurse taking part in Second World War and carrying a weapon appeared in the media. Stalin-era gender policy promoted the mass involvement of women in the work process and social activities (Kivimaa, 2015), the change of their roles and the change of social attitudes, and these were represented in media and visual culture. Nursing was a cult profession during the Soviet era, closely associated with ideology. It was expressed in hundreds of posters, murals and other tools of visual propaganda.

In nursing, this political direction led to the period of suppression and hierarchy, closure, and stagnation of development. The nurses worked under ideological pressure and had to follow the doctors' orders exactly. All the work and training of the nurses was politicized (Kõrran, et al., 2008). The description of the main role of a nurse in publications was astounding. Nurse's chief responsibility was described as "accurately carrying out physician orders" (Kalninš, Barkauskas & Šeškevičius, 2001, p.142). The publications did not mention the independent role of a nurse in the assessment of patients' conditions, planning and application of nursing care (Ernits, et al., 2019).

By the 1980s the health care systems of the Baltic region were lagging far behind Western standards. There was a shortage of employees, medicine and equipment. The ratio of hospital beds and patients was disproportional. The main shortage was of support staff, including nurses and paramedics (Healy & McKee, 1997). The fall of the Soviet Union caused the collapse of the health care system of the time and the system had to restart from scratch (Ernits, Talvik & Tulva, 2019). The new crisis highlighted the need for a new nursing leader and paved the way for arrival of the third Nursing Queen, Ilve-Teisi Remmel (born 1938).

Ilve-Teisi Remmel chose the specialty of a feldsher (that is, emergency treatment and ambulance practice). In 1957, she graduated from Tallinn Medical School and entered work life. Remmel gained her first experiences as a nurse and leader in Soviet times. In photographs from that time, Remmel, appearing as a Soviet-era boss, sits at a large table and wears a headdress typical of the era and profession.

When the time of awakening came in the end of the 1980s, the radical changes in nursing began. When the borders were opened, international co-operation could resume, especially with the Finnish and Swedish nurses. Again, it was possible to talk about the Nursing Queens Florence Nightingale and Anna Erma. Ilve-Teisi Remmel organized conferences dedicated to Nightingale and Erma and numerous meetings to introduce their ideas (Remmel, 2020). Continuous self-improvement and international training, which had only been possible since 1989, ensured success for Remmel in various positions: feldsher, nurse, head nurse and leading specialist in the field of nursing (Talving, 2020; *Kõrgkooli auliige,* n.d.). Being an active developer of nursing, Remmel consistently supported bringing the training of nurses to the level of higher education. The renewal of nursing became her life's work (Talvik, Tulva and Ernits, 2020a).

Remmel herself has participated in various nurses' forums. Her activities have been echoed in Estonian health specialty journals, and Remmel's professional work has been reflected in the 80th anniversary book of Tallinn Health Care College (Talving, 2020). Ilve-Teisi Remmel achieved the highest that could be achieved in the field of nursing. She was a member of the board of the Estonian Nurses Association (ENA) from 1967 and in 1988–2002 she was the chairwoman of ENA. From 1990–1993 she was the president of the Baltic Nurses Association, and from 1999 to 2015 she was a member of the board of the Estonian Council of Health Care Managers. From 1998–2002 the chairman of the Health and Social Work Professional Council and since 2003 a member of the Tallinn School Health Council.

Since the beginning of the nineties, when there was a difficult transition period in Estonia, Remmel has helped many people in need, participating in charity through a Christian organization (Remmel, 2008). Faith and commitment have played an important role in Remmel's life and her contribution to the development of Estonian nursing is meaningful. Like the aforementioned queens, Ilve-Teisi Remmel has received national recognition and her diverse activities have been widely noticed. Remmel is an honorary member of the two health care colleges of Estonia. The Order of the Red Cross was conferred upon her in 1999 and in 2006 she was awarded the Order of Honorary Citizen of the City of Tallinn for organizing nursing care in Tallinn (Talvik, et al., 2021).

Coda

The main goal of this essay was to describe how the Nursing Queen archetype rose and was created, with specific attention to Estonia. The key people and the course of their lives were placed in their social and cultural context. Media representation offer opportunities to discuss the cultural peculiarities of the story of Estonian nursing against the background of the archetype of being a queen.

Florence Nightingale became a leader and reformer of nursing firstly because of the many prerequisites of nature and the environment, including religion, origin, and a very thorough and varied education. Secondly, the time when she was born created the preconditions and at the same time required a person with such qualities to be further noticed. She fought to free herself from the restrictions imposed on women by Victorian society, and carried out a complete revolution in nursing. Her legacy comprises a very large number of written texts that are of interest even today. Media coverage contributed greatly to her becoming a figurative queen. What made Nightingale a Queen were her intelligence, energy, and determination that allowed her to work passionately and with great determination.

Florence Nightingale's ideas were eventually represented globally. Nightingale created a school that carried a whole system of values as a symbolic capital that combined the upbringing, education, and behavioral culture that nursing school students had to embrace and follow. Equally strong was the nursing culture in Estonia created by Anna Erma and Anette Massov, which also included, in addition to nursing activities, norms of behavior, attitudes, principles of being a nurse and being a responsible person. Evidence of this culture is noticeable in various cultural products, texts and images that date back to that time and have now reached the general public. This nursing tradition developed constantly until the Soviet era lowered and ruined it. In the 1980s, a gradual liberation began, the ideas of the Western world penetrated through the Iron Curtain, and this gave the opportunity to act and created a favorable surface for the third Estonian nursing leader, Ilve-Teisi Remmel. It was possible to start changing the status of the nurses again. Society needed a new health hero and the media helped to create it.

The ideas of Nightingale have been developed in Estonia for over 100 years. In 1875, as an elderly and experienced advisor, Nightingale wrote to her graduates the following lines, what became an important credo of her life's work: "A woman with a healthy, active tone of mind, plenty of work in her, and some enthusiasm, who makes the best of everything, and, above all, does not think herself better than other people because she is a 'Nightingale Nurse,' that is the woman we want" (Nightingale & Nash, 1914: 108). This credo has influenced many generations of nurses and helped to create a meaningful frame for their activities.

During times of change, societies need symbolic figures, strong personalities, whose behavior is worthy of being exemplified and whose activities become archetypal. Nightingale's ideas about patient-centered care were represented in the winds of change in Estonian society and achieved sustainable development under the leadership of the Queens of Estonian nurses. The awakening of new potential leaders in nursing, health care and other areas of society is relevant and very possible in the current context of a pandemic, when we, as a society are facing a situation we have never known before. The role of the media in a chaotic situation is very important. People are waiting for evidence-based explanations and possible solutions to the situation, and the media is able to provide these. There is always a part of the past in the future, and so future leaders need a legacy from the past leaders to induce a different kind of change in society.

References

A.H.L. (1974) Anna Erma: In Memoriam. *Vaba Eesti Sõna*, 1 August, 31: 11.

Andrews, R.J. (2019) Florence Nightingale Is a Design Hero. May Her Light Forever Shine Bright. *Medium*, 15 July, [online]. Available at: https://medium.com/nightingale/florence-nightingale-is-a-design-hero-8bf6e5f2147 [Accessed 15 June 2020].

Anna Erma, n.d. [manuscript] Tallinn: Estonian Health Museum.

Bauer, M.W., and Gaskell, G. (1999) Towards a Paradigm for Research on Social Representations. *Journal for the Theory of Social Behavior* 29, 2: 163–185.

Bourdieu, P. (1993) *The Field of Cultural Production. Essays on Art and Literature* (R. Johnson, ed.). Cambridge: Polity Press.

Bourdieu, P. (2003) *Praktilised põhjused. Teoteooriast* (translated by L. Tomasberg). Tallinn: Tänapäev.

Dijk, T.A. van (1998) *Ideology: A Multidisciplinary Approach*. London: Sage Publications.

Dijk, T.A. van (2005) *Ideoloogia: Multidistsiplinaarne käsitlus*. Tartu: Tartu Ülikooli Kirjastus.

Ernits, Ü., Puusepp, K., Kont, K.-R., and Tulva, T. (2019) Development of Estonian Nursing Profession and Nurses' Training: Historical, Political and Social Perspectives. *Professional Studies: Theory and Practice* 5, 20: 9–27, [online] Available at: https://svako.lt/uploads/pstp-2019-5-20-2.pdf [Accessed 21 August 2020].

Ernits, Ü., Talvik, M., and Tulva, T. (2019) Nursing Education in the Wind of Changes: Estonian Experience. In: *Proceedings of the International Conference on Research in Education, Barcelona, Spain.* Diamond Scientific Publication, 1–14, [online] Available at: https://www.dpublication.com/wp-content/uploads/2019/05/icreconf-60-174.pdf [Accessed 21 August 2020].

Evans, M., n.d. *Mary Evans Picture Library. The Widest Range of Historical and Cinema Images for Editorial and Creative Use,* [online] Available at: https://www.maryevans.com/ [Accessed 19 August 2020].

Florence Nightingale. A Life from Beginning to End (2018) Hourly History.

Frank, G., and Lange, B. (2015) *Sissejuhatus pilditeooriasse. Pildid visuaalkultuuris.* Translated by K. Kaugver. Tallinn: Tallinna Ülikooli Kirjastus.

Hall, S. (1997) *Representation: Cultural Representations and Signifying Practices.* London: Sage Publications/Open University.

Hallett, C.E. (2020) Nightingale, Florence: Visions and Revisions. In: Sironi, C., and La Torre, A. (eds.) *Proceedings of International Conference on the History of Nursing,* 13–15 February 2020, Florence, Italy, 139–145. [online] Available at: http://www.florence2020.org/download/conference-proceedings [Accessed 7 December 2020].

Healy, J., and McKee, M. (1997) Health Sector Reform in Central and Eastern Europe: The Professional Dimension. *Health Policy and Planning* 12, 4: 286–295.

Hiebert, R.E., and Gibbons, S.J. (2000) *Exploring Mass Media for a Changing World.* London: L. Erlbaum Ass. Publishers.

Jung, C.G., von Franz, M.L., Henderson, J.L., Jacobi, J., and Jaffé, A. (1968) *Man and His Symbols.* New York: Dell.

Kalnins, I., Barkauskas, V.H., and Šeškevičius, A (2001) Baccalaureate Nursing Education Development in Two Baltic Countries: Outcomes 10 Years After Initiation. *Nursing Outlook* 49, 3: 42–147.

Kikas, T. (2018) Annette Vilhelmine Massov (Massow). *Geni, 13 January,* [online] Available at: https://www.geni.com/people/Annette-Vilhelmine-Massov/6000000008495367869 [Accessed 10 July 2020].

Kivimaa, K. (2015) Naiste Rollid ja õigused kui riikliku propaganda osa. *Feministeerium,* 29 October, [online] Available at: https://feministeerium.ee/naiste-rollid-ja-oigused-kuiriikliku-propaganda-osa/ [Accessed 23 August 2020].

Kiviranna, R. (1939) Rahvusvaheline teenetemärk Tallinna halastajaõele: kes oli Florence Nightingale? *Eesti Kirik,* 20, 773: 7.

Kõrgkooli auliige Ilve-Teisi Remmel., n.d. Tartu Health Care College Website, [online] Available at: https://www.nooruse.ee/et/korgkoolist/ajalugu/auliikmed/ilve-teisi-remmel [Accessed 10 July 2020].

Kõrran, T., Onoper, A., Pruuden, E., Roots, E., Ruul-Kasemaa, K., Saluvere, T., Sarv, H., and Õunapuu, M. (2008) *Sammud käänulisel teel: Eesti õenduse arengutest 21. sajandini.* Tartu: Eesti Õdede Liit.

Lewis, J.J. (2019) Biography of Florence Nightingale, Nursing Pioneer. *ThoughtCo. Humanities: History & Culture,* 21 July, [online] Available at: https://www.thoughtco.com/aboutflorence-nightingale-3529854 [Accessed 16 June 2020].

McQuail, D. (2000) *McQuaili massikommunikatsiooni teooria.* Tartu: Tartu Ülikooli Kirjastus.

Monuments and Memorials to Florence Nightingale, 2020. Wikimedia Commons, 7 March. [online] Available at: https://commons.wikimedia.org/wiki/Category:Monuments_and_memorials_to_Florence_Nightingale [Accessed 25 January 2021].

Nightingale, F. (1859) *Notes on Nursing. What It Is and What It Is Not.* Reprint 2018. Foreword by V.M. Dunbar, preface by M.B. Dolan, New York: Dover Publications.

Nightingale, F., and Nash, R.N. (1914) *Florence Nightingale to Her Nurses: A Selection from Miss Nightingale's Addresses to Probationers and Nurses of the Nightingale School at St. Thomas's Hospital.* Reprint 2007. London: Macmillan.

Otsasoo, M. (1940) Vestluses Anna Erma'ga. *Eesti Naine* 3: 39–40.

Põder, M. (1997) Esimene ja seni ainuke Florence Nightingale'i medali pälvinud eesti õde—Anette Massov. *Eesti Õde* 2: 18.

Rahvusvaheline teenetemärk Eesti õele, kes ravinud haavatuid kolmes sõjas (1939) *Uus Eesti*, 129, 13 May, [online] Available at: https://dea.digar.ee/cgi-bin/dea?a=d&d=uuseesti19390513.2.95 [Accessed 17 August 2020].

Reinart, H. (2019) Eesti haiglaõdede esiema. *Postimees, Arter*, 11 May 12–14.

Remmel, I.-T. (2008) Kui jõuluajal on teistel kõigil keegi…. *Teekäija*, 12, [online] Available at: http://teek.ee/index.php/teemad/8-persoon/442-kui-jouluajal-on-teistel-koigil-keegi [Accessed 21 August 2020].

Remmel, I.-T. (2020) *On the Development of Nursing in Estonia*. Interviewed by T. Tulva. [Telephone interview, recording, transcription]. Tallinn: 6 June.

Renders, H., de Haan, B., and Harmsma, J. (2017) The Biographical Turn: Biography as Critical Method in the Humanities and in Society. In: Renders, H., de Haan, B., and Harmsma, J. (eds.) *The Biographical Turn: Lives in History*. New York: Routledge, pp. 3–11.

Sarapuu, B. (2020) Daam lambiga viis ellu revolutsiooni kätepesus. *Postimees, Aja Peegel*, 6 May, pp. 1–4, [online] Available at: https://leht.postimees.ee/6966189/daam-lambiga-viis-ellu-revolutsiooni-katepesus [Accessed 12 May 2020].

Seibert, S. (ca. 2012) *Henrietta Rae*. Sartle: Rogue Art History, [online] Available at: https://www.sartle.com/artist/henrietta-rae [Accessed 7 December 2020].

Selanders, L. (2020) Florence Nightingale: British Nurse, Statistician, and Social Reformer. *Encyclopædia Britannica*, [online] Available at: https://www.britannica.com/biography/florence-nightingale [Accessed 16 June 2020].

Shetty, A.P. (2016) Florence Nightingale: The Queen of Nurses. *Archives of Medicine and Health Sciences* 4, 1: 144–148.

Sooväli, E.-M. (1998) Õenduse ajalooline ülevaade maailmas ja Eestis. *Eesti Õde*, 1: 18–19.

Starks, T.A. (2017) Propagandizing the Healthy, Bolshevik Life in the Early USSR. *American Journal of Public Health*, November, 107, 11: 1718–1724.

Talvik, M., Tulva, T., and Ernits, Ü. (2020a) Florence Nightingale'i pärand ja selle peegeldused Eesti õenduse teerajajate tegevuses. In: T. Tulva, M. Talvik, K. Puusepp, Ü. Ernits and P.E. Routasalo (eds.) *Eesti õendus ajas ja muutumises: Teadus- ja õppemetoodiliste artiklite kogumik*. Tallinn: Tallinna Tervishoiu Kõrgkooli väljaanded, A, pp. 43–72, [online] Available at: https://ttk.ee/sites/ttk.ee/files/js/16.10.20_TTK_Odede_kogumik_1-140_veeb.pdf [Accessed 7 December 2020].

Talvik, M., Tulva, T., and Ernits, Ü (2020b) Nursing in Estonia and Its Initiators in the Context of Florence Nightingale's Ideas. In: Sironi, C., and La Torre, A. (eds.) *Proceedings of International Conference on the History of Nursing*, 13–15 February 2020, Florence, Italy, pp. 79–80. [online] Available at: http://www.florence2020.org/download/conference-proceedings>= [Accessed 7 December 2020].

Talvik, M., Tulva, T., and Ernits, U. (2021) Representation of the Nursing Queen Archetype in the Context of Social Changes in Estonian Society. *Folklore: Electronic Journal of Folklore*, 82. Tartu: Folk Belief and Media Group of the Estonian Literary Museum, Institute of Estonian Language USN.

Talving, S. (ed.) (2020) *Kuldlõige: Tallinna Tervishoiu Kõrgkooli kaheksa kümnendit*. Tallinna Tervishoiu Kõrgkool, Statusprint.

Wagner, W., Duveen, G., Farr, R., Jovchelovitch, S., Lorenzo-Cioldi, F., Markova, L., and Rose, D. (1999) Theory and Method of Social Representations. *Asian Journal of Social Psychology* 2: 95–125.

When Nurses Go Wrong

Not My Nurse

Pessimism in Representations of Nurses in 1970s Cinema

VICTORIA N. MEYER

Introduction

Since Florence Nightingale's Victorian-era reforms, professional nursing has projected an image of compassionate, skilled care, and nursing leaders have worked to craft a positive image of the profession. The rising popularity of film as entertainment and information source since the turn of the twentieth century provided a whole new avenue of crafting an image of nursing. However, the influence of nursing professionals on media portrayals had declined by the 1950s, contributing to a complicated and strained relationship between popular culture images of nursing and nurses' self-perception. This tension culminated in the late 1960s as nurse characters in films often appeared as uncaring, inhumane, or sex-obsessed in direct contrast to the compassionate image maintained by the profession. Both the American public and nursing profession rejected these portrayals as neither the nurses they were nor the nurses they wanted. In this essay, I will explore the nurse characters of films from the late 1960s and 1970s as manifestations of widespread pessimism, uncertainty, and resistance to authority in American society, as well as tensions over transformations in medicine broadly and nursing as a highly gendered profession. These films emphasize the diverse influences outside of cinema and the profession, leading to nursing imagery's mutable and constructed nature.

Celluloid Nurses

There has been a growing literature on nurses and cinema since the 1970s. Nursing scholars have dominated as broader studies of film and medicine focus on doctors, hospitals, and biomedical imagery. Analysis of nurses in the media has been rooted in defense against a perceived devaluation of the profession and calls on fellow nurses to protest derogatory portrayals and promote positive, realistic imagery. In particular, focusing on memorable characters, such as Nurse Ratched from *One Flew Over the Cuckoo's Nest* (1975) and Margaret "Hot Lips" Houlihan in *M*A*S*H* (1970) (see Susan Hopkins' essay in this collection), research has characterized the long 1970s (stretching from 1967 to 1979) as the nadir of nursing in American cinema. Two of the most influential scholars on nurses in cinema, Philip Kalisch and Beatrice Kalisch, have repeatedly characterized the late 1960s and 1970s as bringing about "the complete destruction of the once proud and noble film image of the nurse" (Kalisch et al., 1982: 610). Early works dating from the mid–1970s to the early 1980s extended feminist scholars' work on the negative stereotypes of women in film to the adverse impact on nursing. Viewing film as a defining influence on American popular thought and the primary source of health information for the masses, nursing leaders declared the necessity of rehabilitating cinematic portrayals of nursing. As media scholar Julia Hallam assessed, the literature has routinely criticized the media "for promoting false myths and fantasies" and correlated negative images of nurses to widespread resistance to medicine (Hallam, 2002: 21). Repairing the portrayals of nursing would improve the field's stature, attract desirable students, and empower nurse activists to effect broad changes in healthcare.

Therefore, much of the literature on cinematic nursing has evaluated nurse characters as either positive or negative, good or bad for nursing. Connecting specific characters to stereotypes, including the angel of mercy, handmaiden of medicine/physicians, virtuous woman in white, sexy nurse, battle-ax, and sadist, is useful but encourages absolutist evaluations (Darbyshire et al., 2005: 69–82). Recent research has also questioned designating characters as good or bad based on heavily gendered ideas as inconsistent metrics reflecting the scholar's understanding rather than universal standards or the film's particular historical context (McAllister, 2018; Hallam, 2001). We will continue to use the stereotypes prominent in the literature but seek to show how emphasizing them as positive or negative obscures the convoluted relationship between popular thought and film imagery.

This essay re-examines nurse characters in films of the long 1970s in their historical and cinematic context. Films can influence popular culture but also reflect society. Scholars such as Joseph Turow and Rachel Gans-Boriskin assert that changes in popular culture products allow insight into widely held views about health and medical professionals (Turow et al., 2007). The "world of artificial contrivance" of movies does not directly reenact real-life (Wijdicks, 2020: 24). Films do, however, provide a window into how society interprets real-life experiences. If the image of nurses declined as precipitously from the late 1960s and 1970s as scholars claim, this would indicate a significant readjustment in society leading up to and during this period.

While the 1970s are often dismissed as a disappointing period between the outburst of liberal, progressive activism in the sixties and neo-conservatism's triumph in the 1980s, this era had more than disco fever. Events like the Vietnam War, economic recession, exploding health care costs, Women's Liberation and other civil rights protests, and the Watergate scandal created a widespread sense of disillusionment, uncertainty, and cynicism in the United States. Belief in progress faltered, and many Americans felt leaders had betrayed their confidence in the country's institutions. We cannot understand the decline in the presentation of nursing without accounting for the totality of the context rather than just medical or gender issues. Examining the broader context helps us explain why complicated and even unflattering nursing images emerged and struck a chord with audiences.

There is also an extensive scholarship on American cinema in the 1960s and 1970s. The late 1960s to mid–1970s were a time of fluctuation and experimentation in the film industry that led to a Hollywood renaissance labeled "New Hollywood" or American New Wave. Many of the young directors who first helmed a picture during this period, such as Martin Scorsese, would come to define Hollywood filmmaking in the following decades. Film scholars have deconstructed many films with settings in medicine or characters identified as medical professionals. Nevertheless, beyond the extensive discussions of Nurse Ratched and "Hot Lips" Houlihan, film scholars' works have not comprehensively engaged with the medical imagery nor engaged with the literature coming from nursing academics.

These divisions in the literature have created gaps in our understanding of the period's imagery of nursing and medicine more generally. This essay integrates perspectives from film scholars, historians, and nurses to create a more coherent analysis of nursing images in the long 1970s. Accommodating perspectives and information will allow us to understand better how broader shifts in American society, as well as events specific to medicine and the nursing profession, connect to the unflattering portrayals of nursing in cinema. These films reflected a general pessimism about authority and institutions and skepticism about the potential for progress. As medicine in the early twentieth century often embodied hopes of improvement, the shift in perceptions led to critiques of the period and a less receptive audience.

I focus on films released between 1967 and 1980. Most of the films are American in origin due to Hollywood's overarching dominance on these film industries through the 1970s. However, movies from other English-speaking countries, including Britain and Australia, are also included. I will analyze films that identify nursing with a primary or significant supporting character in the narrative. However, films that rely on nurses' images in the background to add realism to a medical narrative also reflect popular perceptions of nursing. The genres encompass melodrama, drama, thriller, noir, comedy (inclusive of dark comedy, satire, and parody), exploitation films, and horror. Comedy, dramas, and exploitation films were significant forces in the film industry and, therefore, predominate in the essay.

Sexuality and the Nurse

Popular American culture continues to gender the nursing profession as feminine. Consequently, nurse characters in films are likely to reflect or comment on the dominant social views of women and related attitudes towards women and sex. The sexy nurse or bombshell stereotype thus provides an opportunity to examine gender notions of work and sex. However, this stereotype requires the scholar to focus on the context and eliminate personal or social biases. The sexy nurse archetype also has a long history, reaching back to the emergence of nurse characters in movies.

Nevertheless, to the profession's frustration, the sexy nurse character gained a higher level of visibility across film genres in the 1960s and 1970s. The notorious Margaret Houlihan of *M*A*S*H* embodies this gendering of both nursing and sexual behavior. The surgeons mockingly nicknamed her in *M*A*S*H* as "Hot Lips" following a prank in which they broadcast her lovemaking to the entire military camp. Moreover, nursing scholar David J. Stanley found that the number of films with the sex kitten nurse stereotype doubled from eight in the 1960s to fifteen in the 1970s (Stanley, 2008).

To better understand the imagery of nursing and gain insight into the popular views of the profession, we must go beyond compiling the numbers of sexy nurse characters in films to contextualize and interpret the use and implications of that association. The display and reference to sexual activity, particularly outside the bounds of marriage, took on new dimensions in the late 1960s and 1970s, reflecting changing societal mores and generational, cultural conflicts. Consequently, we must ask if this increase in references to sex was unique to nursing, how the gendering of nursing overlapped with gendered ideas about sex, and the overall perspective of the film on sexuality.

Sex was undoubtedly a factor in movies before the 1970s, and the sexy bombshell character certainly took over the screens by the 1950s, from Bettie Paige to Marilyn Monroe. With the physically intimate interactions between patient and nurse required for proper nursing care, there has been a long tradition in films and novels of associating the nurse and sex. It is not surprising then that this stereotype continued into the 1960s and 1970s to dominate many pop culture references for nursing by the 1980s. Though sexuality has a long screen tradition, there were vital differences in content and presentation in how sex and nursing were portrayed in cinema before the late 1960s. The contrast is rooted in the extensive censorship system of American films created in the 1930s that lasted until the late 1960s.

With rising concerns about the film industry's morality during the interwar period, the American film industry opted for self-monitoring with the establishment of the Motion Picture Producers and Distributors of America (now known as the Motion Picture Association of America). By 1930, this collective had created a program of self-censorship, known popularly as the Hays Code. From 1934 to 1966, the Hays Code controlled films' content before release to prevent sex, swearing, violence, race, crime, and drugs from reaching mass audiences. The intent was to promote traditional morality, treating movies as fables for adults and children alike, teaching how to be productive, moral, and obedient citizens.

When films did display loose morals, the plot ended either with the character getting their just punishment as in *Vigil in the Night* (1940) or a redemptive character arc as in the 1951 Italian film *Anna*. *The Nun's Story* (1959) is also a strong example of the desexualized, if still attractive, nurse. Gaby is an intelligent, strong-willed young woman who enters an order of nursing nuns. There could be no more recognizable rejection of sexuality than a nun's habit. The movie explicitly links her religious vocation and dedication to her nursing of patients. Ultimately, although she leaves her order, Gaby retains the beatific association as a nurse, reinforcing the classic stereotype of the nurse as an angel, a secular saint devoted to others. Significant also is that the film promotes an image of nursing as all-consuming and takes priority over other aspects of living. Such stories have previously earned the approval of scholars for the positive portrayal of nursing (Kalisch et al., 1982).

Additionally, we can see the Hays Code's impact and its buttressing of traditional gender stereotyping dominant after the Second World War in *Not as a Stranger* (1955). Kristina Hedvigson is a curvy bombshell with bleached blonde hair. Despite her sexy appearance, the narrative repeatedly downplays her sexuality, with Kris saying that she is not "sexy" like the other nurses. More significantly, while Kris is recognized as an excellent nurse and nicknamed "the Swedish Nightingale" by her coworkers, her goal is expressly to become a wife and mother. She quits nursing once married, implying a dichotomy between domesticity and nursing, even though earlier nursing leaders promoted training programs as furnishing the skills required for motherhood. Since she adheres to traditional post–World War II gender roles idealizing domesticity, Kris can look like a sexy nurse but still be a "good girl."

Hollywood continued to project the unrealistic ideals of a "true woman" into the 1960s, widening the gap between film presentations of nurses and a rapidly changing society reading Betty Friedan's monograph *Feminine Mystique* (1963). Friedan asserted that forcing women to choose "true womanhood" in the home over a profession for which they were educated caused a loss of self. Films emphasizing nursing as a vocation only until marriage reinforced an expectation that nurses would transfer their nurturing skills to the home once married, reinforcing an expectation against which an emerging cadre of nurses chafed, viewing nursing as a life-long profession. It was not until the 1970s that married women with young children began to work full-time outside the home, further complicating the gendering of professionalism and associations of "nurture." These nurses faced particular economic difficulties, however, as the 1947 Taft-Hartley Act prevented unionization of the profession. Nursing lacked the power to agitate for wages commensurate with their education, skills, and duties.

Movie screens did not reflect these developments in nursing and society broadly until the Hays Code collapsed by 1966. Declining movie attendance due to increasing competition with television weakened the code's application by the early 1960s. Both industries increasingly focused on the growing youth market of people under age twenty-five. In order to differentiate films from television, directors pushed the boundaries of the Hays Code. In the 1960s, there was a flourishing "B" film industry, known as exploitation films, providing images of sex and violence with limited moral discussion to an adolescent and primarily male audience. By 1967, major studios and mainstream directors attempted to stave off the recession hitting the film industry and appeal to audiences by ignoring the code. The economic depression rendered the censorship system defunct. The Motion Picture Association established a new rating process in November 1968 that evaluated a film's content and suitability for different age groups. This classification allowed for truly adult films to be produced and led to an explosion of sex and violence across American movie screens. In the fall of 1970, the *Newsweek* associate editor Frank Trippett labeled the period the "Age of Great Disrobing," complaining that "Public sex pops up everywhere…" (Trippett, 1970).

Nursing scholars have lamented cinema's sexualization of nursing, linking it to the rapid decline of nursing's status. However, this sexualization has a different implication when examined in its historical context. Without the suppressive Hays Code, sex became omnipresent, and bombshell characters of the late 1960s were realigned to contemporary practices and views of sex and gender. As these had been shifting rapidly in the previous decades, this realignment produced a striking difference. For example, before the 1960s, only fifty percent of women had sexual intercourse before marriage. By 1980, eighty percent of women had intercourse before marriage and experimented with more partners. While nurse characters in films decreased after the 1950s, nursing scholars have contended that sexually-active women with an occupation in movies between 1966 and 1984, were frequently a nurse (Kalisch et al., 1987: 166–67). Considering that nursing, along with teaching, remained the primary profession for women through the 1970s, it would not be surprising to see nursing appear. The Kalischs calculated that thirty-two percent of films during the 1960s and 1970s with a significant nurse character contained some sexual relations, rendering nurses "the sexual mascots of the health care world" (Kalisch et al., 1982: 611).

Alternatively, with widespread visibility of sex on screen and in public life and the emphasis on cinematic realism, it would have been striking if films involving nursing had not been sexualized to some extent. This was problematic because it accentuated the oppositional relationship between nursing and sex or any other social pursuit in the profession's identity and imagery of the 1950s. Could nurses be shown as sexually active and still professional? With the misogynistic slant to many films and continuing one-dimensionality of most female characters, this friction remained unresolved in the 1970s. Nevertheless, among the hundreds of sexploitation films made quickly and cheaply during this time, the number of features with nurse characters overall was less than the thirty sexploitation films released in 1971 alone (Mark, 2007: 50–51).

Moreover, if we compare the new "sex kitten" nurse roles appearing in the 1960s and 1970s to other films in the same period—as opposed to nursing films from the 1940s and 1950s—changes in nurses' imagery are in line with general cinematic and social trends. Film scholar Jonathan Kirshner explains that the emphasis on sexuality in the 1970s was an expected result of opening the floodgates on movie-making regarding sex (Kirshner, 2016: 85). Initially audiences received this positively until the neo-conservative shift dominated society by the early 1980s. A question that emerges is whether sexual actively inherently undercuts identity as a nurse or depends on film and character development?

The films reflected changing mores among men and women through the 1960s and into the 1970s. Sexuality was not just a reality of the everyday and private life. The liberal political movements of the late 1960s emphasized celebrated that "the personal is political," an approach expanded by the Women's Liberation Movement through the 1970s. Second-wave feminism sought to disconnect sex from reproduction and emphasize the individual. In 1962, Helen Gurley Brown had popularized the idea of a "nice" single girl with an active sex life in her book *Sex and the Single Girl* (1962). Complicated adult relationships outside of marriage began to appear on film screens by the late 1960s, reflecting and normalizing the practices of younger generations. The number of unmarried couples living together jumped by fifty percent between 1970 and 1980 (Friedman et al., 2007: 12). Sexual behavior was no longer a primary factor in an unmarried woman's moral status, creating a conflict with the characterization of equating sexuality as contradictory to the nursing profession.

Under the new rating system, directors could craft films for adult viewers wrestling with sexuality and its implications in their own lives. Sexuality could be the brunt of the joke, a source of anguish, or a means of social critique. Many of the films then that take advantage of the new permissibility of sex in mainstream production offer conflicting images and statements on women as nurses and women's sexuality. In an interesting reversal is a feminist film on nurses with an exterior of pure exploitation. *The Student Nurses* (1970) is a sexploitation flick centered on four young, pretty nursing students. As required by the genre, it includes female (and male) nudity, as well as several sex scenes. The character Priscilla has a sexual encounter during a drug-induced trip leading to pregnancy and then an abortion. With plenty of shock value, the plot touched on the counter-culture coming and feminist issues. Priscilla's decision to have an abortion is linked to her desire to be a nurse but controlled by faceless males representing the health care system. Mirroring the locus of many 1970s films, Priscilla faces a morally complex question in which there is no clear right answer.

The movie shows the abortion procedure done by a medical resident in the students' apartment, but significantly Priscilla receives no punishment for her actions. The Hays Code's morality would have required a negative outcome from death to damaged health to reinforce Christian moral authority. Instead, Priscilla recovers quickly, graduates from her nursing program, and is last viewed walking into the hospital in her nursing uniform. While the topic of abortion remains controversial, director Stephanie Rothman intended to shock the audience while engaging with feminist discourses about sex and work. Even while catering to the male gaze to attract an audience that demographically skewed young and male, Rothman presents four young, complex women entering the workforce on their terms.

The tension between modern views of sex and conventional nursing portrayals appears further in the blaxploitation film *Coffy* (1973). The titular character is a nurse who rushes from her first revenge killings to her shift as an operating nurse. The fact that she cannot concentrate during surgery is not because of her sexuality or her race, as a surgeon describes her as a superior nurse. Coffy struggles because she had just betrayed her nursing commitment to save lives by killing two people. Coffy continually wrestles with her desire for revenge, her duty to help others, and the morality of violence. The identification of Coffy as a nurse then was not to demean the stature of nursing but was essential in setting up the quandary of nurture versus revenge. Director Jack Hill relied upon the popular view of nurses as self-sacrificing and caring to underscore the disconnect between Coffy and the world in which she lived. Hill also employed the virginal association of the nurse's white uniform for shock value when thugs later violently rip open her uniform, exposing her bare breasts. The film's extreme misogyny is not a reflection of views about nursing but a racist objectification of women.

Alternately, comedy and horror films played on the sexy nurse's extremes for laughs, subverting conventional expectations about the relationship between sexuality and appearance. While *Not as a Stranger* profited from displaying but denying Kris's sexuality, Mel Brooks's Hitchcock parody *High Anxiety* (1977) plays up the disparity. The head nurse of the psychiatric hospital in which the film is set perverts the conventional image of nurses as caring, virginal, and beautiful. Nurse Diesel is a scowling, old woman with a harelip and exaggerated, conelike breasts. In earlier films, Nurse Diesel might have embodied the sexless crone matron or battle-ax. Instead, Nurse Diesel not only has an iron grip on the hospital administration but also a sexual grip on a chief physician with light BDSM sex play. The gap between the sexy nurse and sexless crone assumed in films previously makes for laughs when combined, even though at the expense of Nurse Diesel.

Examining the sexual politics at play in the representation shows that some 1970s directors, in their quest for realism, translated portrayals of the sexist and harassing situations women of all occupations commonly faced at work. It was only in the 1970s that society began to acknowledge the common sexual harassment of women at work as an issue. Groups such as the National Organization of Women (NOW) worked to ensure enforcement of Title IX of the Civil Rights Act of 1964 prohibiting sexual and racial discrimination. The much-maligned sexual escapades and cruel jokes of *M*A*S*H* represented the difficulty of being a military nurse. Nurses in

Vietnam even reported having to be "virtually confined to the quarters ... with guards outside to protect them from male servicemen" (Roberts, 1990: 143). While the presentation of nurses as willing participants to the sexual escapades in *M*A*S*H* is problematic, to say the least, it portrays the pressure on these nurses to be both professionally and socially available. When questioned in 2009 about the presentation of women in *M*A*S*H*, director Robert Altman responded that he was "showing the way I observed that women were treated" (*M*A*S*H* 2009 DVD commentary).

It was not until the early 1970s that nurses began speaking out about the discrimination they experienced (Roberts, 1990: 187). While the dominance of sex in movies did little to improve women or nurses' situation, a direct link between the struggles of the nursing profession and sexualization in movies has not been demonstrated. We cannot assume the direct influence on public perceptions for this or earlier periods (Hallam, 2000: 46). Scholars writing in the 1970s and 1980s viewed the sexualization of nursing through the lens of professionalization and oversimplified the dynamics of sexuality and nursing present in films.

Monstrous Women

The association of nurses with sex affected another frequently unflattering stereotype: the battle-ax matron. The battle-ax has a long history, emerging as a binary opposite to the angelic nurse stereotype in early films. Battle-axes were traditionally nurses in authority positions, older spinsters who strictly enforced professional standards and practices. Being a "battle-ax" had positive connotations when the label emerged in the nineteenth century, describing determined and forceful women. Yet, by the twentieth century, the term marked an aggressive and domineering woman. By the 1940s, the battle-ax image, such as in the 1943 *And the Lamp Still Burns*, was a woman who had failed—bitterly—at fulfilling her obligations of true womanhood and had become a petty tyrant. This definition reflects post-war emphasis on women's return to domesticity. Through the 1950s, though, the battle-ax made up only a minority of nurse characters and was rarely a featured role. Instead, films of the 1940s and 1950s frequently emphasized nursing as a heroic act and placed nurses in romantic plotlines.

Positive images of nursing authorities as knowledgeable and kind professionals continued into the 1970s in films such as *The Student Nurses* (1970), *Johnny Got His Gun* (1971), and *Carry On Matron* (1972), which poked fun at the battle-ax stereotype. While the public as patients would have wanted to see a kind, caring nurse dedicated to their care, more complex cinematic portrayals reflected the changing healthcare they experienced. Overall, the battle-ax stereotype of nursing increased in the 1970s, and these characters took on more significant roles in films. This increasing visibility could reflect concern about the expansion of hospitals after World War II that increased access to medical care, overwhelming hospital staff. The national total of hospitals increased from 253,000 to 1.7 million just between 1957 and 1963 (Keeling et al., 2018: 293). Therefore, by the late 1960s, the work of nurses had changed drastically. The importance of bedrest decreased as treatment relied on quick intervention, such as surgery and new medicine. Bedrest had been a primary aspect of nursing care that, once replaced with technology and new products, revealed deep divides within the nursing profession over the nature of nursing and its distinction from medicine (Roberts, 2001).

For many Americans, nurses had become nothing more than "needle bearers" (Sandelowski, 2000: 102–103). With changes in medicine, the primary task of nurses became administering shots prescribed by a doctor: a painful and unnerving experience for many patients. Nurses then were not those who comforted but those who worked as the physician's agent and caused pain. While some nurses clung to the Florence Nightingale model of the nurse as a skilled caregiver fully dedicated to the patient and subservient to the physician, other professional nurses had been agitating for greater authority and education. This disagreement came to the fore with the increasing specialization of nurses from cardiac to ICU care and the creation of the nurse practitioner role.

Nursing continued to evolve with an accelerated discussion of education after the 1972 Briggs Report recommending multiple levels of training and status for nurses. More diverse training programs emerged from the Bachelor of Science in nursing to the registered nursing programs graduating technical or practical nurses and even nursing assistants. The new, complex hierarchy of nursing further obscured the core nature of nursing work. Professional nurses with a bachelor's degree infrequently worked directly in caring for patients, bolstering the idea of nurses as uncaring and rigid. If nursing was not about care, a skill naturalized as feminine and maternal in Western society, were nurses denatured women, unfit mothers?

Moreover, in an era then when women were increasingly working outside the home and entering professional occupations at higher rates, tensions over these questions and changes elevated the battle-ax image and frequently morphed it into a monstrous mother. The most iconic portrayal of the battle-ax as castrating mother is Nurse Ratched in *One Flew Over the Cuckoo's Nest* (1975). Critics' reviews abounded at the time of the film's release about the on-screen representation of the sadistic, cold rule of women and monstrous mother. However, initially, in the film version,

Ratched appears as the ideal nurse in her starched white uniform, a red lip, perfectly coiffed hair, and a soft voice and kind smile, but the film's anti-hero, McMurphy, soon reveals the cracks in this facade. The dissonance between Ratched's appearance and actions reproduced a widespread concern in the 1970s about how authorities, including governments, lied to the public. The release of the Pentagon Papers in 1971 detailing the government's intentional deception of the public about the Vietnam War and Nixon's Watergate scandal, which erupted in 1973, revealed the casual misrepresentation of authority figures and their betrayal of a sacred duty. The disclosure in 1972 of the Tuskegee Syphilis Study further demonstrated the potential danger of misguided officials and uncontrolled institutions to the public. Deception by those entrusted with the public's health constituted a personal nightmare and a humanitarian crisis. Ratched is an extreme example of what happens to patients when care is not the locus of nursing's professional work, despite expectations. Indeed, Ratched's battle with the film's anti-hero, patient Randall McMurphy, reveals her to be incapable of genuinely meeting a patient's needs.

Moreover, Ratched as the monstrous battle-ax embodies the institution—the Big Machine—which is itself uncaring with different priorities other than the patient. This identification of the monstrous battle-ax with the organization of health care differs from earlier battle-axes in film. For example, in *The Snake Pit* (1948), a matron in one of the psychiatric wards, Miss Davis, is a cruel and authoritarian nurse with no empathy for patients or staff. Davis, however, is just one among many competent and caring nurses that make up the asylum and is emotionally disconnected from the patients, making no claims of maternal or feminine care. Ultimately this makes her less dangerous than a monstrous mother figure like Ratched. Ratched believes she is doing the best for the patients even though her actions serve her authority rather than patients' needs. Many critics remarked that the film version of Ratched was a more ambiguous villain than in the novel because she is someone who believes in methods and accepts the goal of nursing but is unable to see how far she has deviated from the nursing ideal (Arnold, 1975).

Nor is she wrong. Nursing scholars Deborah Boschini and Norman Keltner interviewed nurses of different generations in 2009 and found that Ratched does many things right in her nursing for the period and even contemporary psychiatric nursing (Boschini et al. 2009). Rules are still essential for an effective therapeutic environment, and Ratched uses methods and practices reflective of the setting in the 1960s to manage patient care in the ward. This realism in Ratched's portrayal, following cinematic trends of the 1970s, raised the possibility of viewers' own care. The contradiction evident in Ratched's ability to care despite her professionalism points not just to public anxiety about healthcare but also about the increasing number of women working in professional fields outside the home.

Technology, though, was also rapidly changing nursing in other ways as medical corporatization led to large hospitals and rising costs by the early 1970s. Private insurance, as well as Medicare and Medicaid, made hospitals the site of modern medicine but also a business leading to bed shortages as well as nursing shortages. Gone were the large wards of earlier hospitals, replaced with private or semi-private patient rooms modern patients demanded, making observation from a central location impossible for nurses. Nurses became more reliant on various technological devices to track physical indicators and spent less time interacting with patients. This shift led to a view by the 1960s that the nursing profession had an empathy problem (Muff, 1982: 338–340). This point is driven home in the dark comedy *The Hospital* (1971). A young nurse finds a male resident dead and naked in a patient's bed. Showing no discernible reaction, she takes a peek at his genitalia and then strolls back to the charge nurse's station to report the death. The charge nurse reacts with nothing more than irritated confusion. If the death of one of their own initiated no urgency or emotion, patients would not either. Films like *Cuckoo's Nest* and *The Hospital* with a negative view of healthcare and medical professionals converted the classic stereotype of the nurse as handmaiden to a physician into the nurse as henchman for a corrupt and greedy system of medicine.

The thriller *Coma* (1978) brings this to life with the pairing of a corrupt, egotistical physician and his supervising nurse as a perverted nurturer. While the Chief of Surgery, Dr. Harris, rants that society had abdicated decision-making about life and death issues to "us, the experts. The doctors." Nurse Mrs. Emerson monitors the coma patients at the mysterious Jefferson Institute. Emerson expounds on the benefits of the technology employed to attentively "care" for the patients and later fondly looks down at one coma patient before kissing his forehead. She then moves on to direct a black-market auction for patients' organs. This emotional dissonance between nurse as caregiver and nurse as a cog of an evil machine is jarring and monstrous. She is not just an authoritarian nurse; she has lost her humanity. This disconnect appeared in discourses within nursing but also in broader debates about whether medicine had embraced science and technology too fully and had abandoned its humanity (Imber, 2008: 120). By the 1950s, sociologist Hans Mauksch had already recognized that as front-line professionals who most consistently determined patient care through a multitude of interactions, nurses were expected to be the most humane and bore the brunt of mistakes by other practitioners (Roberts, 2001). Consistent portrayals of burned-out nurses who have stopped caring were a larger indictment of healthcare.

Nor were they unrealistic. Nursing scholars in the 1970s and 1980s began to examine the high turn-over rate among nurses, seeking how to solve the situation when faced with constant nursing shortages. The reality of continued low pay, long hours, hard work, and the under-appreciation of nurses in practice was at stark odds with the positive images of nursing in films of the 1940s to early 1960s. Scholars such as Janet Muff pinpointed that the gap between expectations of nurses entering the profession and reality frequently lead to burn out, marked by emotional detachment leading to dehumanization and disregard for patients (Muff, 1982: 339). The profession in the 1970s split on whether widespread use of technology had driven nursing from its roots in feminine care, as theorized by nursing leader Hildegard Paplau, or technology, helped distinguish nursing skills from medical skills in a healthcare system increasingly focused on bio-medicine (Sandelowski, 2000: 130). As on many other issues during the period, the profession was divided on the nature and presentation of nursing, making it more concerned and sensitive to outside criticism and negative portrayals.

Conclusion

We cannot characterize nurses' imagery in films of the long 1970s as positive, nor simply label them as negative. Nurse characters were a mix of complex, contradictory images reflecting the pervasive pessimism, uncertainty, and malaise of American society in the 1970s. During this period, cinema emphasized the flaws in humanity, deconstructing the image of an absolute hero and complicating the ideas of villains. As contemporary events demonstrated, conventional "good" people might inflict damage, and conventional "bad" guys might be lurking behind a white uniform, military garb, or politician's smile. The images of nurses we have are of flawed characters, treated both seriously and humorously. Inviting audiences to mock, fear, or dismiss nurse characters did not raise nursing's status as a profession in society. However, it effectively exhibited the massive social and cultural transformation since just the Second World War and the goal of cinema to show humanity, flaws, and all.

Previous cinematic representations of nurses founded on stereotypes of good and bad resisted society's complex humanity and messy realities. Differences with previous stereotypes like the angel in white moreover exposed underlying problems in nursing's identity at the time. Ideals of self-sacrifice and nurturing solidified impossible standards for nurses. The mass expansion and corporatization of the health care industry accelerating by the 1960s only further exacerbated nursing's dilemma. The gap between the real and the ideal increased the likelihood of dissatisfaction with nursing, even as nursing itself reorganized and moved away from direct bedside care of patients to administrative and technology-based monitoring. Divisions within nursing reached a peak in the 1960s as disagreements over the purpose and nature of nursing skills and the different training and occupational designations created a void in the profession and dissatisfaction amongst patients. Without a clear message from the profession itself, the media reflected the scattered and conflicting views of nursing, exaggerating the more negative or disturbing elements of nurse stereotypes, reflecting tensions over changing gender roles, professions, and the purpose of health care.

Films and Television Productions Referenced

Anna (1951) Lux Film.
Carry On Matron (1972) Rank Organisation.
Coffy (1973) American International Pictures.
High Anxiety (1977) 20th Century Fox.
The Hospital (1971) United Artists.
Johnny Got His Gun (1971) World Entertainment.
M*A*S*H (1970) 20th Century Fox.
Not as a Stranger (1955) United Artists.
The Nun's Story (1959) Warner Bros.
One Flew Over the Cuckoo's Nest (1975) United Artists.
The Snake Pit (1948) 20th Century Fox.
The Student Nurses (1970) New World Pictures.
Vigil in the Night (1940) RKO Radio Pictures.

References

Arnold, G. (1975) Pain, Not Laughter Rules the Roost in Cuckoo's Nest. *The Washington Post*, December 1975, C1.
Boschini, D., and Keltner, N. (2009) Different Generations Review *One Flew Over the Cuckoo's Nest*. *Perspectives in Psychiatric Care* 45, 1: 75–79.
Darbyshire, P., and Gordon, S. (2005) Exploring Popular Images and Representations of Nursing. In: Daly, J., Speedy, S., and Jackson, D. (eds.) *Professional Nursing: Concepts, Issues, and Challenges*, Springer Publishing Company, pp. 69–92.
Hallam, J. (2000) *Nursing the Image: Media, Culture, and Professional Identity*. London: Routledge.
Imber, J. (2008) *Trusting Doctors: The Decline of Moral Authority in American Medicine*. Princeton, NJ: Princeton University Press.
Kalisch, P.A., and Kalisch, B. (1982) The Image of the Nurse in Motion Pictures. *The American Journal of Nursing* 82, 4: 605–611.
Kalisch, P.A., and Kalisch, B. (1987) *The Changing Image of the Nurse*. Menlo Park, CA: Addison-Wesley Pub. Co.
Keeling, A.W., et al. (2018) *History of Professional Nursing in the United States*. New York: Springer Publishing.
Kirshner, J. (2016) *Hollywood's Last Golden Age*. Ithaca: Cornell University Press.

Mark, M. (2007) 1971: Mores and the Exploitation of Excess. In: Friedman, L. (ed.), *American Cinema of the 1970s*. New Brunswick, NJ: Rutgers University Press.

McAllister, M. (2018) Tainted Love: Gothic Imaging of Nurses in Popular Culture. *Journal of Advanced Nursing* 74: 310–317.

Muff, J. (1982) *Socialization, Sexism, and Stereotyping: Women's Issues in Nursing*. St. Louis: Mosby.

Roberts, J., and Group, T. (1990) *Feminism and Nursing*. Westport, CT: Praeger.

Roberts, J., and Group, T. (2001) *Nursing, Physician Control, and the Medical Monopoly*. Bloomington: Indiana University Press.

Sandelowski, M. (2000) *Devices & Desires: Gender, Technology, and American Nursing*. Chapel Hill: University of North Carolina Press.

Stanley, D. (2008) Celluloid Angels: A Research Study of Nurses in Feature Films 1900–2007. *Journal of Advanced Nursing* 64, 1: 84–95.

Trippett, F. (1970) What's Happening to Sexual Privacy. *Look*, Oct. 20.

Turow, J., and Gans-Boriskin, R. (2007) From Experts in Action to Existential Angst. In: Reagan, L. (ed.) *Medicine's Moving Pictures*. Rochester: University of Rochester Press.

Wijdicks, E. (2020) *Cinema, MD*. Oxford: Oxford University Press.

Lesbians, Nymphomaniacs and Enema Specialists

Nurses, Horror, and Agency

MARCUS K. HARMES, MEREDITH A. HARMES
AND BARBARA HARMES

Introduction

Nursing is the healing profession, established by Florence Nightingale on high-minded principles, to comfort and treat the sick. Films of her life and career, especially in the wards at Scutari, made in 1915, 1936 and 1951 showed her as this source of comfort (see Richard Bates's essay in this collection). Similarly, hospitals are (or should be) places of safety and healing. What therefore are the messages to take from those media texts, primarily films, which situate menace not only among the ranks of the nursing profession but in the putatively safe spaces of hospitals? Pursuing these points, and focusing on the unsettling juxtaposition of the horrific and the healing, this essay examines instances of horror where nurses, nursing and places of healing become sites of horror. It takes examples from English-language film and television productions extending from the 1970s to the present. The starting point emerges from the notable instances of nurses involved in horror in 1970s cinema especially the exploitation cinema characteristic of the decade, and proceeds through works, both well-known and obscure, to interpret the activities of nurses situated in horror. As McAllister and Brien note, what they call the darker or "shadow side" of nursing inheres with the traumatic and profane, but does have value by ensuring that a more complex and un-sanitized vision of nursing does exist (2020).

The presence of nurses in horror films testifies to recurring ways nurses and nursing are stereotyped. These have been reduced to "six major nursing stereotypes: angel of mercy, handmaiden to the physician, oman in white, sex symbol/idiot, battleaxe, and torturer" (Darbyshire and Gordon, 2005: 74). However, even more specifically, it is asserted "If nursing iconography has an enduring stereotypic image, it must surely be the nurse as angel." Horror scenarios speak directly to some but perhaps not all of these, as the angel of mercy may ameliorate horror but the torturer may perpetrate it. But to what extent may the participation of nurses and nursing in horror repackage or recalibrate these stereotyped perceptions? The stereotype is contingent on the setting, as the caring environment of the ward contextualizes the Angel of Mercy.

The effect of any of these stereotypes is to reduce the agency of nurses, making them subordinate to other authorities. What agency therefore is shown by nurses in either resisting or enacting horror? Following the Second World War and in subsequent decades, information emerged that both endorsed and shattered expectations of nurses as healers. In terms of endorsing, the work of war heroines sustaining and caring for combatants aligned with pre-war reputations and filmic representations, representations that had already modulated into stereotypes. But these stereotypes are challenged by the ways actual nurses shockingly broke the bounds of conventional behavior during and after the Second World War. This essay brings together the actual and the fictional iterations of nurses committing horrifying acts, or caught in circumstances that horrified. It considers the particular contribution of horror films to the cinematic impression of the nursing profession, locating in these films a possibility for agency unobtainable in other scenarios.

The Nurse and Exploitation

To begin, the junction of horrific connotations and practices with the apparently high minded intentions of the nursing profession is articulated in horror films made across decades. Hospitals provide an evocative environment; places with bright hygienic spaces where treatment takes place can sit alongside the sinister environment of the morgue, or dark corridors where predators may lurk. The instruments for life saving surgery can be easily misappropriated for torture or murder and the easy manner in which the place of healing modulates into a place of horror provides an environment for the nurse in horror. The ozploitation horror movie *Patrick* (1978) brings the perverse together with the healing, as the movie begins with an unusual job interview between the stern matron of the private Roget Clinic and an aspiring young nurse. The Matron's insistence on rigid standards and her intrusive questions about the young nurse's private life set the scene for an even stranger turn in the conversation, when the Matron insists that

"We're not interested in restless housewives who resign at the first threat of a soiled bedpan." For a 1978 movie the line is indicative of real-world parameters for nursing, which was still a mostly female profession and one that re-admitted married women. Further, the Matron suggests that she has found that a private clinic seems to attract "certain types" of people and proceeds to deliver a disturbing taxonomy of perverse nurses. "Lesbians, nymphomaniacs, and enema specialists, zoophiliacs, algolagniacs, necrophiliacs, peadophiliacs, exhibitionists, voyeurs" are among the perverted members of the nursing profession the Matron has encountered. "Disease like God moves in mysterious ways," she notes, for "it can don the mask of perversion and spread like cancer through a hospital staff." This early scene in *Patrick* is framed and shot to present a striking contrast; on the wall of the Matron's office hangs a print of Florence Nightingale in her guise of the "Lady with the Lamp" in the hospital ward at Scutari. The iconography is not remarked on by the characters, being a silent participant in the scene, but this participation is telling, as the most high minded foundational and high minded moment in the history of nurses watches over a strange taxonomy of the all the different types of perversion that can infect a nurse and the nursing profession.

Patrick is far from being the only horror film to insist on the location of the perverse and horrifying among the ranks of the nursing profession and in a hospital but the Matron's long, clinically detailed and comprehensive taxonomy of weirdness is among the most extensive moments in a horror film where many ways nurses can go wrong are enumerated. The Matron's long list of weird and often sexual perversions of behavior testify to *Patrick*'s classification by film and cultural historians as an "ozploitation" film, and therefore as a product of a distinctive type of disreputable film making in the horror genre that found sexually charged potential in various institutional scenarios, often involving women in positions of uniformed authority. Among others are the nunsploitation, whipsploitation, women in prison, Nazisploitation and hagsploitation films made across the 1960s and 1970s. Central to many of these of course are sexualized women, especially women whose erotic transgressive actions are offset by and masked by (at least temporarily) a traditional or even sacerdotal outer layer, such as the nun's habit, the prison wardress's uniform, or the nurse's cap and cape.

Exploitation films often cross their own boundaries, and while not all horror films set in hospitals and featuring nurses are exploitation movies, many exploitation films find both horror and deviance in a medical institutional setting. Horror films that include nurses traverse different types, although the insistence on the traditional but transgressive iconography of the uniform of cap, dress and cape that defines the exploitation film carries across types. Nurses appear in horror films that present supernatural forms of evil (*Scream and Scream Again*, *Silent Hill*), or are grounded simply in an innate human ability to cause harm to others (*One Flew Over the Cuckoo's Nest, Misery*). As noted elsewhere in this volume, the traditional iconography of the nurse's cap and cape has mostly disappeared from actual nursing (see Tatiana Prorokova-Konrad's essay), but the traditional appearance remains essential to nurses in horror in particular. A virginal white uniform and veil transformed by vivid red blood is striking imagery. The traditional cap is essential to the juxtaposition of the grotesque and the nursing profession in *Silent Hill*'s nurses. Anachronistically, the cap is worn by sadistic nurses in *Nursie* (2004) and *Nurse 3D* (2013).

Nurses Who Kill

Sensationalist and tabloid media from time to time have reported on real-life cases of individual nurses who kill, including those who may be cases of Munchausen by Proxy syndrome, or people in a care giving capacity who cause harm to their patients, including pediatric nurses (Repper, 1995). By 1972, the unethical Tuskegee Syphilis Study experiments entered public knowledge, together with the knowledge that it was a nurse who had coordinated the abusive and harmful treatment of scores of African American men, most of whom were poor and uneducated.

However the possibility that nurses could harm and kill entered popular consciousness earlier than Tuskegee, especially after the Second World War. Rationalizing and explaining the fact that nurses could harm not heal gained a distinctive focus and necessity in the years following the Second World War. This war, like the First World War, was marked by the enlistment of female nurses to care for combatants. However the Second World War revealed other dimensions of the nursing profession, these not as laudatory. The participation of not only physicians but nurses in the atrocities of death camps, ranging from sterilization to inhuman experiments leading to murder, became clear after the war.

The war had provided many occasions to celebrate members of the nursing profession, as care givers to combatants but also as heroes (or more accurately in most cases heroines) in their own right. Even these reputations were occasionally subject to censorship to ensure there was no association between the profession and the sexual, including the decades-long suppression of the fact that Japanese troops had not only massacred army nurses on Banka Island in 1941 (an act that was always in the public domain) but had also sexually assaulted them. Heroism in the face of

Japanese military aggression harmonized with popular depictions of nursing in a way that sexual assault did not. As Summers and Summers point out, after the First World War and until after the Second World War, nurses in films were pragmatic, heroic, and, if young nurses, not battle-ax matrons; they were also romantic interests for handsome young male physicians (Summers and Summers, 2014: 35). Importantly, Summers and Summers also adduce that nurses were portrayed as unskilled, therefore deferential to male medical authority, needing strict layers of supervision from older sisters and matrons and the male doctors. The portrayal of the profession was therefore positive in terms of nurses as healers, but limited their agency by downplaying their intelligence and ability. That presentation points to the significance of less positive portrayals, where nurses do not heal, but are, however, exercising some agency.

The heroism (even if not all details were made available) of some nurses is one dimension of the profession during and after the Second World War. Another, however, was that nurses killed. The de-Nazification programs following the war, as well as war crimes trials and the documenting of the work done in concentration camps, revealed that nurses had been enthusiastic rather than reluctant participants in ethically compromised medical schemes. These included the forced euthanasia of children and adults with mental and physical disabilities. As Benedict and Kuhla (1999) point out, understanding the role of nurses as active rather than reluctant killers has lagged behind an understanding of the role of medical doctors in enacting genocide, and there has not been a large-scale effort at bringing killing nurses to justice equivalent to the Belsen Trial in 1945, which included the Nazi doctor Fritz Klein among the accused, or the "Physicians' Trial" (or Doctors' Trial) at Nuremberg in 1946 (although one of the doctors on trial was a female) (Freyhofer, 2004: 71). Much research into medicine during the Third Reich and the experiments in death camps and the medical culture coordinated by the Ministry of the Interior has focused on physicians rather than nurses (Kater, 1987).

Nonetheless the actions of Nazi nurses actions eclipse anything that could be imagined in a horror film. As noted by the medical historian Barbara Heggen, nurses under the Nazi regime participated in a "widespread campaign of killing," taking place in hospitals rather than death camps (2015). Indeed, in some instances the nurse transitioned into the death camp wardress and Irma Grese, notorious as the "hyena of Auschwitz" and active also at Bergen-Belsen, began as a nurse before becoming a concentration camp guard (Kater 2009: 70). The nursing profession in Nazi Germany was an important profession, intrinsic to core ideologies and practices related to motherhood, race and eugenics, and where nurses and midwives came to play pivotal roles in the implementation of race purity policy in cooperation with public health authorities (Lisner and Peters, 2014: 174). Professional training and professional education inculcated particular attitudes to people with mental and physical illness, including children, as well as people of mixed-race heritage. When questioned and tried as non-military personnel following the defeat of Nazi Germany and the end of the Second World War, some nurses denied direct responsibility, using the explanation and excuse used in tribunals such as Nuremburg that they had followed orders and would have received a punishment if they had disobeyed orders (Benedict, Lagerwey and Shields, 2014: 68). In this instance, the orders were those which had come from Nazi physicians. Their explanation displaces responsibility but also displaces agency.

Similarly, the few interviews and the deposition made by Nurse Eunice Rivers, the community nurse involved in the now notorious Tuskegee Syphilis Study across many decades, included statements in what Susan Reverby calls the "taking-orders voice." Reverby's detailed investigation of not only the Study but Rivers' different accounts, the different interpretations of her accounts, and the intersections between Rivers, caring, nursing, and race, notes that part of Rivers' defense when questioned was to claim that she did as she was told and did not do anything she was not told to do (Reverby, 2009: 176).

Scholarship on actual historical examples of nurses who have killed or harmed, including on a large scale, stresses the importance of context. McFarland-Icke's large scale study of the nursing profession during the Third Reich makes that point, stressing that moral decisions took place within a distinctive historical context, which included among other things the mainstream medical acceptance of eugenics not only in Nazi Germany but in the medical profession globally, the inculcation of nationalist party politics, and the introduction of stringent race laws requiring medical reinforcement (Zukas, 2002).

It is precisely this historical and scientific context that many film accounts of horrifying or harmful nurses lack. Precisely because horror films featuring nurses are often exploitation pictures, they are cut-off of from a meaningful historical or cultural context. Instead the action takes place in a type of exaggerated or even supernatural reality of its own. The nature of that hyper reality resonates with a further point about the context, not only of nursing practice, but also of nursing malpractice. As Field (2007: 292) notes, "the media has clearly shaped the construction of the nurse who murders baby patients as among the most evil of human beings." Shaping that discursive construction is a media with a reading or viewing public. In the case of real life nurses who may harm patients, including babies or the elderly, there are contextual consequences including high levels of public hatred. Nurses enacting horrific deeds in film, especially in the hyper reality of an exploitation film, can be remote from any such response or backlash.

When Nurses Go Wrong

In horror scenarios, nurses are part of the fabric of film narratives and themes defined by menace. The irony and the significance is that the inversion of a cornerstone of practice and identity—that nurses heal not harm—can in fact invert another misconception that nurses exist as largely passive and non-essential members of a nursing team, compared to the medical doctors. Although the agency is misdirected to causing harm not healing, horror films can in fact invert a number of stereotypical assumptions, endowing nurses with a degree of agency they are otherwise perceived as lacking. It was noted above that horror films involving nurses often fit within the category of sexploitation films, a category within which sit mutually reinforcing types. One example is the low budget supernatural horror film *Nurse Sherri* (1978), which has elements of slasher cinema as well as blaxploitation, in addition to the exploitative potential of nurses (Clark, 2013: 195). Elements of the plot, including voodoo ritual and terms such as "honky" pinpoint its intersection with contemporary Blaxsploitation in American cinema, especially drive-in and grindhouse. The film's plot concerns a young white nurse, dating a young doctor, who is possessed by the spirit of an occultist, who dies on the operating theater table and vows revenge on all the medical personnel who were present. The vengeful spirit uses the nurse as his agent. The nurse character therefore occupies an unusual place in any discussion of agency. She plots and violently kills a number of them, impaling a surgeon with a pitchfork, and deluding her boyfriend the doctor, but she does so as the tool of a male spirit. The film ends with the spirit gone but the nurse's sanity fractured. She is locked in a cell in an asylum, while male doctors observe her, comment on her, and discuss her medical history and prognosis. Her agency, temporary and due to male control, is gone. The film exploits the nursing profession. The nurses in general exist for the gratification of male doctors and male patients. One nurse sexually services a patient, others become or already are the romantic playthings of male doctors and patients. The nurses of *Nurse Sherri*, in virginal white uniforms and demure caps, sit squarely in an exploitative tradition as objects of desire. Other nurses in the horror genre, less traditional in appearance and appeal, have a more dynamic agency as well.

In 1978, Australia contributed a further ozploitation (in addition to *Patrick*); *The Night Nurse* is set not in a hospital but in the grand home of an aged and retired opera singer, cared for by two private domiciliary nurses. One is elderly, disapproving and (so it is later revealed) demented and murderous and the other is young. Both nurses gain agency from the context of horror they are in. The older enacts a complex and perverted caring relationship with her elderly patient, dressing up and impersonating the patient's long dead friends at bizarre dinner parties but, once the costumes come off, regaining her subordinate status as a nurse and servant, no longer fit to sit at the table as a guest. The younger nurse enters this bizarre environment, actively investigating the mysteries she encounters and unmasks a killer. Here however comes a twist; her agency is demonstrated one last time when, having discovered the complicity of her employer in decades of murder and deceit, she leaves the mansion and her patient, criminal but elderly and disabled, to her fate. Throughout the film, her sense of agency has contributed to the young nurse's willingness to investigate, but at the very end, her decision to leave and her judgmental action in leaving her patient helpless and alone, has meant the agency involved the abrogation of nursing care and responsibility.

Significantly, horror narratives create opportunities for storytelling to toy with and subvert what are in other genres (or in exploitation features such as *Nurse Sherri*) stable interactions between authoritative males and subordinate female nurses. The character of Annie Wilkes in *Misery* (a 1990 adaptation of Stephen King's 1987 novel) embodies several types of nursing identity. When first seen, from the perspective of her injured patient Paul Sheldon, Wilkes seems a capable and caring nurse. As is established, she has successfully extricated him from a car accident scene, dressed his wounds, administered a drip through a cannula, and she explains events in a calm and rational voice. She is in fact the embodiment of the caring profession. However the character draws off other more horrific nursing identities, her backstory including her notorious reputation that she was a maternity nurse who murdered children.

In addition, a darker sexual frisson is apparent in the interactions between the female nurse and the male patient. Sheldon's legs are injured, leaving him helplessly bedridden, the actual injuries to his legs leaving him figuratively emasculated as he becomes weakened and subordinate to female authority. His weakened physicality is apparent in other ways. Nurses should and do cross personal boundaries, such as helping incapacitated patients to bathe or toilet themselves, and they should do so in respectful and dispassionate ways (McAllister and Brien 2020). Wilkes carries out these physical responsibilities but in a manner that shifts from the professionally detached to the transgressive, such as her almost exultant collection of her patient's urine, which she then waves around in a flask. The broad contours of this story recur in the American horror *Nursie* (2004), which additionally is structured and plotted to toy perversely with the traditional notion of "playing doctors and nurses." A sadistic nurse controls and torments a young male doctor. The plot emulates *Misery*'s narrative of a car accident victim putatively cared for by a nurse and the traditional white uniform and cap is anachronistically present as a signifier of horror.

Perverse sexual agency inheres in other iterations of horrific nursing. Nurse Ratched's control of the patients in Salem House in *One Flew Over the Cuckoo's Nest* (1975) includes physical means such as subjecting them to disruptive therapies and her control over their medications. However her dominance is also sexual, extending to the mental and physical destruction of Billy Bibbit. What should be his moment of triumph after bedding a woman for the first time becomes a demeaning and humiliating end of his life after Ratched catches him and threatens him. The moment of transformation of sexually proving himself is immediately undone by Ratched's exploitation of that sexuality.

Particular examples illustrate dynamic agency in surroundings defined by menace and horror. Rupert Goold's adaptation of *Macbeth* in 2010 was filmed in England but thematically evoked the Romanian dictatorship of Nicolae Ceaușescu. Macbeth begins in the aftermath of a battle and film stays faithful to that narrative but in a setting updated to evoke the repressive dictatorship in Eastern Europe, the scenes take place in a war-damaged hospital. As such, the weird sisters, the witches, whose prophecies are so critical to the narrative, are re-imagined as the nursing sisters of the battlefield hospital. Clad in the traditional uniform, including the cap, these nurses represent the ultimate in nursing agency. They inspire and provoke each of Macbeth's actions as he schemes and murders his way to be the ruler. These nurses therefore direct fates and futures; dynamically, they also revel in carnage and carrion flesh.

Nurses interacting with supernatural agencies and forces recur in other contexts. The 1970 British horror film *Scream and Scream Again* wove together elements of political Cold War thrillers with science fiction and horror derived from sadistic medical experiments. Among the sadists is a nurse, attired in cap and white uniform, who is an eerily silent member of staff in a chillingly quiet hospital. The only patient is a man who has each of his limbs amputated. The nurse taunts and torments as he gradually diminishes physically and loses his mind to hysteria. The sexualized antics of Sister Mary Eunice in *American Horror Story: Asylum* (2012) draws on the longer history of nuns as nursing sisters, but also contributes satanic possession and forthright sexuality to the depiction of a nursing sister's ambitious and inexorable rise.

Science fiction and the supernatural intersect in ways that showcase nurses in horror. *World Enough and Time*, a 2017 episode of *Doctor Who*, was steeped in the medical. Much of the plot took place in the wards, operating theatres and corridors of a hospital, in which a nurse is seen working alongside a surgeon. Having a male surgeon and female nurse endorses long-standing gender based stereotypes. Much else is also familiar, including the nurse's generally officious and bustling demeanor, her starchy uniform and neat white cap, and even her large proportions, and her demeanor, dress and size cumulatively recall the dominant matronly stereotype associated with Hattie Jacques from four *Carry On* films, and to an extent the "battle-ax" stereotype of the senior ranks of the nursing profession. Contextually, the nurse's *mise-en-scène* is a fully functioning hospital. There are gowned and robed patients connected to medical equipment such as drip stands. Nightingale wards, metal framed screens, frosted glass windows, and swing doors further evoke a post-war NHS hospital, and their fictional iterations such as the sets built at Pinewood Studios to create the hospital scenes in the *Carry On* films. However outside the hospital is a hazy, polluted dystopian world, seemingly at odds with the comfortably familiar environment within the hospital. The setting signaled much that is "normal" regarding nursing and its context. The nurse is however the antithesis of a carer, a contrast signaled explicitly by her callous actions. She mocks, bullies and taunts the sick. Most shockingly, she turns down the vocal synthesizer of a stricken patient who was pleading that he was in pain. This particular scene is written to subvert expectations. The patient cries in pain and the nurse comes to see what the problem is. However instead of ameliorating the pain, the nurse ensures the patient will not be able to further articulate need or distress. Critically, the nurse in *World Enough and Time* takes medical actions that are cruel but dynamic, and imbued with agency not passivity. The hospital's operating theatres are not healing the sick through treatment; rather they are converting people via bio-mechanical surgery to become Cybermen. This nurse neither cares for nor heals, but she does not take orders. Importantly she is seen working alongside the male surgeon as his equal, not his subordinate.

The nurse in *World Enough and Time* owes aspects of her demeanor and appearance to a fictional nurse, the Matron of the *Carry On* films. The horrific nurses of *American Horror Story* owe aspects of their creation to real-world nurses. Miranda and Bridget Jane lure and murder elderly patients. The plotting of their storyline echoes the real-world killer nurses Catherine May Wood and Gwendolyn Gail Graham, both arrested in 1988 and sentenced in 1989 for killing elderly patients (Sobsey 1995). The adaptation of a real-world crime to the narrative and supernatural environment in *American Horror Story* has implications for the presentation of nurses and the nursing profession. Crucially, the killer nurses are also same-sex lovers, an affront to almost all nursing stereotypes that one way or another situate a nurse as a female attracted to or sexually at the service of, a male superior. Alternatively, the stereotype of the battle-ax matron strips all sexuality away, insisting that an older, plainer woman is asexual, as insisted on in the preposterous wooing scenes in *Carry On Matron*.

The Healing Profession

The agency of nurses is horror films, and because they enact horror, is not an absolute impression and is complicated in two particular ways. One is that films that make nurses horrifying are offset by horror films featuring nurses, but where the nurse takes on a more obviously healing capacity. In terms of internal chronology, the late Victorian-era setting of *The Elephant Man* (1980) is an early portrayal of the nursing profession, including in this instance the matron and nursing sisters of the London Hospital where the titular "Elephant Man," Joseph Merrick, had lived and been not only cared for but studied. The hospital's Matron, Mrs. Mothershead, is characterized as dispassionate, but in a way that makes her stern dispassion positive, in that she is prepared to treat and care for Merrick when others recoil. Mrs. Mothershead characterizes her care as "I bathed him, I fed him, and I cleaned up after him. And I see that my nurses do the same. And if loving kindness can be called care and practical concern, then I did show him loving kindness, and I am not ashamed to admit it." *The Elephant Man* may in fact resist classification as a "horror" film, although the black and white cinematography, the Victorian setting including the freak show and the insistence on the abject evoke many of the tropes of British horror films, placing the film alongside rather than within the horror genre. The black and white *mise-en-scène* in particular evoked earlier films which essayed the association of the hospital, the Victorian era, and the horrific including *Corridors of Blood* (1958) and *Jack the Ripper* (1959).

In films set in the present day, the nurse can again be amidst scenes of horror but maintain a reassuring presence. *Visiting Hours* (1982) takes place mostly around the wards and theatres of a modern hospital in Montreal. A psychopathic killer stalks and murders the staff and patients, however the nursing sisters are sources of comfort, not causes of menace. The character of young nurse Sheila Munroe comforts people who are frightened, admires and upholds a campaign for women's rights, and is eventually targeted by but is also a survivor of the psychopathic killer. A similar point can be made about *Patrick* (1978). The horror lies with the patient, the psychokinetic Patrick, who is simultaneously comatose and paralyzed but also dangerously active and interventionist in people's lives, using his mental powers to maim and kill. The young nurse by contrast is a caring and competent presence in the clinic, doing her utmost to care for patients in dangerous circumstances.

The other are those occasions when nurses themselves are subjected to horror. Similar themes prevail. The hospital setting and often the traditional iconography of the nurse, especially the cap and cape, should be images that reassure. Instances of storytelling such as *Green for Danger* (1946), *Halloween II* (1981), *Hospital Massacre* (1982) and *The Exorcist III* (1990) turn hospitals into places of menace and the nurses into victims. In *Hospital Massacre* and *Halloween II*, nurses at the county hospital in Los Angeles and Haddonfield Memorial Hospital respectively are among the victims of the serial killers, including in *Halloween*'s Michael Myers. Similarly, supernatural horror violates the safety of a hospital in *The Exorcist III*, when a nurse is murdered and dismembered. The juxtaposition of the traditional iconography of the cap and the uniform was noted above in the context of narratives such as *Nursie* and *Silent Hill*, where the traditional appearance of the nurse offsets her perverse actions. The traditional iconography can also contribute to the appearance of victimhood. *American Horror Story*'s first season included the home invasion narrative of the murdered nursing students Gladys and Maria. The latter was compelled by a serial killer, one with a particular hatred of nurses, to don the cap and uniform before her murder. The incident was suffused with sexual danger, the student nurse anticipating that she would be raped and fearfully telling the killer she was a virgin. The white uniform and cap contribute to the sense of sexual and physical danger.

Conclusion

Nurses and nursing recur in horror, not least as the uniformed nurse is an intrinsic aspect of exploitation. Where films can exploit they can also deliver agency and this essay has suggested that the narrative impulses in horror can be a way for nurses to appear with greater agency than is possible or apparent in other types of storytelling. That agency frequently subverts the higher minded intentions of actual nursing, and may therefore impose its own limitations, as the nurses with agency can be constrained, in narrative terms, to the roles of tormenter and killer, their horrifying actions accentuated by their juxtaposition with the clean, starched and demure uniforms. These uniforms, including the cap, are often retained anachronistically in horror as visual signifiers of the profession and as a means to offset the mayhem with the traditions of healing. However as this essay noted, nurses in horror, or at least in horrific settings, perform other narrative functions, sometimes as victims but also sometimes as healers and carers, and horror can deliver a variety of agencies to a profession that otherwise subsists on screen within a host of stereotypes.

FILMS AND TELEVISION PRODUCTIONS REFERENCED

American Horror Story: Asylum (2012) FX.
Doctor Who: World Enough and Time (2017) BBC.
The Elephant Man (1980) Paramount Pictures.
The Exorcist III (1990) 20th Century Fox.
Halloween II (1981) Universal Pictures.
Macbeth (2010) BBC.
Misery (1990) Columbia Pictures.
The Night Nurse (1978) Gemini Productions/Channel 7.
Nurse Sherri (1978) Independent-International Pictures.
Nurse 3D (2013) Lionsgate.
Nursie (2004) Jatrac/Tre Boucher.
One Flew Over the Cuckoo's Nest (1975) United Artists.
Patrick (1978) Filmways Australasian Distributors.
Visiting Hours (1982) 20th Century Fox.

REFERENCES

Benedict, S., and Kuhla, J. (1999) Nurses' Participation in the Euthanasia Programs of Nazi Germany. *Western Journal of Nursing Research* 21, 2: 246–263.
Benedict, S., Lagerwey, M., and Shields, L. (2014) Psychiatric Nursing During the Era of National Socialism. In: Benedict, S., and Shields, L. (eds.). *Nurses and Midwives in Nazi Germany: The "Euthanasia Programs."* London: Routledge, pp. 48–70.
Clark, R. (2013) *At a Theater or Drive-In Near You: The History, Culture, and Politics of the American Exploitation Film.* London: Routledge.
Darbyshire, P. (2009) Heroines, Hookers and Harridans: Exploring Popular Images and Representations of Nurses and Nursing. In: Daly, J., Speedy, S., and Jackson, D. (eds.) *Contexts of Nursing: An Introduction.* Elsevier Health Sciences, pp. 51–64.
Darbyshire, P., and Gordon, S. (2005) Exploring Popular Images and Representations of Nursing. In: Daly, J., Speedy, S., and Jackson, D. (eds.). *Professional Nursing: Concepts, Issues, and Challenges.* New York: Springer Publishing Company, pp. 69–92.
Field, J. (2007) Caring to Death: A Discursive Analysis of Nurses Who Murder Patients, University of Adelaide Ph.D.
Freyhofer, H.H. (2004) *The Nuremberg Medical Trial: The Holocaust and the Origin of the Nuremberg Medical Code.* Berlin: Peter Lang.
Heggen, B. (2015), *Ethical Questions Raised by "Nazi Nurses" Still Relevant*, The Drawing Room, ABC Radio, https://www.abc.net.au/radionational/programs/drawingroom/ethical-questions-raised-by-nazi-nurses-still-relevant/6619214.
Kater, M.H. (1987) The Burden of the Past: Problems of a Modern Historiography of Physicians and Medicine in Nazi Germany. *German Studies Review* 10, 1: 31–56.
Kater, M.H. (2009) *Hitler Youth.* New Haven: Harvard University Press.

Lisner, W., and Peters, A.K. (2014) German Midwifery in the "Third Reich." In: Benedict, S., and Shields, L. (eds.). *Nurses and Midwives in Nazi Germany: The "Euthanasia Programs."* London: Routledge, pp. 164–197.

McAllister, M., and Brien, D.L. (2020) *Paradoxes in Nurses' Identity, Culture and Image: The Shadow Side of Nursing.* New York: Routledge.

Repper, J. (1995) Munchausen Syndrome by Proxy in Health Care Workers. *Journal of Advanced Nursing* 21, 2: 299–304.

Reverby, S. (2009) *Examining Tuskegee: The Infamous Syphilis Study and Its Legacy.* Chapel Hill: University of North Carolina Press.

Sobsey, R. (1995) *Violence and Disability: An Annotated Bibliography.* Ann Arbor: University of Michigan.

Summers, S., and Summers, H.J. (2014) *Saving Lives: Why the Media's Portrayal of Nursing Puts Us All at Risk.* Oxford: Oxford University Press.

Zukas, A. (2002) Nurses in Nazi Germany. *The European Legacy: Toward New Paradigms* 7, 5: 653–655.

Scary Women

Nurses, Power Relations and Regimes of the Visual

Ronja Tripp-Bodola

Introduction

This essay discusses fictional representations of nurses in visual media, from Miloš Forman's *One Flew Over the Cuckoo's Nest* (1975) to Ryan Murphy's *Ratched* (Netflix, 2020–present). It focuses on excavating the underlying power relations, gender politics and visual regimes with which the narratives are imbued. Arguing that nurses are a ready means for gendered projections and phantasmagoria that prompt control strategies such as abjectification (Kristeva, 1982; Creed, 1993), the trope of the evil nurse is intricately linked to heteronormativity and misogynist strategies (Butler, 1993; Butler, 1999). With younger nurses, those politics spawn voyeuristic and sado-masochistic fantasies catering to the male gaze. As they get older and are deemed unattractive, they become "scary women" (Sobchack, 2004). Nurses share certain hyper-gendered qualities with mothers and nuns that further account for their ambiguity in the cultural imaginary: they all embody the essentialist positive feminine characteristics such as nurturing kindness and providing physical and spiritual remedies that make us feel better when we are most vulnerable. And yet, nurses differ from both which, as I will argue below, makes them prone to become an abject monstrosity.

Nurses are intricately linked to multiple oppressive systems such as patriarchy, ageism, ableism or educational hierarchies in the health care system. Traditionally, the horror genre toys with dark revenge fantasies of the suppressed, yet nurses go beyond the shock value and simple inversion of power relations. The examples taken from movies, TV shows, streaming content and video games will illustrate that they are explicitly viewed as empowered, not least because of their power over those in their care, and thus prompt violent responses. However, as the visual *dispositif* (Foucault, 1977) has shifted and gazes diversified significantly over the last decade, this response has changed. As I will argue below, more recently the approach to the figure of the empowered nurse has become more integrative by exposing heteronormative mechanisms of repulsion and thus rendering them impotent.

Visual Regimes and Intersectional Identities

The visual regimes affecting nurses on the screen go beyond representations. In reference to Christian Metz's coinage, and Martin Jay's discussion of the term "scopic regime" (Jay, 1988), the term implies the power relations and *dispositifs* connected to systems of oppression related to race, class and gender as they govern their visual presentation. Beyond acting, makeup, or cinematography, this includes well-established concepts such as the "male gaze" (Mulvey, 1975) as well as practices of looking, such as scopophilia or voyeurism.

Most of the pop cultural representations are still rooted in a particular historical precursor to nursing that took shape in the second half of the nineteenth century and is synonymous with the name of Florence Nightingale. Demographically, nurses in Western cultural imaginaries have been female, middle-class and white, and these demographic aspects translate smoothly into visual representations. In addition, the conspicuous uniform including cap and cape became a shorthand in visual culture for that prototypical identity, if not a fetish. Florence Nightingale, who was herself unmarried and had unusual levels of agency and impact for a Victorian woman, advocated for women to be able to work outside the home without any stigma (Michie, 1987: 33–34) and paved the way for nursing to become a middle-class occupation. As far as the social status is concerned, the TV show *Call the Midwife* (BBC One, 2012–) is a good example for this: the clash between the middle-class midwives and the working class women they serve is one of the major plot-driving factors. Another example that features class prominently is *Nurse Jackie* (Showtime, 2009–2015) which portraits the titular protagonist as an emancipated, down-to-Earth breadwinner and contrasts her to her extremely wealthy, but out-of-touch doctor-friend.

In the United States, the racial bias was further perpetuated by the white supremacy strategies of the Red Cross (Jones, 2013: 54–56), the Flexner report (Sullivan and Mittman, 2010) and other segregationist policies.

To this day, nurses of color and male nurses are still portrayed as out of the norm, if included at all. The characters are subject to parody or are presented in stereotypical terms, for example the characters Laverne and Carla in *Scrubs* (NBC, 2011–2010), Thor in *Nurse Jackie*, or the entire premise of "Nurse Focker" in *Meet the Parents* (2010, dir. Jay Roach). The nurses of color are mostly female matrons—unattractive, often overweight, older—or dominating matriarchs as a cliché of Latinx cultures. Male nurses are associated with queerness or are assigned effeminate qualities.

Intersectionality is the notion that our social identities comprise several overlapping factors that potentially subject us to discrimination. While the racial and social status of mainstream nurses might render them privileged, nurses in pop culture are connected to a less privileged position with regard to gender, education, ageism and ableism. As McAllister and Brien point out, this leads to "challenges [that] involve struggles with personal, institutional and systemic manifestations of power, hierarchy and control" (2020: 2). In all of these aspects of their identity, they are presented as ambivalent. They are part of the "biopower" (Foucault, 2003: 239–264) and at the same time they are expected to be what Foucault called "docile bodies" (Foucault, 1979: 135–169; Wildman, 2014). They have direct power over those in their care but its legitimacy is precarious and can tip easily into abuse of power or violence as the boundaries are notoriously hard to define in a profession "where touch is an important component of care" (Gallop, 1999: 43). They are medically educated, but are considered "less than" doctors, as women, they are "less than" men, and as older women they are "less than" younger women. Most importantly for the following argument, though, is that they are "less than" the figures of femininity at the core of heteronormativity—the virgin saint or the mother.

Again, the show *Call the Midwife* (see also Morag Martin's essay in this collection) serves as an illustrative example. While the show's focus is on the poverty and living conditions of the dock workers and their families in the East End of London, as well as the young nurse's maturation as she navigates these conditions, the show reveals the specific place that nurses inhabit in the realm of femininity. The midwives are unmarried, single women who do not have children. They are part of a convent of nuns, who are by definition virginal. The show paradigmatically locates the young midwives between the virgin ideal and proto-feminine mothers. However, they are middle-class and thanks to Florence Nightingale's proto-feminist activism, working outside of the home and are thus not considered prostitutes (Michie, 1987: 67). This independence finds its visual correlative in their bicycles which also marks them as progressive women, and poses a potential threat as they operate outside of patriarchal control.

This is shown at the very beginning of the pilot episode (2012, dir.

Philippa Lowthorpe). The opening scene has the main protagonist Jenny Lee arrive at the docks. With a swagger in her walk and bright red lipstick, she walks through the workers who all turn their heads and leer at her. A few scenes later, she is wearing her uniform that substitutes her individual identity with a mere occupational function. As she is still wearing a skirt and not trousers, she has transformed into a gendered, but non-sexual entity. She forfeited her femininity and now flies under the radar of the male gaze which provides her with more freedom and power. In this scene, Jenny changes from a sexualized woman into the functional vessel that only serves that core femininity of motherhood.

Abjectification of Nurses

Thus she becomes the *chora*, the vessel that receives and brings into the world without having any other feature or quality (Kristeva, 1982: 13–15; Butler, 1993: 41–42). In feminist readings of the Platonic *chora*, and particularly in Butler's queer theory, the *chora* and the abject are blended (Butler, ibid.). Julia Kristeva reads the mother as the first, original abject figuration, but argues that her threat is domesticated and controlled by the symbolism of the Virgin Mary (Kristeva, 1977; Covino, 2004: 21–22), while the nurse is neither.

This is the tipping point between the stereotype of the docile and demure, "good nurses" like Jenny Lee in *Call the Midwife*, and scary women such as Annie Wilkes in Rob Reiner's *Misery* (1990) or in the show *Castle Rock* (Hulu, 2018–2019). Certainly, nurses are linked, through their occupation, with gore or the abject, with death, decay and bodily functions, but that does not turn them into abject monsters. Just because they clean bedpans or work in a hospice does not mean they are neither subjects nor controllable objects, but an *abject*, created to consolidate another subject's identity:

> The forming of a subject requires an identification […], and this identification takes place through a repudiation which produces a domain of abjection, a repudiation without which the subject cannot emerge. This is a repudiation which creates the valence of "abjection" and its status for the subject as a threatening spectre [Butler, 1993: 3].

Nurses in visual culture become abject in the moment they incorporate everything that the heteronormative ideal of the virgin/mother is not: they are old, unattractive, gay, barren, promiscuous, uncaring and/or abusive. Additionally, the abject is closely linked to sexism, homophobia, and racism. By "the repudiation of bodies for their sex, sexuality, and/or color is an 'expulsion' followed by a 'repulsion' that founds and consolidates culturally hegemonic identities along sex/race/sexuality axes of differentiation" (Butler, 1999: 170).

Butler (1993: 41) claims that they "displace the feminine at the moment they purport to represent the feminine." Nurses are not mothers, they are assigned femininity outside of that "essential" femininity, they become the abject, just as the lesbian is the abject in a phallocentric world (ibid.). First the subject expels the "not me" to form its own identity, then it is repulsed by, and scared of it. As a classic horror trope, it needs to be purged from a purified, sacred society:

> [The] abject is also the non-objectality [sic!] of the archaic mother, the locus of needs, of attraction and repulsion, from which an object of forbidden desire arises...[A]bject can be understood in the sense of the horrible and fascinating abomination which is connoted in all cultures by the feminine or, more indirectly, by every partial object which is related to the state of abjection.... It becomes what culture, the sacred must purge, separate and banish so that it may establish itself as such in the universal logic of catharsis [Kristeva, 1982: 317].

The abject, "scary" figure of the nurse, along the lines of Kristeva's psychoanalytic reading, is neither an object that can be dominated, nor an externalized *doppelganger*, but something that used to belong to the subject and now is rendered *unheimlich* (Kristeva, 1991: 182–183) and considered repulsive. In Butler's deconstructivist rendering, the abject is part of the non-phallocentric subjectivization and is linked to lesbianism. In the following, we will encounter examples of both, the heteronormative and the queer-deconstructivist version of the nurse as abject.

Nursing Monstrosities: Fragile, Silent Hill *and* Nurse 3D

In Jaume Balagueró's *Fragile* (2005), Amy Nicholls, an attractive, single nurse takes over the post at an almost abandoned hospital. She takes care of the few pediatric patients who have not yet been transferred to the new facility after certain supernatural events drove off the previous night nurse. Amy soon learns about the urban legend of "Charlotte," a ghost who allegedly lives in the abandoned upstairs ward. She is said to be responsible for unexplainable fractures and other injuries that are forcing the children to stay at the hospital as they cannot be transported elsewhere. Charlotte communicates through alphabet blocks, appears to the orphan Maggie, and Amy finds a photograph that says "Charlotte and Mandy, 1959" which shows a hospitalized girl with a nurse. Amy and the audience are led to believe that Charlotte is the girl in the picture. The big reveal of the movie, however, is that Charlotte is the old, childless nurse who breaks the child's bones to be able to continue to care for her. After her Munchausen Syndrome by Proxy is exposed, she turns her own body into an abject monstrosity by screwing the metal orthodontic braces into her bones, and falls to her death in an elevator shaft.

Charlotte is the abject antagonist to the kind, mild-mannered and much younger Amy, who emotionally connects with the terminally ill Meggie. While Charlotte wants to control the children in her care, Amy develops a motherly love that strives to protect Meggie. The showdown finally shows Charlotte for the ultimate shock value. It is less the mutilation than her old naked body that makes her one of Sobchack's scary women. Specifically, it is her old breasts—*mammae*—that are exposed in the restraining medical device which points to the opposite of nurturing motherhood and is its abject counterpart. It is significant in this regard that both Meggie and Amy grew up orphans, so are motherless. Amy does not have a child of her own, she is single and probably past her child-bearing years. However, it is suggested that her love for the child transcends death. The play-in-play structure of Disney's *Sleeping Beauty* and the "true love's kiss" that can wake even a comatose girl points here to a feminist twist. While *Fragile* conventionally externalizes and exorcises the future horror of the old spinster nurse for Amy, she is also as powerful as Prince Charming. The movie transposes the male dominance over a petrified, controlled women's body, the same logic that Charlotte's braces follow as well, onto a maternal love that is literally meta-physical. Neither Amy nor Maggie need a man to find true love or to father a child. At the same time, the parallel between their relationship and Charlotte/Mandy illustrate the split off abject horror that is inherent in nursing: The Munchausen by Proxy trope cuts both ways as it reveals both the potentially abusive side of nursing as well as the performative aspect of nursing and its importance for identity formation: nurses depend on someone to care for; it constitutes their entire *raison d'être*.

In the Konami's *Silent Hill* video game franchise (1999–2012), the abusive power and correlation with the abject of disease or pain spawns two variants. Related to *Fragile*, in the first *Silent Hill* (1999) and *Silent Hill 3* (2003) the female protagonists are girls, Alessa or Heather as her alter ego, who were hospitalized in the past. Their memories of horrific pain after Alessa's mother burnt her almost to death as part of a cult ritual creates the fantastical Puppet Nurses (Alessa in *Silent Hill*) or more human-seeming nurses (Heather's in *Silent Hill 3*). They are "puppets" as part of the executive arm of her mother's cult. They bring pain and are connected to memories of torture. In the game, they become adversaries to fight the player at the hospital with scalpels, but are not part of the character's journey and they can thus be avoided. The trauma they represent is re-imagined as the wounds they inflict on the player.

Significantly, these nurses look more like the old-fashioned variant with cardigans over conservative blouses and skirts that cover the knees and the traditional nurse's cap. This stands in stark contrast to the so-called Bubble Head Nurses in *Silent Hill 2* (2001) and other variants that are rooted in the male protagonists' subconscious. These nurses are wearing tight, low-cut uniforms and ultra-mini skirts. They are long-legged and busty. Their sex-appeal, however, is mixed with the abject: their uniforms are stained with blood and what looks like excrement, their legs look varicose, their limbs are distorted and constantly twitching or writhing. Most notably, however, their faces are obscured by bandages, only their bloodied jaws and teeth are exposed, referencing symbolically the *vagina dentata*. The clash of sexual desire and the abject is rooted in the protagonist James' experience of his wife Mary's slow death and decay, and his suppressed, unfulfilled desires that came with it.

The Bubble Head Nurses stand for his wife Mary and the desire for her that waned as her illness progressed and she became increasingly aggressive. Accordingly, these nurses are more aggressive than their precursors, and it is hard to avoid them as they are part of his journey. Significantly, they fight him with a weapon similar to his, a phallic steel pipe. They are not only a threat, but are also the revenge to his phallocentric egotism that led him to kill his sick wife who was never able to bear his child. The nurses need to be kept at bay and killed off from a distance. If that is not possible, they need to be struck down and kicked when they are already on the ground. The sexual fantasy meets the suppressed bad conscience, which is intricately linked to fear of castration and other sado-masochistic fantasies that make the Bubble Heads a favorite of Halloween cosplay.

While Charlotte is the ghostly manifestation of abuse, and the Bubble Head Nurses are monstrous projections in the hell of James's own making, Doug Aarniokoski's *Nurse 3D* (2013) stars a real-nurse protagonist, who takes the sado-masochistic fantasy to an extreme. An attractive, highly sexualized head nurse tortures and punishes the men who cheat on their wives, and stalks a young nurse who she drugs at some point to have sex with her. The movie caters in every way to the male gaze and fantasies, including lesbian sex that is marked as abusive if not violent. It also plays on the trope of the hysterical woman, taking revenge on men. It turns out that she used to be hospitalized in a mental institution for killing her violent father, and subsequently took on the identity of the nurse who took her in. The movie is the prototypical example for, and parody of the figure of the nurse who is interlocked with the abject, fear of castration, mental health, lesbianism and pornographic, sado-masochistic fantasies. It also shows the other hallmarks of the "scary nurse" in pop culture, that places her outside of a socially accepted femininity of heteronormative relationships and motherhood. This culminates in the movie's poster of Abby in the sado-masochistic fantasy uniform, riding a gigantic syringe like a broomstick.

Beyond taking stock of these clichéd elements, the movie serves as the extreme example of a pervasive pattern. Even groundbreaking shows like *Nurse Jackie* that featured a capable, emancipated and complex nurse as the main protagonist, turned her opioid addiction into something that made her a morally bad character in terms of heteronormative femininity. Although in scrubs and middle-aged, she abuses the power she has over men, she is neither a good wife, nor mother. As breadwinner and as seductress, she is a threat to the men around her. However, she is an excellent nurse nonetheless, and above all, the show renders her a person, a fallible human being. However, the "heterosexist economy that disempowers contestatory possibilities by rendering them culturally unthinkable and unviable" (Butler, 1993: 111) is still at work, and the show remains moralistic in outlook.

After the above examples had aired, streaming services were soon to dominate the markets—a tendency that was exacerbated by the 2020 pandemic, as well as socio-cultural change, most notably the #MeToo Movement. Like other new media before it, the streaming industry has shaped viewing habits as well as content. Apart from its *dispositif* more comparable to TV than cinema, streaming content for the most apart is free of overt sponsorship, operates outside institutional politics of the broadcasting systems and democratized gazes as well as forms of life (McDonald and Smith-Rowsey, 2016; Johnson, 2018). It is certainly no coincidence that after *Nurse Jackie* and the Me Too–Movement, two of the most notorious nurses returned to the screen at practically the same time. In the following, I will compare the two originals, *Misery* (1990) and *One Flew Over the Cuckoo's Nest* (1975) with their imagined prequels to excavate the subtle power relations between the two most famous scary nurses and the populations they serve.

Annie Wilkes, Psychiatric Nurse

> ANNIE is standing beside the bed. She wears off-white and seems very much like a nurse. A good nurse. She has pills in her hands.
> —Goldman, 1990: n.p.

Watching the second season of *Castle Rock* (2019), the homage to Rob Reiner's 1990 iconic *Misery* is evident and the (reverse) continuity tangible. Yet, the show provides a depth and layering to the notorious Annie Wilkes that is significant in terms of gender and abjectification. The same is true for Mildred Ratched's imagined backstory. Yet, while Nurse Ratched takes care of, and sadistically abuses vulnerable psychiatric patients, Annie herself is a patient with an obscure, undiagnosed mental illness. She is delusional, at times psychotic, obsessive-compulsive, then again violently depressed. Her unpredictability and uncontrolled rage while she wields complete power over her patient Paul Sheldon is what makes her a scary woman, a threat to the male protagonist.

The camera supports these moments with low angle shots as she towers over her immobile patient. The streaming show captures a similar threat by expressing her rage in her unnatural, mechanical gait when she approaches. Additionally, both old and young Annie Wilkes are rendered unattractive and unfeminine in a way through several means: her old-fashioned hairstyle, her body shape (overweight in the older version, no curves in the younger), her clothing and lack of makeup, her style of speaking, the holier-than-thou moralism and anachronistic mannerisms, and above all her childishness. She is not a mother, although she poses as one in *Castle Rock*. Her shrewdness is almost grotesque, as, for instance, she lives with a sow she named Misery after the titular protagonist of Paul's novels. Thus, her power does not derive from sexuality, but the opposite: She represents the abject, pitiful, overlooked woman who is only participating in Paul's world by proxy of his books.

The beginning of the movie has a cool, handsome and affluent, best-selling author almost die in a car wreck during a blizzard. Annie rescues him from certain death, and nurses him back to health. She has an ulterior motive: to make him stay with her as she is his stalkery "number-one fan" (Goldman, 1990: n.p.). She is portrayed as emotionally unsound and silly in her girlish infatuation with the worldly Paul. Annie is completely powerless in Paul's universe, until she controls the limits of his world: while he is unable to move, most of the scenes show Paul bedridden or in a wheelchair, the shots are either on him, or point of view shots from his perspective. Accordingly, the majority of scenes are filmed in his room, limiting his and the audience's view. Stephen King's novel and Rob Reiner's movie reimagine Alfred Hitchcock's *Rear Window* (1954) with the male gaze turned onto itself and the caretaker not as a beautiful ally, but an abject aggressor. It is the phallocentric fear of the revenge of the undesirable, men-hating woman.

Annie's horror arises from her absolute control over the emasculated man. She is constantly visually fractured and she is hardly ever shown in total, evading a fixating gaze. The scene that introduces her in the movie first shows her legs, her hands on the crowbar, her arms dragging Shelby out of the car. She carries him through the deep snow and uphill, but her face is obscured by the body over her shoulder. She could pass for a man, and she is stronger than Paul. In addition to her strength, his first sight of her shows that she possesses everything in her private ward that helps her to control him, specifically the drugs she feeds him as pain killers. Her care and help actually render him immobile. When he tries to escape, she "hobbles" him so he cannot run away like her husband did. The only reason she puts him in a wheelchair is so that he can write a new novel under her directive. The typewriter symbolically represents her ambivalent care and his dependence on her: As the machine is missing the character "N," she has to fill those in the manuscript. He is completely dependent on Annie, who is now in control of the stories he tells.

The story centers on the acts of writing and reading, and the inherent gendered power relations. Paul, as a writer of romance novels, is the maker of his female characters, and has the power to "kill his darlings" (King, 2001: 222) as he does with Misery Chastain. In a reveal conversation with his agent, she claims that he uses his characters, then drops them, suggesting that this is how he treats women. It is also pointed out that he exerts a huge influence on women like Annie. Annie, on the other hand, correlates her voracious reading to her long hours of nightshift nursing. The demure, docile body of the good nurse intersects here with the quiet female reader. This dynamic is dramatically changed by the accident. Their first encounter shows Annie performing CPR, thus breathing life into him, "You hear me—Breathe! I said breathe!!!" (Goldman, 1990: n.p.). After she brings him back, he becomes a character in her story.

They are competing storytellers, readers and critics of each other's narratives throughout their encounter. Annie's power lies in her ability to conjure up and control narratives. Both Paul and the viewer only have the information she provides. As Paul finds her photo album filled with newspaper clippings, he becomes the shocked reader of her past auteurship of horror stories that involve her as an Angel of Death, responsible for killing children. Furthermore, early in the film, Paul, with a writer's alertness to narrative consistency, catches some inconsistencies in her accounts, he also interrupts her reminiscing and he patronizes her several times, to which she angrily responds: "I know that, Mister Man—… I'm not stupid, you know" (Goldman, 1990: n.p.). In a similar situation, she throws the writing paper into his lap, revealing the connection between the phallocentrism of his writing, as well as the castration threat she poses.

The power relations of writer and reader, phallocentrism, the nurse and the abject tie young Annie with her notorious older version. Her backstory explains her character while making significant changes: whereas the movie narrates the events from the male writer's perspective, the TV show presents Annie's story and is often told from her point of view. Here, the fragmented shots express her fragmented reality and disrupted perception. The first episode, "Let the River Run" (dir. Greg Yaitanes), introduces teenage Annie first as the proverbial babe in the woods. The prosodic shots are interspersed by dark screens that accentuate the sounds, mostly a clicking typewriter, which lend rhythm to the scene and acoustically mark the connection to *Misery*: We hear Annie panting, then we see a close-up of her bloody hands on a banker's box, labeled "The Ravening Angel." A typewriter clacking, then a bloodied shirt, a close up on her bloody face and wide blue eyes, frantically glancing over her shoulder as she is haunted by the typing sound. As the typewriter's carriage return zings to a new line, a new scene starts: The camera zooms in, and the box gives an ominous shake. From the start, Annie is constructed to be the haunted victim and it seems that the real threat is in that box.

What is in that box is her father's creation—her baby half-sister Evangeline/Joy, labeled as the novel he wrote. The baby and the novel merge into one from the phallocentric angle of creation. This is revealed in episode 5, "The Laughing Place" on which the entire season hinges. The viewer sees her in grade school. She is bullied because of her dyslexia so she hits another child. As the principal suggests having her screened by a psychiatrist, the parents are outraged. Her mother, a severe, aging nurse, thinks she is pure and perfect; her father, a failed writer and narcissist with a history of mania critiques their approach. Both parents have paranoid streaks, and they don't want her numbed or "brainwashed." The father becomes Annie's entire world as he homeschools her. Against the dismissal of the mother, the father makes Annie an accomplice in his writing of the novel "The Ravening Angel." He makes her his first reader and critic but teaches her little else. Though he is more loving than her mother, the relationship to her father is marked by emotional abuse, blind admiration and inappropriateness.

The reading tutor, Rita, a young, beautiful and self-confident woman, transforms Annie into a positive, healthy and potentially independent teenager. Though her father moves out, she rejects her mother's pessimism, depression and alcoholism, and is ready to go to college. Yet, her subjectivization is not completed as her continued extreme fixation on her father suggests. Her Electra complex is further complicated by her mother trying to kill them both in a murder-suicide. As her father moves back home, she learns he has had an affair with Rita, and that they have a child together. Annie, now enraged by their betrayal and lies, has a psychotic breakdown when the triangle of desire between father and (new) mother is reiterated. She inadvertently kills her father who is spiked on a bannister post, and stabs Rita with a pair of scissors, then takes the baby. Instead of severing ties with the mother to abjectify her, Annie becomes her. Annie takes on her mother's strict, moralistic persona and becomes a parody of the nurse and mother figure she represents, down to emulating her phrases.

She reenacts this traumatic patricide with phallic weapons when the "dirty birdie" landlord is threatening her and Joy ("Let the River Run"). The scene shows her in the kitchen, in child-like pajamas, dishing out ice cream for herself. When he approaches her, she shoves the scoop down his throat. Annie kills him but he returns, like all her past skeletons. This is what she has in common with the other female characters in the show. Her story of personal haunting is mirrored by a white soldier being haunted by his killing of a Somali mother, and the entire town is haunted by its genocidal past. Annie and her female antagonists are united in their fight against the casually misogynistic patriarchs of the town. While the movie gravitates towards its phallic center, literally Paul's crotch as he stuffs everything he thinks might come in handy into the front of his sweatpants, the show focuses on the female characters' perspective and their struggle against patriarchal dominance. However, while the black female doctor succeeds, nurse Annie fails and remains stuck in her infantile stage of her Electra complex. In a scene of dramatic irony she drowns Joy, who just completed her subjectivization successfully and was about to "emancipate" herself. Annie, who has lost her status of motherhood, sublimates this by becoming Paul Sheldon's "number-one fan" as she says in the very last scene of the season.

Mildred Ratched, Psychiatric Nurse

> "Your mother and I are old friends, you know that."
> —*One Flew Over the Cuckoo's Nest*, 1975

While young Annie Wilkes is directly linked to the original, the prequel to Nurse Ratched differs significantly from the character as portrayed in the movie. The character in *One Flew Over the Cuckoo's Nest* is as flat in affect as her imagined younger iteration but this is where the similarities end. The horror of the original adversary to cocky, manic narcissist Randle McMurphy is rooted in a very specific power dynamic. It is manifest in the nurses' station that functions as Ratched's panoptic surveillance booth and as her seemingly impenetrable fortress. It is expressed by her access to, and frequent use of the PA system, her control over the TV, her supervision in group therapy, dominating the discourse. As such, Nurse Ratched's power is institutional as well as systemic. Furthermore, she takes care of a very vulnerable patient population, which makes her real or perceived manipulations all the more upsetting. As a powerful female controlling a group of men, McMurphy challenges her threat to their masculinity, particularly when he thinks she is abusing her power. She is explicitly linked to Billy's mother, more blatantly in the movie version than the script, but Lawrence Hauben's original is more revealing: "I don't want your mother to believe something like this but what am I to think?" (Hauben, 1975: n.p.). By treating Billy's mother as a victim of her son's actions, and conflating what the mother believes and what Ratched thinks, she punishes Billy for expressing his sexuality.

This sadistic response is a sublimation itself. It occurs at the climax of the movie after Nurse Ratched—or Big Nurse, as she is called in Hauben's script, discovered that McMurphy entered and symbolically penetrated her sanctum, as he defiled the nurses' station in a night of drunken debauchery. This blatant deconstruction of her power makes evident the sexual frustration that she causes for McMurphy as she keeps him locked up and away from his girlfriends. She depicts the severe mother, while at the same time presenting an austere, but attractive woman whose whole expression and demeanor is mirrored in the screened off nurses' station: she is detached, in full control and out of reach. Her speech is deliberate, her facial expression motionless. While her apprentice at her side, young Nurse Pilbow, is an attractive and round-eyed novice, Ratched wears no make-up, and her face is curiously grey and hard. She represents the totalitarian and at times absolutist power that lies behind the impenetrable boundary which McMurphy tries to dismantle (Gross, 2018).

The perspective, that some read as anti-feminist (Munoz 2013) in addition to capturing the dehospitalization of U.S. mental health (Rondinone, 2020), shifts from movie to show. Instead of the rage of an emasculated McMurphy or the quiet rage of entire indigenous people rendered powerless by systemic racism as represented by Chief Bromden, her younger version becomes a titular heroine in her own right. Her detached and inaccessible source of power follows a similar logic as the show uses the aesthetics of 1940s movie stars to convey it: She appears to be hyperreal, luminous, out of reach. She is also manipulative and unscrupulous, and in episode 1 she drives a patient to commit suicide. Clearly, her notoriety and the fascination with the graphic side of 1940s psychiatry were enough for the producers of the *American Horror Story* to make this spinoff.

The show's aesthetic is akin to *American Horror Story*'s visual regimes and what Alberto Garcia described as the emerging "bright noir" (2018). The filters, colors and set design are all domineered by the visual paradigm of a "society of spectacle" (Debord, 2012). The mental health aspects such as the lobotomy, hypnosis, multi-personality patients and lesbianism are on the same plane as degradation of the human, commodity fetishism, and the spectacle of politics. Everything follows the dictum of the spectacle, including abject bodies populating the scenes, the torture and the gore. One example which affects only male characters is the frequent amputations in lieu of actual castrations that occur in the show.

Mildred Ratched, in this version, becomes a luminous simulacrum of her movie version, a copy with no original. In Butler's sense she also becomes a parody, a pastiche of elegant 1940s women, including nurses and lesbians. The entire nursing staff is white and female (with the exception of one disfigured male), and the characters are color-coded. The older women are dark-haired, witch-like tricksters, the young blonde nurses are promiscuous. Ratched herself as morally ambivalent, bisexual and highly manipulative is the only redhead. Her age is obscured. She is neither young nor markedly middle-aged. Like her predecessor, her looks are a mirage, a projection screen for everybody around her, as well as for the viewers.

Younger Mildred is not powerful because of her (sublimated) sexuality or her institutional power, but her intrigues and the knowledge they provide her with. She uses it to blackmail other characters to achieve her goals. What makes this show interesting, despite the conventional abject horror and clichéd notions about mental health, is the perspectival change on heteronormative power relations, and the anti-phallocentric tendency of gazes. Firstly, those relations are starkly gendered and, by means of slapstick elements, clearly marked as parodies of well-known stereotypes. It is also a contemporary comment on the 1940s sexual politics the show presents. The clinic director is a short man with a Napoleon complex, the head nurse is dominating. The castration threat here is exposed as an uncompelling cliché when old Nurse Bucket muses that he probably doesn't ask her out because she is too strong and powerful. At the same time, the director is portrayed as a charlatan: incompetent, clueless and completely dominated by the women around him. By contrast, Nurse Bucket shows real leadership and takes over after the doctor is murdered and comments on the antiquated hiring practices, "I hired a woman doctor, isn't that incredible?" ("Mildred and Edmund," dir. Daniel Minahan) Moreover, similar to *Nurse Jackie* this show offers the broad range of nurse stereotypes such as the Angel of Mercy, hand-maiden, battle-ax, and naughty nurse (Ferns and Chojnacka, 2005: 1028), but all of them transgress heteronormative boundaries: the demure handmaiden is not at all the docile body that she is supposed to be, and Mildred as an "angel of mercy" kills several severely injured soldiers during the war while the show does not morally dismiss the act. Mildred is shown to be a capable nurse, even while she is euthanizing her patients.

In a similar vein, the role of homosexuality in *Ratched* is ambivalent but errs again on the side of parody, that is, not of the lesbians but of homophobia. In a scene of suppressed homosexual desires, a male patient who is known to "stab" men as a sublimated act of penetration, roofies the director with the medication he is about to receive himself. After taking the medication, the doctor has a psychotic episode and amputates the patient's limbs so he cannot stab anyone anymore. Likewise, Mildred at first violently rejects the notion of lesbianism, then helps the affected patients to escape while she boils the man alive who tells her she was the "worst 'lay' [he] ever had" ("Angel of Mercy: Part Two," dir. Michael Oppendahl).

> What is "unveiled" is precisely the repudiated desire, that which is abjected by heterosexist logic and that which is defensively foreclosed through the effort to circumscribe a specifically feminine morphology for lesbianism [Butler, 1993: 86].

She subsequently starts a relationship that is remarkably respectful and stands in stark contrast to the visual regime of scopophilia the show promotes: both women are middle-aged, and their relationship loving, harmonious and not explicitly sexual. In short, the lesbianism here is not presented as abject, but as anti-phallocentristic, overcoming the stigma of the abject.

From Mothering Nurses to Nursing Mothers

> So this horror of the abject body is [...] linked with the body of the mother, but with an even more radically other mother [...]
>   —Covino, 2004: 21

In her essay "Scary Women," Vivian Sobchack quotes Simone de Beauvoir: women are "haunted by the horror of growing old ... when the first hints come of that fated and irreversible process" they would feel "the fatal touch of death itself" (2004: 42). Sobchack is quick to point out that de Beauvoir's lament is "by today's standards problematic" (ibid.) as it underscores the mid-twentieth-century phallocentrism. Contemporary visual culture would render even Sobchack's argument as outdated when considering shows like *Ratched* and its bright noir, or films like *Fragile* that suggests an anti-biologistic form of motherhood as equally viable.

In a changed socio-cultural climate and changing visual dispositif with a proliferation and globalization of content, diversified identities and alternative gazes have affected gendered tropes and stereotypes. At the same time, there is a conservative tendency to re-introduce another variant of the monstrous-feminine. The symbolic order "can maintain itself only by maintaining its borders; and the abject points to the fragility of those borders" (Oliver, 1998: 56). While the narratives of nurses have been slowly changing over the last decade, transgressions of heteronormative boundaries have become more frequent. This prompts a counter narrative that aims at the original site of the abject: At the same time that nurses become complex human beings, and with nuns seemingly out of the picture with notable exceptions such as *Dracula* (Netflix, 2020). Certain mother figures are back in focus.

The most prominent trope involved in the more recent negative portrayals of mothers is the Munchausen Syndrome by Proxy, which has become popular over the last decade in fiction and nonfiction. It is at the center of *Sharp Objects* (HBO, 2018), *Ma* (2019, dir. Tate Taylor), *Run* (Hulu, 2020, dir. Aneesh Chaganty), or *The Act*, one of many shows, movies and documentaries about DeeDee Blanchard (Hulu, 2019). The fascination with the trope and its anti-feminist impetus follows the same logic as the abject in our above examples, and is paired with another staple of pop cultural othering—mental health. While mothers in the narratives discussed above are marked as blatantly absent, it is interesting that nurses and mothers are often portrayed as antagonists in stories about Munchausen: one who sickens and one who heals. And it is indicative of the abject scary woman that it seems interchangeable who takes on which role.

Films and Television Productions Referenced

The Act (2019) streaming, Hulu.
Call the Midwife (2012–present) BBC.
Castle Rock (2018–2019) streaming, Hulu.
Dracula (2020–present) streaming, Netflix.
Fragile, Frágiles (2005) Castelao Producciones S.A.
Ma (2019) Universal Pictures.
Meet the Parents (1990) Universal Pictures.
Misery (1990) Columbia Pictures.
Nurse Jackie (2009–2015), streaming, Showtime.
Nurse 3D (2013) Lionsgate
One Flew Over the Cuckoo's Nest (1975) United Artists.
Run (2020) streaming, Hulu.
Rear Window (1954) Paramount Pictures.
Scrubs (2001–2010) NBC.
Sharp Objects (2018), streaming, HBO.
Silent Hill (1999) Xbox 360 [Game]. Konami, Tokyo.
Silent Hill 2 (2001) Xbox 360 [Game]. Konami, Tokyo.
Silent Hill 3 (2003) Xbox 360 [Game]. Konami, Tokyo.

References

Butler, J. (1993) *Bodies That Matter: On the Discursive Limits of "Sex."* New York: Routledge.
Butler, J. (1999) *Gender Trouble: Feminism and the Subversion of Identity*. New York: Routledge.

Covino, D.C. (2004) *Amending the Abject Body: Aesthetic Makeovers in Medicine and Culture.* New York: State University of New York.

Creed, B. (1993) *The Monstrous-Feminine: Film, Feminism, Psychoanalysis.* London: Routledge.

Debord, G. (2012) *Society of the Spectacle*, 2nd edition. Eastbourne: Soul Bay Press.

Ferns, T., and Chojnacka, I. (2005) Angels and Swingers, Matrons and Sinners: Nursing Stereotypes. *British Journal of Nursing* 14, 19: 1028–1032.

Foucault, M. (1977/1980) The Confession of the Flesh. Interview. In: Gordin, C. (ed.) *Power/Knowledge Selected Interviews and Other Writings*. pp. 194–228.

Foucault, M. (1979) *Discipline and Punish: The Birth of the Prison.* London: Vintage.

Foucault, M., et al. (2003) *Society Must be Defended: Lectures at the Collège de France, 1975–76* (trans. David Macey). New York: Picador.

Gallop, R. (1998/1987) Abuse of Power in the Nurse-Client Relationship. *Nursing Standard (Royal College of Nursing (Great Britain)* 1987), 12, 37: 43–47.

García, A.N. (2018) The Rise of "Bright Noir." In: Hansen, K.T., Peacock, S., and Turnbull, S. (eds.). *European Television Crime Drama and Beyond, Palgrave European Film and Media Studies.* Basingstoke: Palgrave Macmillan, pp. 41–60.

Goldman, W. (1990) Misery. Based on a Novel by Stephen King, Screenplay, Online source: https://www.dailyscript.com/scripts/misery.html (accessed 4 January 2021).

Gross, T. (2018) Remembering Milos Forman, Director of *One Flew Over The Cuckoo's Nest*, NPR, Online source: https://www.npr.org/2018/04/20/604295204/remembering-milos-forman-director-of-one-flew-over-the-cuckoos-nest (accessed 4 January 2021).

Hansen, K.T., Peacock, S., and Turnbull, S. (eds.) (2018) *European Television Crime Drama and Beyond.* Basingstoke: Palgrave Macmillan.

Hauben, L. (1975) One Flew Over the Cuckoo's Nest. Based on a Novel by Ken Kelsey, Screenplay, Online source: https://www.scriptslug.com/assets/uploads/scripts/one-flew-over-the-cuckoos-nest-1975.pdf (accessed 4 January 2021).

Jay, M. (1992) Scopic Regimes of Modernity. In: Lash, S., and Friedman, J. (eds.) *Modernity and Identity.* Oxford: Blackwell.

Johnson, D. (ed.) (2018) *From Networks to Netflix: A Guide to Changing Channels.* London: Routledge.

Jones, M.M. (2013) *The American Red Cross: From Clara Barton to the New Deal.* Baltimore: The Johns Hopkins University Press.

King, S. (2001) *On Writing: A Memoir of the Craft.* London: Hodder & Stoughton.

Kristeva, J. (1974/1986) Revolution in Poetic Language. In: Kristeva, J., and Moi, T (eds.), *The Kristeva Reader.* Oxford: Basil Blackwell, pp. 90–136.

Kristeva, J. (1977/1986) Stabat Mater. In Kristeva, J., and Moi, T. (eds.), *The Kristeva Reader.* Oxford: Basil Blackwell, pp. 161–186.

Kristeva, J. (1982) *Powers of Horror: An Essay on Abjection* (translated by Len S. Roudiez). New York: Columbia University Press.

Kristeva, J. (1982/1986) Psychoanalysis and the Polis. In: Kristeva, J., and Moi, T. (eds.) *The Kristeva Reader.* Oxford: Basil Blackwell, pp. 302–320.

Kristeva, J., and Roudiez, L.S. (1991) *Strangers to Ourselves.* New York: Columbia University Press.

McAllister, M., and Brien, D.L. (2020) *Paradoxes in Nurses' Identity, Culture and Image: The Shadow Side of Nursing.* New York: Routledge.

McDonald, K., and Smith-Rowsey, D. (eds.) (2016) *The Netflix Effect: Technology and Entertainment in the 21st Century.* New York: Bloomsbury Academic.

Michie, H. (1987) *The Flesh Made Word: Female Figures and Women's Bodies.* Oxford: Oxford University Press.

Mulvey, L. (1975) "Visual Pleasure and Narrative Cinema." *Screen* 16, 3: 6–18.

Munoz, M. (2013) "A veritable angel of mercy": The Problem of Nurse Ratched in Ken Kesey's *One Flew Over the Cuckoo's Nest. The Southern Review* 49, 4: 668–671.

Rondinone, T. (2020) The Folklore of Deinstitutionalization: Popular Film and the Death of the Asylum, 1973–1979. *Journal of American Studies* 54, 5: 900–925.

Sobchack, V.C. (2004) Scary Women. Cinema, Surgery, and Special Effects. In: *Carnal*

Thoughts: Embodiment and Moving Image Culture. Berkeley: University of California Press, 36–52.

Sullivan, L.W., and Suez Mittman, I. (2010) The State of Diversity in the Health Professions a Century After Flexner. *Academic Medicine Journal of the Association of American Medical Colleges* 85, 2: 246–253.

Wildman, S. (2014) "Docile Bodies" or "Impudent Women": Conflicts Between Nurses and Their Employers, in England, 1880–1914. *Medizin, Gesellschaft, und Geschichte Jahrbuch des Instituts fur Geschichte der Medizin der Robert Bosch Stiftung*, 32: 9–20.

Eroticizing the Nurse

(Bi/Homo)Sexuality and Monstrosity
in Nurse 3D

Tatiana Prorokova-Konrad

Introduction

The nurse as a cultural construct has acquired multiple meanings through the portrayals offered by film, literature, and other media. Those depictions are contradictory and polar in nature. The nurse can appear as a caregiver and savior, or, on the contrary, as a murderer—both such representations are induced by the fact that a nurse possesses certain medical knowledge that can potentially be used to cure or harm another human. Even more enthralling is a cultural transformation of the nurse into a sex object—a stereotype that seems to have become even more persistent than the first two. Indeed, Sandy Summers and Harry Jacobs Summers (2015) note that media portrayals of nurses are that of "low-skilled handmaidens, sex objects, or angels" (xxiv). Similarly, Margaret McAllister and Donna Lee Brien (2020), commenting on nursing in cultural imagination, observe that "common stereotypes include the angel of mercy, the hand-maiden and the battleaxe" (7). Finally, Jacinta Kelly, Gerard M. Fealy, and Roger Watson (2012) identify two major stereotypes relating to nurses on screen: "the caring mother and the object of sexual desire" (1805). This essay focuses explicitly on the stereotype of the nurse as a sex object, and argues that it is essentially generated relying on the two original visions of the nurse as either a savior or a murderer. Specifically, the essay explores how, by means of eroticizing the uniform, training, and terminology, among other things, the image of the nurse as a sex object continues to perpetuate female oppression but also, more precisely, discriminates against bisexuality and lesbianism, being a creation by and for heterosexual men.

To illustrate the culturally, socially, and politically obscene affects that the image of a nurse as a sex object has on women, sexuality, and gender roles more generally, this essay focuses on Douglas Aarniokoski's film *Nurse 3D* (2013) that tells the story of Abby Russell. Abby is a nurse who not only saves human lives in the hospital where she works, but also, in a rather peculiar way, "helps" women whose partners cheat on them. The nurse seduces these men and then kills them. Most overtly, through Abby, the film employs two stereotypical portrayals of the nurse, namely a sexpot and a savior. Yet, as it does so, the film reinforces the (female) monstrosity of the nurse—the concept that I borrow from Barbara Creed (1993). Her uniform, and also the instruments that she works with (syringes, scalpels, etc.), foreground the idea that this woman is attractive, seductive, yet dangerous. As Abby cleanses the world of men who disrespect their wives and generally treat women as sex objects, her sexuality is brought to the fore. While there are multiple scenes depicting Abby having sex with men, she seems to be truly attracted only to another nurse, Danni Rogers. Abby has sex with Danni once, when Danni is drunk. Although Danni is in a relationship with Steve, Abby does not punish Danni for "cheating" on her boyfriend but, on the contrary, continues to murder men (Danni's stepfather and later also Steve) to become closer to Danni. As depicted in the film, Abby's sexual orientation is thus ambiguous. On the one hand, the multiple scenes where she has sex with men and her attraction to Danni make her appear bisexual. On the other hand, she uses sex as a tool to trap men in order to later kill them, whereas her attraction to and desire for Danni appear authentic, thus making her lesbian. Whether Abby is bisexual or lesbian, the monstrosity that characterizes her portrayal largely underlines the film's interpretation of bisexuality and lesbianism. This essay, hence, argues that while the film emphasizes the existing sex stereotypes about the nurse, it also criminally reinforces the idea that bisexuality and lesbianism are forms of monstrosity.

Eroticized Nurse and Oppressed Gender

The interpretation of the nurse as a sexually available, promiscuous woman akin to a prostitute has been prompted by multiple cultural narratives. While such a view of the nurse may seem to be odd and offensive, it has distinct roots in the traditional image of the nurse. Nursing was and remains an honorable profession. For women, nursing was one way to participate in wars; indeed, women's roles, through various activities, including nursing, in multiple world and local conflicts should not be underestimated (Fowler and Deacon, 2020: 3). The image of the nurse—from her

uniform to her professional behavior—has undergone significant transformations over time. Earlier images of nurses can be easily compared to those
of nuns: "Often called 'sisters' (as British nurses still are), [nurses'] lives
were indeed similar to those of nuns. Forbidden to marry, they were clois-
tered in 'nurses' homes' on hospital grounds, where every aspect of life was
strictly disciplined" (Doris Weatherford in Donald and MacDonald, 2014:
222). They were also veiled. Such a tight association of nurses with nuns has
not only classified nurses as a special cast but also impacted, if not generated, an (a)sexual image of the nurse. The nurse has become largely equated
with a *woman*, thus gendering nursing as an almost exclusively women's
profession. But most importantly, the nurse has come to stand for a woman
who is timid, virgin, and untouched/not-to-be-touched (her association
with a "sister" suggests familial relationship based on devotion, care, and
help, rather than provokes any sexual attraction, which could ultimately be
interpreted as a form of incest). Clearly, however, nurses are not nuns: for
example, they do not give the vow of chastity. The earlier views on the nurse
as a nun, yet the one that can potentially engage in a sexual relationship and
marry another individual, generate a certain sexual type of a woman: if she
wants to, a nurse, unlike a nun, can indeed engage in a sexual relationship.

Sexualization of nurses is also a direct outcome of the misinterpreta-
tion of the actions that are required to be taken by nurses on a daily basis.
In order to inspect a patient or carry out a specific manipulation, the nurse
has to engage in a close tactile contact with that person that crosses boundaries of personal space. The practice and process of nursing through these
manipulations has been turned into "a metaphor for sex": "Having seen and
touched the bodies of strangers, nurses are perceived as willing and able
sexual partners" (Fagin and Diers in Darbyshire, 2014: 59). Similarly, McAllister and Brien (2020) elaborate on the complex nature of nursing: "Nurses
are … permitted to transgress numerous personal and human boundaries. They access patients' bodies in extremely intimate ways, and they are
privy to intensely personal thoughts, feelings and confessions. They are also
immersed in the same feelings and tensions that can overwhelm patients,
such as fear, anxiety, fatigue and helplessness" (5–6). Sexualization of
nurses and nursing as such thus is directly connected to the primary tasks
that every nurse performs. Notably, nurses are viewed as much more desirable sexual partners than, for example, prostitutes, because "the cleanliness
of their white uniforms and their professional aplomb" make them appear
"safe" (Fagin and Diers in Lupton, 2012: 125).

Nurse 3D is one such vivid example of how the cultural imagining
of the nurse as a lascivious woman is not just a preferred interpretation of
the nurse, but is the one that is largely based on the nurse's expected role
of a savior and the feared role of a murderer (in case the nurse decides to

use her medical knowledge to do harm). Abby—the film's main character—performs two different roles. By day, she is a nurse in a hospital, helping people and saving lives. At night, however, she becomes a merciless murderer. Abby is clearly disgusted with men who cheat on their partners, and they become her main target. Already in the opening scene, the viewer sees how Abby punishes such men—the scheme that she applies to all her victims, with slight variations. Thus, at the beginning of the film, she meets a man in a nightclub, seduces him, and—because he was ready to cheat on his wife, instead of refusing Abby's invitation—cuts open his femoral artery before throwing him off the roof. An even more detailed scene of her murdering an unfaithful husband is shown later in the film, when Abby seduces her psychiatrist Larry; the man turns out to be a stepfather of her friend Danni, who is also a nurse. Again, Abby seems to give a chance to Larry: to ignore her or, to have sex with her. Larry chooses the second option and from then on becomes Abby's prey. Wearing a tight, revealing white dress, black tights, stiletto shoes, a black tight necklace, black leather gloves, and a red lipstick, Abby is a dominatrix in this scene. She gets into Larry's car, and as they are slowly driving, the voiceover (narrated by Abby) sums up the situation for the viewer: "And so the dedicated husband, esteemed author, learned educator, and renowned therapist took me to an alley to fuck." The car stops and Larry suggests going to a nearby hotel, whereas Abby signals that she is fine with staying in a car. Her necklace turns out to be a tie that she skillfully uses to tighten Larry's hands. While Larry is kissing her, she takes a large syringe out of her bag and injects him with "4 cc's of vecuronium," a medication that causes muscle relaxation. The dose that she injects, however, quickly paralyzes Larry. As Larry sits on the driver seat with an open mouth, unable to move, his saliva starts dripping out of his mouth. Abby, with due care, takes a napkin and cleans his face. Soon, she leaves the car, letting it drive to the main road and thus causing a car accident in which Larry dies.

This scene recreates the dual meaning of the nurse as a savior and a murderer: both roles are based on the fact that Abby is a trained medical nurse. Her superior knowledge of medication and her ability to use a syringe become her major weapons: she knows exactly how much vecuronium she should inject to make sure her plan works out. She uses her skills several times more in the film, when she puts drugs into Danni's drinks; later, when she injects the human resources employee Rachel with some medication; and, of course, in the opening scene briefly mentioned above, knowing how to injure the man so that he bleeds to death. Yet she also performs a traditional role of a nurse as a savior in the scene with Larry. Note, for example, how diligently she is caring for the paralyzed man, cleaning saliva off his chin. Abby obviously does not need to do that, considering that she knows that in a few minutes Larry will be dead anyway. Yet she behaves like a good nurse, helping her patient. She is disgusted with him as a man and a human being, but she views nursing as a job that must be done no matter who her patient is. Finally, in a more metaphorical sense, Abby is a savior in the scene for she rids the world of unfaithful men, thus, as she believes, helping women.

Abby's appearance rather curiously contributes to her image as a nurse. She essentially looks as a vintage nurse. The way her hair is done and the carefully placed cap on her head along with the impractical uniform that she wears that reveals her legs and breasts and accentuates her buttocks certainly reinforce her sexual attractiveness. Abby's cap is a deliberate anachronism given nurses in western hospitals no longer wear the cap. Strippers as nurses do, however, meaning the traditional symbol is now sexualized. However her uniform also conveys the meaning of a good nurse—a medical worker who is in the hospital to take care of patients and to perform her tasks diligently. Abby rather ambiguously defines what it means to be a nurse earlier in the film, underlining the multifaceted nature of the profession, as she views it: "This job is more than sticking thermometers in butts and looking pretty. It's our job to take care of the problems, not make the problems." Here, Abby comments on rather basic medical skills that every nurse should have, including "sticking thermometers in butts." Her comment on a nurse "looking pretty" can be interpreted in two ways. On the one hand, Abby might refer to the general appearance of a medical worker who starts his/her new working day: a clean individual in a freshly washed uniform. On the other hand, she might, of course, also foreground the problem of sexualizing the profession, accentuating that a "real" nurse is a woman that fits certain beauty standards. Interestingly, Abby's rather casual reference to a nurse's appearance as "pretty" suggests that being sexy and beautiful is not an extraordinary phenomenon but rather an ordinary, integral part of the profession. Abby, however, largely simplifies, if not distorts, nursing by her comments on both basic medical skills and on the appearance of nurses. Evidently, on a daily basis, nurses do much more than only "sticking thermometers in butts"; numerous other complicated and stressful tasks fill up their work schedule. The comment on "looking pretty," if interpreted as a reference to sexualization of women in the workplace, is clearly an outcome of gender inequality and harassment. When considering these words as a reference to a "clean" appearance of a medical worker, they are also rather contradictory, for it is obvious that the work that nurses perform can easily lead to their uniforms becoming quickly dirty, where their general appearance after having assisted at a complex operation or after a stressful night shift might differ dramatically from the images of eroticized nurses that Nurse 3D offers to its viewers.

After all, real nursing differs considerably from the routine performed by young, model-looking girls, with nicely done hair, fresh make up, and snow-white revealing uniforms depicted in *Nurse 3D*. In real life, nursing is about dealing often or regularly with various "abject situations":

> Many nurses have … found, or find, themselves in a range of abject situations: witnessing misery, pain, torture, death or slow and painful human decline. In delivering routine health care, nurses regularly encounter anxiety, fear, sorrow, anger and even violence. They come in intimate contact with—smelling, seeing and touching—wounds that bleed and leak. They deal with bodily decay and excreta. This association with the abject constitutes a familiar, but often unspoken, dark side of nursing's everyday work [McAllister and Brien, 2020: 5].

The stereotype of the good, diligent nurse—perhaps the most traditional, original interpretation of what it means to be a nurse and most akin to Florence Nightingale's intentions—has rather degrading effects on nursing as a profession and individual nurses. As McAllister and Brien (2020) observe: "the trope of the good nurse simplifies and obscures the complexity of contemporary nursing" (9). To specify:

> In reality, individual nurses often act in ways that defy this notion, but the idea of the good nurse is so prevalent that it is widely accepted not only by patients but within nursing itself and so, when nurses fail to live up to the stereotype, they are sanctioned [9].

Basing its images of sexualized nurses on traditional stereotypes of the good nurse and the bad nurse, hence, *Nurse 3D* promotes distorted images of nursing as a profession and nurses as workers. To "'actively break away from the stereotype of the good nurse,' is thus a crucial task for nurses in real life but also for those who create images of nurses on page and screen" (McAllister and Brien, 2020: 9). Recognizing the distorted and discriminating nature of the good-nurse stereotype can also help minimize and potentially eliminate the widely spread images of nurses as sex objects.

Yet Abby's line where she explains what nursing is concludes as follows: "It's our job to take care of the problems, not make the problems." This equivocal observation can be interpreted in two ways. On the one hand, nurses can solve various problems literally: if they have a patient that needs to be treated in a certain way, they do it in order for the patient to get well. On the other hand, Abby emphasizes the traditional meaning of the nurse as a savior. Abby understands this role of hers in a rather broad way: she takes care of patients in the hospital where she works, but she also intervenes in situations that, as she believes, demand her participation. When she murders unfaithful men, she performs the role of a problem-solver and a protector of those (women) who find themselves in unjust situations, even if they are unaware of that.

One of such problems (along with cheating men) is sexual harassment in the workplace that some nurses experience. The hospital where Abby works is an example of a place where a doctor abuses his dominant position to have sex with nurses. Dr. Morris (Judd Nelson) is described by Abby as follows: "That doctor, pig-face Morris. He loves breaking in the new girls. You could see the bulge in his pants." Sexual harassment in hospitals has a long history. Gender inequality that patriarchy has created worldwide can be illustrated by the example of the relationship between the (male) doctor and the (female) nurse. Gender stereotyping has dramatically influenced nursing. The doctor-nurse relationship has been largely compared to that of a husband and a wife in the Victorian time: "Nurses, like women, were seen as natural subordinate, responsible for others and naturally caring" (Sellman and Snelling, 2017: 260). Because in the mid-twentieth century, gender division in hospitals became particularly apparent, with men being doctors and women nurses, "nurses as sex objects" has become a dominant cultural stereotype (260). The sexual connotation implicit in "playing doctors and nurses" is based on the culturally and socially shaped male doctor/female nurse relationship. Importantly, the situation has not changed much since then, as sexual harassment in the workplace remains an issue in practically all professions, which continues to sustain the stereotype of "women as sex objects" from the 1960s–'70s (260). The recent sex scandals that were uncovered with the help of the #MeToo movement is a vivid yet tragic illustration of the ongoing sexual exploitation of women and of gender inequality more generally.

In *Nurse 3D*, Abby's actions reflect these realities as she tries to protect Danni—a younger colleague who has just started to work at the hospital—from, as she believes, two major sources of harassment in the hospital: the paramedic Steve (Danni's boyfriend) and Dr. Morris. Dr. Morris, indeed, sexually abuses nurses at the hospital and makes it clear to Danni that there is a way to make him forget about her unprofessional clumsiness and inability to react quickly that everyone could witness when the first badly injured patient was delivered to the hospital. In turn, Steve is viewed through Abby's eyes as a *potential* cheater and abuser. Abby's stance on men is rather straightforwardly articulated at the beginning of the film, when she is portrayed hunting for another victim: "My name is Abigail Russell. I look like a slut. But don't be fooled. This is merely a disguise to lure the dangerous predators who walk among us. This is their jungle, their breeding ground. And tonight, I'm on the hunt. These are the cheaters. The married, lying scum. They are like diseased cells, cultured in alcoholic petri dishes that destroy unsuspecting families and infect millions of innocent vaginae. There is no cure for the married cock. Only me. The nurse." And this is primarily the sort of "problems" that Abby believes she, *being a nurse*, should deal with, which she inscribes within specific medical terms, such as the pedantically correct Latin plural for vagina. While it might look as if Abby simply hates men, particularly those who cheat on their partners, in principle, she views cheating as a form of illness that she, as a nurse, simply ought to cure. Murders are thus, in her view, simply necessary medical procedures carried out in order to make the world a safer, *healthier* place.

Sexual abuse of nurses is the problem that not only affects specific individuals but also largely impacts nursing as a profession. It both shapes the cultural image of the nurse as a sex object and is a direct outcome of spreading such an image. Scholars note: "Much of global society continues to regard nurses as sex objects. A 2006 Agence France-Presse item reported that a recent poll had found that 54 percent of British men had sexual fantasies about nurses—more than about any other profession" (Summers and Summers, 2015: 155). In turn, "the staggering global prevalence of the 'naughty nurse' image" produces specific effects, too: "such social contempt discourages practicing and potential nurses, undermines nurses' claims to adequate resources, and encourages workplace sexual abuse—a major problem for real nurses" (xxviii). Quite oddly, McAllister and Brien (2020) see a positive aspect in sexual images of nurses, for they claim that "the associations of desirability, fondness and familiarity that feed into the idea of nurses as 'sexy' are positive in terms of the public's view of nursing and, thus, it may be possible for these aspects to strengthen nursing's identity and place within the social world" (12). Promoting a positive image of nursing through nurses as sexual objects only deeply roots the discriminating stereotype and, in principle, sustains gender inequality. Thus, instead of attempting to find positive aspects in the overtly discriminating image, it is more productive to work toward an erasure of such an image.

Sexualization of nurses is believed to happen in part because of "anxiety and fear of a loss of dignity" (McAllister and Brien, 2020: 51). To specify, the patient who finds himself/herself in a vulnerable position compared to the nurse caring for him/her, in a way, compensates his/her loss of power through sexualizing the nurse. Turning the nurse into a sex object makes the patient superior and the nurse inferior in such a situation. In this regard, the scene when Abby kills Dr. Morris is particularly curious to examine. Dr. Morris is shown lying on a surgical table to which he is tightened, unable to move. As Abby appears, she starts to undress slowly. In the end, the only clothes item that she wears is a bra. Abby wants to murder Dr. Morris because he cheats on his wife; but, in principle, she punishes him for sexually abusing nurses. In the scene, the roles switch from the doctor (Dr. Morris) and the nurse (Abby) to the doctor (Abby)—as it seems at first sight—and the patient (Dr. Morris). From an inferior nurse—the way Dr. Morris sees her—Abby turns into a doctor being ready to operate on Dr.

Morris. She thus acquires the type of power that Dr. Morris normally has. Crucially, however, Abby is heavily sexualized in the scene: the camera lingers on her naked buttocks, and her breasts (although in a bra) are present in practically every shot of Abby. As she prepares to begin the torture, she says to Dr. Morris: "Let me get some toys." Here, the reference is to various medical (surgical) instruments that she needs in order to successfully perform the torture. Calling the instruments "toys" suggests that Abby views the situation as a sexual game—or, she simply adapts the situation to the one that is familiar, and more pleasant for Dr. Morris.

Because Abby is so overtly sexualized in this scene, it might be more accurate to argue that Abby does not play the role of a doctor but, on the contrary, she remains the nurse-as-a-sex-object—the only way Dr. Morris views nurses—only this time she is given the power that the doctor usually has. The scene thus explores what happens when the sexually abused victim becomes the abuser, whereas the abuser turns into the victim, thus reinforcing the horror of the problem of sexual harassment and abuse that some nurses face. McAllister and Brien (2020) claim that "the depiction of a nurse as sexually desirable and available is … unrealistic and sexist" (51). This is arguably what the scene attempts to convey, too. The film, therefore, demonstrates that the kind of problems that nurses have to deal with at work include not only work-related matters but also various gender- and sex-related issues, sexual abuse and harassment being among them.

Monstrous Nurse and Repressed Sexualities

Abby's obsession to perform the role of a good nurse by curing not only actual diseases but also metaphorical, including cheating men whom she considers as such, largely intersects with the images of a monstrous nurse and a sexualized nurse. Murdering her victims mostly applying her medical knowledge, she turns into a bad, monstrous nurse—a direct opposition of a good nurse. At the same time, her overt sexualization, if not hypersexualization, brings to the fore the issue of sexuality as such. The primary concern of this section is then how the stereotype of the monstrous nurse not only challenges the image of the nurse as such but also directly affects Abby's sexuality, as represented in *Nurse 3D*.

Abby is classified by scholars as simultaneously "an attractive female nurse" and "a sadistic, sexually aggressive killer with severe psychological issues" (Summers and Summers, 2015: 170). In addition, the way she looks is compared to the way nurses appear in pornography (McAllister, Brien, and Piatti-Farnell, 2018: 313). Through her sexual objectification, Abby's femininity is emphasized. At the same time, committing various acts of violence, Abby is also represented as an empowered, masculine woman. Abby's portrayal continues a long history of violent women on screen: from the 1940s femme fatale and the 1970s heroine from horror and blaxploitation movies to the images generated in the 1980s, when violent women became a ubiquitous cinematic phenomenon (Neroni, 2005: 21, 27, 33). Certainly violence does not make Abby an exclusively masculine woman, just as violence (alone) does not stand for masculinity. But I refer to Abby as, at least to some degree, a masculine woman, drawing on Hilary Neroni's (2005) theory of violence and masculinity:

> Violence itself doesn't entirely make up masculinity, but it is also not possible to entirely erase violence from masculinity. One cannot separate ideas of masculinity from violence in our society—which is why, for example, a woman committing violence is inevitably at some point referred to as masculine…. The intertwined nature of violence and masculinity is one of the reasons the violent woman is so threatening: she breaks up this symbolic relationship between violence and masculinity [45–46].

The contrast between sexualized femininity and empowered masculinity is apparent in the character of Abby. The acts of violence that she commits help her turn from an inferior sexualized object to a powerful individual. After all, as Judith Halberstam has formulated in *Female Masculinity* (1998), masculinity has been equated with "power," "legitimacy," and "privilege" (2). And being a masculine woman, Abby gains the privileges of the masculine world. Barbara Creed's (1993) concept of a woman castrator can help define Abby's identity. A woman castrator "seeks revenge on men who have raped or abused her in some way" (Creed, 1993: 123). Abby herself has not been raped or explicitly abused. But when she was a child, she witnessed her father cheating on her mother and then physically abusing her mother. It is since then that Abby has developed a particular type of hatred toward married men who cheat on their wives and thus betray their children, too. Abby takes on the "*twin* roles" being both a castrator and a castrated woman, yet her dominant identity is that of a "deadly and dangerous" castrator (Creed, 1993: 127–28; italics in original). Abby avenges the pain that her father caused her, the abuse that he perpetrated on her mother, but also the unfaithfulness of selected men to their partners more generally. The goal of a woman castrator is to "castrate and take the place of the masculine subject" (Butler, 1998: 426). Abby tries to teach the cheating men that their gender does not give them the right to humiliate and lie to their wives.

Sexism can, however, be noticed not only through the images of nurses as sex objects but also through the powerful masculine Abby in the moments when she murders men. Scholars have already identified a dramatic difference between action heroes and action heroines, when the former can have any kinds of imperfections, from speaking with an accent to being "just plain ugly," whereas the latter seem to be obliged to be sexually attractive (Schubart, 2007: 5). As I have summed up elsewhere: "Women on screen are not covered in blood, they do not sweat, they always have fresh makeup and clean clothes, no matter how long and hard they fight" (Prorokova "Female Masculinity," 2016: 41). Similarly, Abby always remains sexy, including when she is covered in blood: her revealing uniform and provocative lingerie (or its absence) ensure the woman remains sexually attractive through the course of the whole film. Certainly, violent women on screen can be interpreted differently: on the one hand, their use of "masculine violence" suggests gender equality, yet on the other hand, being forced to look and behave in a way that can sexually arouse a heterosexual man, these characters remain distinct symbols of gender inequality (Schubart, 2007: 6). Combining femininity and masculinity, Abby manages to "articulate" gender—the term that I borrow from Yvonne Tasker (1993)—in a complex way (18). Nevertheless, her portrayal is not liberating and empowering for women, but rather it suggests that a woman can please or withstand a man only with the help of her sexual attractiveness.

Abby's sexual involvement with multiple characters throughout the film raises questions regarding her sexual orientation. Indeed, her promiscuity helps reinforce the stereotype of a "naughty nurse" that Abby personifies (Summers and Summers, 2015: 159). But it also makes the viewer question Abby's sexual orientation: is she heterosexual, bisexual, or lesbian? This essay views Abby as a bisexual or lesbian (the ambiguous portrayals of the character make it impossible to be sure). It is crucial to note, however, that when I draw attention to Abby's promiscuity to examine her lesbianism or bisexuality I by no means suggest that lesbians and/or bisexual individuals are characterized by promiscuity. In the context of the film, promiscuity, however, reveals that Abby has sex with individuals of various genders. Yet having sex with men is considered part of a plan to seduce married men and then murder them. The only character that Abby seems truly attracted to, if not obsessed with, is Danni. This obsession is based on Abby's desire to have Danni's full attention; but she is also obviously sexually interested in the young nurse. The crucial scene in the film is when Abby drugs Danni at a party and then later has sex with her. She uses the photographs from that night to blackmail Danni—but her main aim is to separate Danni and Steve. Moreover, Abby often is depicted staring at Danni, including, for example, the scene in the shower. As she is looking at Danni washing herself in a hospital shower, the voiceover communicates Abby's thoughts: "As I watched Danni's little round ass—the same one that I had eaten the night before, prior to finger-fucking her to six orgasms— and when I saw those tacky $10 flowers from dickless little Steve, I couldn't control myself." Her sexual attraction to Danni is obvious; but it is also apparent that she wants to take the place of Steve as Danni's sexual partner. By diminishing Steve's male potency, which is conveyed through the words "dickless" and "little," Abby attempts to suggest that she is more powerful, and a better sexual partner—after all, she caused Danni's "six orgasms" the night before. It is difficult to say, however whether Abby is bisexual or lesbian, as the film does not develop the character of Abby sufficiently, focusing primarily on her being a good/monstrous/sexualized nurse. If Abby is bisexual, the film makes a contribution to the short list of cinematic portrayals of bisexual characters—indeed, scholars note an evident absence of bisexual characters on screen (Ward, 2020: 119). If she is lesbian, then the film offers another, rather ambiguous portrayal of a lesbian woman. Cherry Smyth (1990) observes: "Lesbian sexuality has been repressed, rendered invisible and impotent by society" (154). Portrayals of lesbian sexuality are thus significant contributions that help shape cultural image of lesbianism and, ideally, promote diversity. As I have argued elsewhere, "In film and literature, the inclusion of the issue of lesbian love in general and that of lesbian sex in particular clearly demonstrates the social and cultural willingness to accept lesbian sex as a norm and denounce its deviation, as it was believed earlier" (Prorokova "Sex and/as Liberation," 2019: 328). That is, however, hardly the case with *Nurse 3D*.

Whether Abby is lesbian or bisexual, her sexuality is compromised by numerous stereotypes. First, she is mentally ill, as becomes clear toward the end of the film. Her obsession with Danni could be the result of her illness. If the film suggests that she becomes interested in a woman because she is mentally ill, then it directly borrows the stereotype about gays and lesbians from the mid-twentieth century, when homosexual individuals "were commonly classified as mentally impaired people, who were responsible for the 'perversity' that they desired or practiced. Queerness was viewed as a contagious disease, for gays and lesbians could spoil the body and the mind of a 'decent' person, turning him/her into a mentally impaired one, too" (Prorokova "Alcoholic, Mad, Disabled," 2018: 127). When thinking about homosexuality as a disease, "society labeled lesbians and gays as disabled and interpreted their sexual desires as manifestations of psychiatric and perhaps even of physical impairments" (127). This is essentially what the film does, too, if it suggests Abby is bisexual or lesbian as a result of her psychological problems. Second, Abby's promiscuity—the problem that I have already briefly referred to earlier in this section—portrays bisexuality/lesbianism as a deviant sexuality. Third, her monstrous nature manifests itself through the moments of murdering challenges bisexuality/lesbianism as a positive, normal from of sexuality. The film does not specify whether it communicates bisexuality/lesbianism as a form of monstrosity or not. Fourth, the focus on eliminating (cheating) men—and not women (for example, it remains unclear why Abby does not try to kill Danni who, being in a relationship, have slept with Abby, although, of course, being drugged)—communicates a rather anti-men stance. Here, it is uncertain again whether the film suggests through the character of Abby that bisexual women and lesbians are, in various ways, "against" men. Finally, the images of Abby—and other "dirty" nurses—are essentially recreations of stereotypes from pornography that is created for heterosexual men. If Abby is bisexual/lesbian, her portrayal is constructed in a way to please a heterosexual man, and is thus not only sexist but also largely discriminating against bisexual women and lesbians. In conclusion, it is quite plausible to argue that the film portrays Abby's sexuality ambiguously in order to eroticize the character even more and thus reinforce the stereotype of the nurse as a sex object for heterosexual men.

Conclusion

Nurse 3D sketches out the image of the nurse as a sex object—a largely problematic and dangerous view of nurses that has been promoted by many other cultural narratives and that inevitably impacted the lives of and attitudes toward real nurses. The film does so relying on two other stereotypes of the nurse: a savior and a (potential) murder. Exploring the intricate linkages among the three cultural imaginings of nurses—sex objects, saviors, and murderers—the film not only uncovers the problem of sexual abuse and harassment in the workplace, sexism, and gender inequality, but it also generates these very problems. This is particularly visible through the film's exploration of Abby's sexuality and how it impacts her as a woman and as a nurse. While *Nurse 3D* successfully communicates some of the problems that nurses experience and the issue of women's exploitation more generally, it does nothing to help solve these problems and fight for equality: quite the contrary, it contributes to an already large pool of texts that promote sexism and abuse of women.

FILMS AND TELEVISION PRODUCTIONS REFERENCED
Nurse 3D (2013) Lionsgate.

REFERENCES
Butler, Judith (1998) Prohibition. Psychoanalysis and the Heterosexual Matrix. In: Mirzoeff, Nicholas (ed.) *The Visual Culture Reader*. London: Routledge, pp. 423–27.

Creed, Barbara (1993) *The Monstrous Feminine: Film, Feminism, Psychoanalysis*. London: Routledge.

Darbyshire, Philip (2014) Heroines, Hookers and Harridans: Exploring Popular Images and Representations of Nurses and Nursing. In: Daly, John, Speed, Sandra and Jackson, Debra (eds.) *Contexts of Nursing*. Sydney: Elsevier, pp. 53–70.

Donald, Ralph, and MacDonald, Karen (2014) *Women in War Films: From Helpless Heroine to G.I. Jane*. Lanham, MD: Rowman & Littlefield.

Fowler, Stacy, and Deacon, Deborah A. (2020) *A Century in Uniform: Military Women in American Films*. Jefferson, NC: McFarland.

Halberstam, Judith (1998) *Female Masculinity*. Durham, NC: Duke University Press.

Kelly, Jacinta, Fealy, Gerard M., and Watson, Roger (2012) The Image of You: Constructing Nursing Identities in YouTube. *Journal of Advanced Nursing* 68, 8: 1804–13.

Lupton, Deborah (2012) *Medicine as Culture: Illness, Disease and the Body*. London: SAGE.

McAllister, Margaret, and Brien, Donna Lee (2020) *Paradoxes in Nurses' Identity, Culture and Image: The Shadow Side of Nursing*. London: Routledge.

McAllister, Margaret, Brien, Donna Lee, and Piatti-Farnell, Lorna (2018) Tainted Love: Gothic Imaging of Nurses in Popular Culture. *Journal of Advanced Nursing* 74: 310–17.

Neroni, Hilary (2005) *The Violent Woman: Femininity, Narrative, and Violence in Contemporary American Cinema*. Albany: State University of New York Press.

Prorokova, Tatiana (2016) Female Masculinity: Revenge and Violence in Tarantino's *Kill Bill* Vol.1 and Vol.2. *The Human: Journal of Literature and Culture*. Special Issue "Masculinities on Film." 6: 37–55. Guest Ed. Robert Mundy and Jane Collins.

Prorokova, Tatiana (2018) Alcoholic, Mad, Disabled: Constructing Lesbian Identity in Ann Bannon's The Beebo Brinker Chronicles. In: Donaldson, Elizabeth J. (ed.) *Literatures of Madness: Disability Studies and Mental Health*. New York: Palgrave Macmillan, pp. 127–43.

Prorokova, Tatiana (2019) Sex and/as Liberation: (Porno)Graphic Lesbian Love. In: Jacob, Frank (ed.) *Blue Is the Warmest Color. Pornography: Interdisciplinary Perspectives*. Berlin: Peter Lang, pp. 313–30.

Schubart, Rikke (2007) *Super Bitches and Action Babes: The Female Hero in Popular Cinema, 1970–2006*. Jefferson, NC: McFarland.

Sellman, Derek, and Snelling, Paul (2017) *Becoming a Nurse: Fundamentals of Professional Practice for Nursing*. London: Routledge.

Smyth, Cherry (1990) The Pleasure Threshold: Looking at Lesbian Pornography on Film. *Feminist Review* 34, "Perverse Politics: Lesbian Issues": 152–59.

Summers, Sandy, and Summers, Harry Jacobs (2015) *Saving Lives: Why the Media's Portrayal of Nursing Puts Us All at Risk*. Oxford: Oxford University Press.

Tasker, Yvonne (1993) *Spectacular Bodies: Gender, Genre and the Action Cinema*. London: Routledge.

Ward, Dan (2020) "Your Body Belongs to the State": The Mobilization of the Action Heroine in Service of the State. In: Prorokova-Konrad, Tatiana (ed.) *Red Sparrow* and *Atomic Blonde. Cold War II: Hollywood's Renewed Obsession with Russia*. Jackson: University Press of Mississippi, pp. 112–28.

About the Contributors

Mark **Aldridge** is a senior lecturer in film and television at Solent University, Southampton, who specializes in television history and Agatha Christie. After publishing his monograph *The Birth of British Television* (2012), he combined his interests with the 2016 book *Agatha Christie on Screen* and later wrote a full history of Hercule Poirot for the official centenary book *Agatha Christie's Poirot: The Greatest Detective in the World* (2020).

Richard **Bates** is a research fellow at the University of Nottingham. From 2018 to 2021 he was attached to the UK Arts & Humanities Research Council project "Florence Nightingale Comes Home" (AH/R00014X/1). He is a coauthor of *Florence Nightingale at Home* (2020) and has also published on French history. His monograph, *Psychoanalysis and the Family in Twentieth-Century France: Françoise Dolto and Her Legacy*, will be published in 2021–22.

Sarah **Chaney** is a historian of health and medicine with a background in museum curation and research interests in the history of psychiatry and nursing. She is a research fellow at Queen Mary Centre for the History of the Emotions, and Events and Exhibitions Manager at the Royal College of Nursing. Her monograph, *Psyche on the Skin* (2017), explores the history of self-injury as a psychiatric category. Her research is on the history of compassion in nursing.

Ülle **Ernits** has been the Rector of Tallinn Health Care College since 2005. She obtained her doctoral degree in nursing science at Tampere University (Finland) in 2018 and is a member of the Council of Gender Equality in the Ministry of Social Affairs. As a member of the Estonian Rectors' Conference of Universities of Applied Sciences (RCUAS), she is active in the implementation of the reform and improvement of professional higher education.

Caitlin **Fendley** is a Ph.D. candidate in the history department at Purdue University. Her dissertation examines grassroots population activism in the United States from the 1960s to 1990s. She received an MA in history from Purdue in 2018. She holds a year-long research grant from the Purdue Research Foundation. Her writing has been featured in *The Conversation, The Washington Post,* and in an edited collection.

Julia **Hallam** is professor emerita in communication and media with the School of the Arts, University of Liverpool. She is a media scholar and former nurse who has published widely on representations of nursing and medicine including *Medical Fictions* (Eds. Hallam J. and N. Moody, 1998), *Nursing the Image* (2000) and in book chapters and journals, including, *Journal of British Cinema and Television* (2016) and *Critical Studies in Television* (with Hannah Hamad, 2017).

Barbara **Harmes** lectures in communication at the University of Southern Queensland. Her doctoral research focused on the discursive controls built around sexuality in late nineteenth-century England. Her research interests include cultural studies, postgraduate education, and religion. She has published in the fields of modern Australian politics, postgraduate education, 1960s American television, and her original field of Victorian literature.

Marcus K. **Harmes** has published extensively in the field of popular culture, including *Roger Delgado: I am usually referred to as the Master* (2017), and numerous studies on the church in modern popular culture, book chapters in the collection *Doctor Who and Race*, and articles in journals including *Science Fiction Film and Television*, and *Journal of Religion and Popular Culture*. In 2018, he edited the Handbook for Springer on *Postgraduate Education in Higher Education*.

Meredith A. **Harmes** teaches communication in the enabling programs at the University of Southern Queensland in Australia. Her research interests include modern British and Australian politics and popular culture in Britain and America. She is a coeditor of *Postgraduate Education in Higher Education* (2018) and has published on American television in the *Australasian Journal of Popular Culture*.

Travis **Hay** is a historian of science and settler colonialism. He completed his Ph.D. in history at York University and was a postdoctoral fellow and adjunct professor of indigenous learning at Lakehead University. He is working as a postdoctoral fellow with Community Housing Canada as he teaches with the Seven Generations Educational Institute in Fort Frances.

Susan **Hopkins** lectures in USQ College at the University of Southern Queensland, Springfield campus, Australia. She holds a Ph.D. in social science and a masters (research) in education. Her research interests include gender and media studies, and she has published in *Celebrity Studies* and *Feminist Media Studies*. In 2002, she published her monograph *Girl Heroes*.

Morag **Martin** is an associate professor of history at SUNY Brockport. She coedited with Marianne Delaporte a volume entitled *Sacred Inception: Reclaiming the Spirituality of Birth in the Modern World* (2018). The volume includes her article "Midwifery as Religious Calling." She has articles forthcoming in *Medical History* and in *French Historical Studies* on the education of midwives in obstetrics in nineteenth-century France.

Victoria N. **Meyer** is an assistant professor of history teaching in a liberal arts and multidisciplinary studies program at the University of Arizona. She holds a Ph.D. from the University of Virginia and works broadly in the history of the body and health humanities. Her research interests include public health initiatives related to smallpox, the imagery of disease, and the intersection of gender and disease in the experience of patients and medical practitioners.

Tatiana **Prorokova-Konrad** is a postdoctoral researcher in the department of English and American studies at the University of Vienna. She holds a Ph.D. in American studies from the University of Marburg. She is the author of *Docu-Fictions of War: U.S. Interventionism in Film and Literature* (2019) and the editor of *Transportation and the Culture of Climate Change: Accelerating Ride to Global Crisis* (2020).

Kristi **Puusepp** is an RN and head of the Chair of Nursing at Tallinn Health Care College. She is responsible for having NANDA-I nursing diagnoses translated into Estonian as well as editing and publishing three versions of "NANDA International Nursing Diagnoses: Definitions and Classification" into Estonian. She is the head of the state-wide NNN Estonia Working Group and founding member of Development Center of Estonian Nursing Quality.

Ronja **Tripp-Bodola** received a Ph.D. in English and visual culture studies, and has published widely on intersectionality, biopolitics, and visual ethics in the "long twentieth century." Her work has also focused on medical humanities, and she is developing a medical humanities curriculum for psychiatrists at LSUHSC, New Orleans.

Merle **Talvik** is a cultural researcher, social scientist, educator and the head of research methodology studies at Tallinn Health Care College. She has previously worked at Tallinn University and Estonian Entrepreneurship University of Applied Sciences, led the research work of students and academics, written over 60 scientific publications, and led international projects. She is the editor-in-chief of *The European Journal of Teaching and Education*.

Taimi **Tulva** is a professor emerita at Tallinn University and a guest associate professor at Tallinn Health Care College. She has a Ph.D. in educational and social sciences. From 1993 to 2016, she worked as a social work professor at Tallinn University. She has supervised master's theses and doctoral research projects and authored over 300 articles and many textbooks.

Jeannine **Uribe** is an RN and an assistant professor at La Salle University School of Nursing and Health Professions in Philadelphia, teaching courses in the Doctor of Nursing Practice program and public health nursing in the undergraduate program. She is an assessor, guardian of collections, and tour guide for the Museum of Nursing History, Inc., in Philadelphia.

Index